*The Decline of the
Old Medical Regime
in Stuart London*

The Decline of the Old Medical Regime in Stuart London

HAROLD J. COOK

Cornell University Press

ITHACA AND LONDON

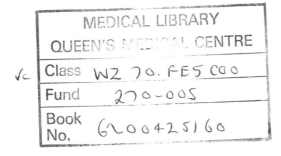

Dedicated to the memory of Eric Kollman,
whose character and knowledge were
an inspiration to many

Contents

Preface   11

Note on Spelling, Dates, and Abbreviations   15

Introduction   19

1. The Medical Marketplace of London   28
     Practitioners and the Medical Marketplace
     Physicians and the Medical Marketplace

2. Knowledge and Power: The London College of
    Physicians   70
     The College of Physicians as a Learned Society
     The College's Public Face
     The College's Regulatory Activity

3. Revolution and Reform: Changing the Enterprise of
    Physic, 1630–1660   94
     The College and the Early Stuarts
     A New Era
     Partial Retrenchment

4. Political Weaknesses and Intellectual Threats, 1660–1672   133
     The College Charter Controversy
     Experimentalism and the Society of Chemical Physicians
     Deepening Divisions and the Widening Threat of the New
       Philosophy

5. The Restoration of the Old Order, 1672–1688   183
     The College and the Common Law
     A Reassertion of Regulation
     The College and James II

Contents

6. The Decline of the Old Medical Order, 1689–1704   210
    In the Aftermath of the Glorious Revolution
    Apothecaries and Their Physician Friends against the "New College"
    A Partial Ending: The Groenvelt and Rose Cases

Conclusion   254

Appendixes
   1. The College of Physicians   265
   2. College Regulatory Activity   276
   3. English Royal Physicians   281
   4. Statutes and Court Cases re the College of Physicians   284

Selected Bibliography   287
Index   303

8

Plates

1. Hans Buling, "The Infallible Mountebank or Quack Doctor," engraving, 1670   37
2. "Magnifico . . . Cunningmanissimo . . . Viro   Iacko Adams de Clerkenwell Greeno. . . ," engraving, 1663   40
3. William Hogarth, "The Company of Undertakers," or "A Consultation of Physicians," engraving, 1736   57
4. After (?) Frans van Mieris I, untitled portrayal of the consultation of a Dutch physician and a patient, oil   64
5. J. Simon, portrait of Sir Theodore de Mayerne, mezzotint   96
6. W. Sherwin, portrait of George Thomson, engraving, 1670   161
7. Portrait of Baldwin Hamey, engraving, 1793   174
8. G. P. Harding, portrait of Charles Goodall, watercolor, 1810   200
9. "The Fashionable Physician Runs over His Rival," engraving, eighteenth century   216
10. "Scene in an Apothecary's Shop," mezzotint, eighteenth century   230
11. "A Description of the Coledge of Physicians," engraving, 1697   245

Preface

This book examines how the medical practitioners of London responded to the intellectual, political, and socioeconomic changes of the age variously called the "scientific revolution" or the "seventeenth-century crisis." As often with literate people of wide and varied experiences, medical practitioners acted and wrote in ways that left a telling record of cultural transformations. The historical evidence about medical practitioners allows us to glimpse some of the interconnections between their ideas and practices, their social and political relationships, and their material goals.

The story told here—based on documents of both a legal/institutional and a literary nature, on archival records and contemporary books, pamphlets, and manuscripts—can better present the various issues at stake in the medical community than could a sociopolitical or an intellectual history alone. By crossing the usual historiographical boundaries of 1641, 1660, and 1689, it also places the revolutions of the day in an extended sweep of time and so makes it possible for us to gauge the effect of these great events on an important group of Londoners.

Not everyone will believe that I have succeeded in satisfactorily describing the changes in medicine in London in the seventeenth century, nor will everyone believe that I have accounted for them well, or well enough. It is my belief, however, that by dealing with large-scale changes in seventeenth-century medicine, the book is able to offer some new insights into the tangled interrelationships of the legal, political, social, and intellectual history of England. I hope to encourage debate on the relationship between early modern medical theory and medical politics in terms of the concrete wealth of human activity rather than in terms of such abstractions as "ideologies" or "climates of opinion."

My debts to many people are such as can hardly be repaid. To the librarians of many institutions and the generations of cataloguers must go many thanks for making available the materials for this book: in particular I thank those at the University of Michigan Graduate Library and Rare Book Room; the Countway, Widener, and Houghton libraries of Harvard University; the British Library; the Public Record Offices (Chancery Lane and Kew); the London Guildhall Library; the House of Lords Record Office; and the Royal Society of London. To the librarians, archivists, and fellows of the Royal College of Physicians, to the Keeper of Manuscripts of the British Library, and to the Wellcome Historical Medical Library, I owe a great debt, not least for giving me their kind permission to publish pictures in their keeping and quotations from their records. I am especially grateful to Geoffrey Davenport, now Librarian of the Royal College of Physicians, and to William Schupach, Curator, Iconographic Collections, Wellcome Institute for the History of Medicine.

Many historians have left their marks on this book, beginning with my undergraduate teachers of history at Cornell College in Iowa, particularly Eric Kollman and William Carroll. Many fine practitioners of the historian's craft made an impression on me at the University of Michigan, where the research for this book was begun. My greatest intellectual debt remains to my graduate adviser, Nicholas Steneck, who taught me much about the history of science and the relationships between systems of thought and their social contexts. His kind encouragement, his support, and his criticism of too-easy conclusions were the sine qua non of this book's beginnings. During later stages of revision and addition, graduate students and colleagues in the departments of the history of science at the University of Oklahoma and Harvard University were invaluable sources of stimulation and criticism.

Abroad, the kind hospitality and the research facilities of the Institute of Historical Research and the Wellcome Institute for the History of Medicine in London, and the Wellcome Unit for the History of Medicine at Oxford, made it easy to consult the published literature and to find other interested minds during the course of three research trips. Funds for my initial research in England were provided by a loan from my parents, John D. and Sybilla A. Cook, when other sources were not forthcoming; a travel grant was made available by the Horace H. Rackham School of Graduate Studies, University of Michigan. Further examinations of archival material were made possible by grants from the Milton Fund and the Clark Fund of Harvard University.

Many people have commented on portions of the manuscript, and I have benefited greatly from their help: Allan Brandt, Jerome J. Bylebyl, Moti Feingold, Michael Hunter, David Lux, Roy Porter, Matthew Ramsay, Hilton Root, Barbara Rosenkrantz, David Sacks, Ellen Smith, and Liba Taub. Early drafts were typed by Valerie Powel and Donna Gold. Some costs incurred in the preparation of the current manuscript were defrayed by a grant from the Clark Fund of Harvard University.

Finally, it is especially to my family and friends who have tolerated, in some instances even encouraged, an interest in history—those from Long Grove, Illinois; Mt. Vernon, Iowa; Ann Arbor, Michigan; Norman, Oklahoma; Cambridge, Massachusetts; and Madison, Wisconsin—to whom I extend my deepest thanks. Four friends and their families in particular sustained me during my days as a graduate student: Francis Couvares, Dennis McNamara, Hilton Root, and, especially, David Lux. In the later stages of the preparation of this book for publication, the encouragement of one person has meant more than she can know: Faye.

HAROLD J. COOK

Madison, Wisconsin

Note on Spelling, Dates, and Abbreviations

The spelling and punctuation in the text have been rendered into modern American English, while the original spellings have been kept in all titles of publications. Transliterations from the Greek to the Latin alphabet in titles have been placed in single quotes. Dates have been modernized by year, but the days remain in Old Style.

The following abbreviations have been used:

Annals: Annals of the Royal College of Physicians.

BHM: *Bulletin of the History of Medicine.*

B.L.:   British Library.

Clark: George N. Clark, *A History of the Royal College of Physicians of London,* 2 vols. Oxford: Clarendon Press, 1964–66.

JHM: *Journal of the History of Medicine and Allied Sciences.*

MH: *Medical History.*

S.P.:   State Papers, Chancery Lane.

Sloane: Sloane Manuscripts Collection, British Library.

Underwood: E. A. Underwood, ed.; C. Wall, H. C. Cameron, *A History of the Worshipful Society of Apothecaries of London. Vol. 1, 1617–1815.* London: Oxford University Press, 1963.

Webster: Charles Webster, *The Great Instauration: Science, Medicine and Reform, 1626–1660.* New York: Holmes & Meier, 1975.

The Decline of the
Old Medical Regime
in Stuart London

Introduction

The social and intellectual possibilities of a culture—the ecology and the economy, the social forms, the religious and cultural notions of a person's relationship to the larger world (or worlds)—all these lie behind medical practice. Examining how medicine changed, and why, can therefore tell us a great deal about the ways in which social and intellectual transformations of a time and place are related.

This book is about how the physicians of seventeenth-century London tried to maintain the dignity of learned medicine by exercising the juridical authority of the College of Physicians, and how they ultimately failed in the face of deeply felt economic, intellectual, and political changes. By the beginning of the eighteenth century the learned physicians had lost their ability to regulate other practitioners. The reasons for their failure illuminate many aspects of seventeenth-century medicine, and about the lived experiences of Londoners, the political transformation of the Stuart Age, and the "scientific revolution."

My sources are the early modern equivalent of trial records for malpractice and illicit practice, editorials in medical journals and the public press, testimony before branches of government and the decisions of those branches, the minutes of medical societies and licensing boards, medical advertisements, and medical treatises.

Telling the story is an impossible task if limits are not established. The first limitation I adopted was to confine the tale to London. London was the heart of the realm and the pacesetter of social and intellectual fashions, but clearly it was not all of England. The second limitation was to organize the narrative around the problems of medical regulation. For although we often think of medical regulation as a "modern" phenomenon, there was an attempt to regulate the medical milieu of early modern London.

The "old medical regime" was legally dominated by a group of men who tried to shepherd other medical practitioners intellectually and politically; that group was an incorporated College of Physicians (by the end of the seventeenth century often called the Royal College of Physicians). The limitations placed on their de jure powers by the House of Lords in 1704 indicate an unraveling of their juridical authority due both to the political transformation of England and to the increasing respectability of new standards of practice often associated with the "new philosophy." Because medical regulation in London was based on a combination of certain political and intellectual attitudes, and because it had social and economic as well as medical ends, it is a subject that can tell us much about the interaction of all these aspects of human activity among medical practitioners and, by implication, among other people.

The learned physicians (a term used throughout to mean university-educated M.D.s) were a fairly new group in England, a product of the intellectual and educational changes of the late fifteenth and sixteenth centuries. To emulate other countries, to encourage medical learning, to tap the advice of learned men, and, probably, to create a network of patronage for physicians close to the court, Henry VIII in 1518 chartered the College of Physicians. The charter was given statutory authority by an Act of Parliament in 1523. The officers of the College were granted the right to judge medical practitioners in London and within seven miles of the City, and to admit to practice those who were qualified. By implication, this made the physicians the judges of good and bad practice: it made the new humanistic medicine of the leaders of the College the standard by which all other practices would be judged. Thus, a standard came into being by which actions could be declared *mala praxis,* a concept earlier unknown in English law.[1] As a royal "innovation" whose members were trying to control other practitioners, the College later became subject to all the political and social vicissitudes of the "century of revolution." As a group of learned men, the members of the College also variously struggled to promote, to assimilate, or to reject the intellectual innovations and implications of

---

[1] I owe this observation to conversations with Dr. Faye Getz. On Bonham's case, in which Chief Justice Sir Edward Coke seems to have first clearly distinguished between malpractice and illicit practice, see my article "'Against Common Right and Reason': The College of Physicians versus Dr. Thomas Bonham," *American Journal of Legal History* 29(1985):301–22.

the new philosophy. The physicians' activities, their hopes and fears, their successes and failures, between 1630 and 1704 can therefore tell us much about the ways in which the intellectual and political culture of the day changed.

Medical regulation in London by the College of Physicians provides the focus for this story, but the story must go beyond a history of the College. Fortunately, George N. Clark has provided a detailed history of the College to which the reader can turn for more information on that institution.[2] Since Clark was concerned only with documenting the internal history of the College, however, I have found it necessary, on the basis of a reading of the College's documents in light of other sources and views, to modify and even, occasionally, to contradict some of his generalizations.

The members of the College formed an exclusive group, a group that did not enroll all the physicians in London, much less the city's numerous other practitioners. Seeing how the College exercised its power by impinging (sometimes forcefully, sometimes indirectly) on the activities of the other practitioners in London is not very fruitful unless we try to understand whom the College was attempting to control, and why. This entails knowing about other practitioners, their activities, ideas, and goals.

Beyond the story of medical regulation by a corporate group, then, lies the story of medical practice in London and the ways in which innovations outside the ranks of the learned physicians of the College forced the College's behavior to change in certain directions. Because the College was a corporate group governed by collective rules and having certain statutory powers and intellectual requirements for entry, its activities were governed by more than the simple sum of the wills of its individual members; its officers in particular could shape its behavior in ways that some other fellows sometimes disliked. But if the College was no mere epiphenomenon "representing" one side of the social and intellectual conflicts of the period, neither was it an unbounded "monopoly" able to exercise its will on others whenever it wished.[3] Some years ago R. S. Roberts set out a fine general guide

[2]G. N. Clark, *A History of the Royal College of Physicians of London*, 2 vols. (hereafter cited as Clark).

[3]Christopher Hill's representation of the College as a Royalist "monopoly" is generally correct for the 1630s, but it depicts the institution too monolithically as a representative of class interests for it to be sensitive to the variety of motivations of its members and its opponents. His work is, however, useful as a starting point. See his *Intellectual Origins of the English Revolution*, pp. 74–84; and idem, "The Medical Profession and Its Radical Critics," in *Change and Continuity in Seventeenth-Century England*, pp. 157–78.

Introduction

to the seventeenth-century medical milieu, showing how important were practitioners and events beyond the College.[4] The ideas and activities of many of these people often affected the College, frequently by helping to change public attitudes toward medicine and authority.[5] Large and complex issues of historical change beyond the story of the College of Physicians itself are therefore at stake in any account of medical regulation; but the various fortunes of medical regulation in London can help us see beneath the thickets of events and controversy.

Chapter 1 discusses the economic medical milieu of London: the "medical marketplace." It outlines the kinds of activities, from selling drugs to giving advice, that could gain a practitioner a living. Because the chapter focuses on the economic activities of London practitioners, it does not attempt to describe the full range of medical practitioners, only those who made a substantial part of their living in medicine from the growing market economy.[6] The chapter emphasizes the competitive nature of medical practice in seventeenth-century London and shows how the physicians were nearly as vulnerable as other practitioners when it came to getting and keeping patients. The physicians have commonly been portrayed as "gentlemen" who were somehow socially removed from the mire of selling their skills,[7] but they did find it necessary to compete with others for patients.[8]

[4]R. S. Roberts, "The Personnel and Practice of Medicine in Tudor and Stuart England," *MH* 6 (1962): 363–82; 8 (1964): 217–34. Also see his "The London Apothecaries and Medical Practice in Tudor and Stuart London" (Ph.D. diss., University of London, 1964). For a published internal history of the Society of Apothecaries that has many useful details, see E. A. Underwood, ed., and C. Wall, H. C. Cameron, *A History of the Worshipful Society of Apothecaries of London. Vol. 1, 1617–1815* (hereafter cited as Underwood).

[5]Many of the "advances" in medical thinking in seventeenth-century England came from outside the ranks of the College physicians. See, for example, Lester S. King, *The Road to Medical Enlightenment, 1650–1695;* Allen G. Debus, *The Chemical Philosophy: Paracelsian Science and Medicine in the Sixteenth and Seventeenth Centuries;* and Charles Webster, *The Great Instauration: Science, Medicine and Reform, 1626–1660* (hereafter cited as Webster).

[6]Also see Margaret Pelling and Charles Webster, "Medical Practitioners," in *Health, Medicine and Mortality in the Sixteenth Century,* ed. Charles Webster, pp. 165–235.

[7]Bernice Hamilton, "The Medical Professions in the Eighteenth Century," *Economic History Review* 4 (1951): 141–69. Geoffrey S. Holmes is only somewhat better on the issue of social rank: *Augustan England: Professions, State and Society, 1680–1730,* pp. 166–235.

[8]William J. Birken has recently stressed the "middling" status of the families from which most physicians came: "The Fellows of the Royal College of Physicians of London, 1603–1643: A Social Study" (Ph.D. diss., University of North Carolina, Chapel Hill, 1977); and idem, "The Royal College of Physicians of London and Its Support of the Parliamentary Cause in the English Civil War," *Journal of British Studies* 23 (1983): 47–62.

The economic and social insecurities of many practitioners, including physicians, were deep because of the nature of the medical marketplace.

Once the vulnerability of the physicians to competition in the realm of therapy is recognized, the ways in which the institutional authority of the College of Physicians was used to protect the physicians' status as learned men become clear. Since university learning was their sole distinguishing mark, the physicians needed to maintain the dignity and supremacy of that medical learning. Chapter 2 therefore details the institutional structure and goals of the College of Physicians and analyzes how its authority was used against others over the course of eighty years. It shows that the public and the College had different expectations of how the College would use its juridical "police" powers. Equally important, the College can be shown to have acted vigorously when the Crown supported it; that is, it took advantage of those times when the Crown was trying to extend its own influence. The College was not a uniformly "weak" institution but one whose strength varied. It often affected the lives of other practitioners significantly in an attempt to maintain a regard for learned medicine.

Chapter 3 begins the narrative, starting during the decade before the civil war and continuing to 1660. Medical regulation under Charles I cost many practitioners much money and anxiety, since the Crown supported the College. But as the political crisis grew, the divisions in the College itself caused the College to move quickly to the side of Parliament, and later to the side of Cromwell.[9] As the College did so, medical regulation was modified, changing from a "monopolistic" protection of the College's licensing powers to a way of punishing medical malefactors brought to the College by the public. But without monopolistic regulation in favor of university learning (except briefly after a new charter from Cromwell in 1656), other practitioners found their voices and spoke out loudly against the College. Members of the College did not take up the new philosophy

---

[9]The account given here somewhat modifies the view of the college as a "Puritan" organization advanced in Birken, "Royal College of Physicians"; idem, "The Puritan Connexions of Sir Edward Alston, President of the Royal College of Physicians, 1655–1666," *MH* 18 (1974): 370–74; and Lindsay Sharp, "The Royal College of Physicians and Interregnum Politics," *MH* 19 (1975): 107–28. The College was, rather, a politically astute group that managed to get along with all the governments of the period.

as a conscious response to such criticism,[10] but many of them did continue to pursue intellectual activities (a great many of which concerned the new philosophy),[11] and their pursuit of the new learning was used in counterattacks on their critics. Many fellows took part in the intellectual activities of Oxford as well as those of London.[12] The period was one of general intellectual ferment, with Continental as well as English, and university as well as nonuniversity, sources. The changes in medical regulation and medical ideas in those decades were the result of complex institutional and intellectual transformations rather than of a single social, religious, or intellectual change.

At the Restoration, however, stronger monopolistic regulation seemed in the offing, as the College obtained a new charter. Other practitioners, particularly the Society of Apothecaries and the Barber-Surgeons' Company, seemingly in association with some of the "virtuosi," managed to block the ratification of the charter in Parliament, leaving the College virtually without coercive power. At the same time, a rival, the Society of Chemical Physicians, was organizing, while the Royal Society was becoming very active and influential; both received courtly patronage, and both gave support to "empirics," or so it seemed to some. The new philosophy that had been promoted by physicians a few years earlier now seemed to many to be an enemy in their midst.[13] The fears of some physicians constituted an important element in the attacks on the Royal Society and the new science of the later 1660s.[14] The several pamphlet wars of the period, often treated separately, ought to be seen as part of the same cloth. The complexity of the interrelationships between institutional and intellectual problems facing medical practitioners is stressed in this chapter, chapter 4.

[10]For this view see Theodore M. Brown, *The Mechanical Philosophy and the "Animal Oeconomy": A Study in the Development of English Physiology in the Seventeenth and Early Eighteenth Centuries;* idem, "The College of Physicians and the Acceptance of Iatromechanism in England, 1665–1695," *BHM* 44 (1970): 12–30; and idem, "Physiology and the Mechanical Philosophy in Mid-Seventeenth-Century England," *BHM* 51 (1977): 25–54.

[11]See Webster; and idem, "The College of Physicians: 'Solomon's House' in Commonwealth England," *BHM* 41 (1967): 393–412.

[12]Robert G. Frank, Jr., *Harvey and the Oxford Physiologists: A Study of Scientific Ideas And Social Interaction.*

[13]Some differences of interpretation and detail will be noticed between this chapter and the interesting earlier work of Charles Webster, "English Medical Reformers of the Puritan Revolution: A Background to the 'Society of Chymical Physitians,'" *Ambix* 14 (1967): 16–41; P. M. Rattansi, "Paracelsus and the Puritan Revolution," *Ambix* 11 (1963): 24–33; and idem, "The Helmontian-Galenist Controversy in Restoration England," *Ambix* 12 (1964): 1–23.

[14]Also see Michael Hunter, *Science and Society in Restoration England.*

The last two chapters chart the course of medical events up to the Rose case of 1703–04, in which the House of Lords overturned the laws and allowed apothecaries the right to prescribe medicines. This is a period that is little discussed by other medical historians. As the Crown's policies became more active, from the ministry of Danby through the Exclusion Crisis and the reign of James II, the College's ability to regulate others was renewed. This period, covered in chapter 5, saw a restoration of older intellectual boundaries between practitioners, as well. Yet after the Glorious Revolution the College was institutionally troubled and intellectually divided. It found some support for regulation from the Whig Junto, but at the same time other practitioners continued to proliferate and to find allies, even among fellows of the College. The apothecaries gained recognition as a "profession," while a divided College of Physicians fought back by founding the dispensary. The "ancients versus moderns" controversy complicated matters further.[15] The gradual failure of the old medical regime was confirmed by the decision in the House of Lords in the Rose case, which ends chapter 6.

This book does not explain medical developments by the rise of a "scientific" approach to the world for two reasons. The intellectual quarrels and transformations of the period called the "scientific revolution" cannot, I think, be subsumed under any one philosophy, whether it be Hermetic, vitalistic, Platonic, Aristotelian, Baconian, experimental, mathematical, mechanical, corpuscular, Newtonian, Cartesian, or any other. All played important parts in the intellectual life of the period; to suggest that one philosophy was most important is too limiting, at least in terms of characterizing the medical debates. The learned physicians faced empirics, defending complex views of health and disease against what they saw as approaches that were too simplistic. Yet neither is the story merely one of empirical approaches to "science" versus the older studies of the texts, for there were also many "empiricisms" in the period. Most physicians wished to defend "learning" in general, as did other well-educated people. Hence, we ought to heed the cautions of the many contemporaries who wished to defend reason and not limit our investigations simply to the rise of "science," which was one among many intellectual changes to affect medical learning.

[15]See Joseph M. Levine, "Ancients and Moderns Reconsidered," *Eighteenth-Century Studies* 15 (1981): 72–89.

Second, the institutional, political, and social changes of the period were at least as instrumental as the intellectual in causing the ups and downs in medical regulation. The institutional story told here tends to conform to a somewhat traditional view of seventeenth-century politics. That is, it seems best to admit that the English Crown did at times try to govern actively by co-opting chartered corporations into its system of administration, a pattern not unlike that of some Continental monarchies of the period, even if in the English case it was opportunistic as much as ideological behavior.[16] The behavior of the monarchical governments during such periods infringed on many people's notions of political right.[17] Such ideas certainly played a role in the two revolutions of the century.[18] The period was one of often vigorous conflict, although, as the "new revisionists" have correctly seen, those conflicts were not simply of the nature of king versus Parliament, and they were often mediated by the royal court and other networks of patronage. The College of Physicians, with its juridical power to sit as a court, was one of the corporations pulled into this pattern of monarchical activity in order to accomplish the wishes of its own officers.

Social changes, too, affected the course of medical regulation in London. The gradual growth of a notion of a "gentleman" that was more a matter of the way one presented one's self than of one's birthright affected relations between medical practitioners, and between medical practitioners and their patients. That is, as the physicians and some of their medical rivals were more commonly accepted

[16]For a particularly good account of the importance of corporations to government, see Brian Tierney, *Religion, Law and the Growth of Constitutional Thought, 1150–1650* (Cambridge: Cambridge University Press, 1982).

[17]See W. H. Greenleaf, *Order, Empiricism and Politics: Two Traditions of English Political Thought, 1500–1700* (Oxford: Oxford University Press, 1964); Howard Nenner, *By Colour of Law: Legal Culture and Constitutional Politics in England, 1660–1689* (Chicago: University of Chicago Press, 1977); Robert Eccleshall, *Order and Reason in Politics: Theories of Absolute and Limited Monarchy in Early Modern England* (Oxford: Oxford University Press for the University of Hull, 1978); Richard Tuck, *Natural Rights Theories: Their Origin and Development* (Cambridge: Cambridge University Press, 1979); Corinne Comstock Weston and Janelle Renfrow Greenberg, *Subjects and Sovereigns: The Grand Controversy over Legal Sovereignty in Stuart England* (Cambridge: Cambridge University Press, 1981); and Harold J. Berman, *Law and Revolution: The Formation of the Western Legal Tradition* (Cambridge: Harvard University Press, 1983).

[18]For another view, which ascribes the revolutions to incompetence and sees them as unimportant in changing the basic way of doing things by "reasonable co-operation" between the king, the Lords, and the Commons, see Geoffrey R. Elton, "The Stuart Century" (1965), reprinted in his *Studies in Tudor and Stuart Politics and Government,* vol. 2 (Cambridge: Cambridge University Press, 1974), pp. 153–63.

26

as gentlemen, their behavior toward one another and toward some of their patients slowly changed. But the suggestion that social pressures determined the intellectual changes during the seventeenth century because they caused certain ideologies to develop is at best an incomplete explanation of the medical transformations in London.[19]

Still, the intellectual history of medicine in the seventeenth century does have a social component. And that social history also has political and economic components. The task of this book is to show how these larger transformations of early modern England affected medical regulation by the learned physicians in London.

[19]For a different view, see the works by Theodore M. Brown cited in note 10, above, and J. R. and Margaret Jacob, "The Anglican Origins of Modern Science: The Metaphysical Foundations of the Whig Constitution," *Isis* 71 (1980): 251–67.

I

The Medical Marketplace
of London

In short, private medical practice is governed not by science but by supply and demand; and however scientific a treatment may be, it cannot hold its place in the market if there is no demand for it; nor can the grossest quackery be kept off the market if there is a demand for it.

A demand, however, can be inculcated.

George Bernard Shaw,
"Preface on Doctors," *The Doctor's Dilemma*

Empirics: Hosts of these uneducated men polluted the English body politic by selling their medical remedies, services, and advice to the unsuspecting public, or so said the learned physicians. Much of the vitriol the physicians directed at other practitioners stemmed from the fact that the public had access to something like a "buyer's market" in medicine, in which the physicians had to compete medically with other practitioners for patients, and in which many members of the public were discerning judges of practitioners—or thought they were.

The social simplicity of the doctor / patient relationship meant that a large variety of practitioners offered medical services, the physicians among them. According to English common law, anyone could practice medicine as long as the patient consented, although if the patient died and the practitioner was not licensed, he could be tried for a felony.[1] The physicians' campaigns in favor of their own ways

[1]Christopher Merrett, *A Collection of Acts of Parliament, Charters, Trials at Law, and Judges Opinions Concerning Those Grants to the Colledge of Physicians London* (1660), p. 66; Edward Coke, *The Fourth Part of the Institutes of the Laws of England: Concerning the Jurisdiction of Courts* (1648), p. 251.

and against the ways of others, then, resulted in large part from the patients' relative freedom to choose the medical practitioners they liked, despite the attempts of some to limit the patients' choices.

Practitioners and the Medical Marketplace

"This week the Lord was good and merciful to me and my family," wrote Ralph Josselin in his diary for January 14, 1649. Every member of his family was basically sound, this clergyman and farmer noted, and yet they had their "distempers." His children had colds, his son Thomas being especially affected, and he himself felt "an heaviness, coldness or moistness in the crown of my head, as if it were rheume, and a pain in my sides, with a little soreness in my bones sometimes in one place and sometimes in another." His wife, pregnant for the fifth time, felt "faint and pained with her child in her back."[2] "But yet," he noted, "through mercy we rest, eat, drink, and walk about within and without doors, though the times are very dangerous in reference to the healths of people."[3]

As this diary entry illustrates, health was precarious in seventeenth-century England, as it had always been. Most of the suffering sprang from nagging illnesses like those Josselin reported for his family during that particularly cold winter of 1648–49. Yet one never knew whether an illness might turn serious and drag one down into the grave, quickly or slowly. The next day's diary entry notes that Josselin "heard of the death of young Mr. Rogers of Taine: Lord, it's thy goodness my wife is not a widow, and my children fatherless."[4]

By the faithful like Josselin who watched for signs of the Lord's favor or disfavor, disease was noted frequently. Yet disease intruded frequently into the letters and diaries of the less religious, also. People did not suffer from illness all the time, of course, and the sufferings of early modern Europeans can be exaggerated. Mortality was clearly higher then than now, particularly among infants, although it was not as high in England as it was on the Continent.[5] And, although harder to measure by far than mortality, morbidity (the prevalence of

[2]She gave birth to a boy in May, but the child died thirteen months later.
[3]The Diary of Ralph Josselin: 1616–1683, ed. Alan MacFarlane, p. 153.
[4]Ibid., pp. 153–54.
[5]Roger Schofield and E. A. Wrigley, "Infant Mortality in England in the Late Tudor and Early Stuart Period," in Health, Medicine and Mortality in the Sixteenth Century, ed. Charles Webster, pp. 61–95; E. A. Wrigley and Roger Schofield, The Population History of England, 1541–1981: A Reconstruction.

disease) was also higher.[6] Hence nagging complaints of ill health are found everywhere in the personal records of the period.

Given their general state of health, people had a desire for frequent medical attention, and English society had developed a wide range of human resources for the ill. One recent estimate by Margaret Pelling and Charles Webster suggests that the ratio of medical practitioners to the general population may have been as low as 1:400, in some places reaching perhaps 1:200.[7] Curers of all sorts attempted to counteract maleficent forces or to bring the patient back into harmony with his or her social and natural environment.[8] Given the frequency of their illnesses and the number of practitioners available, patients often became opinionated judges of the various practitioners.

The most widespread forms of healing were carried out in the home or in the local barter economy. From time immemorial, families, particularly the female members, had cared for their sick and injured. Housewives were expected to know basic medicine, and they kept medicinal remedies on hand.[9] As the proverb had it, "Kitchen physic is the best physic."[10]

Local oral traditions and symbolic as well as herbal treatments were accepted by most people as being of at least some value. Most of the practices are difficult to document, but herbal remedies clearly left their mark on the common names of many English plants: "pilewort," "wound wort," "sneeze wort," (*wort* meaning "plant" or "herb" in Old English), "deadly nightshade," "henbane," and other names were derived from the plants' medicinal properties.[11]

[6]For one account of morbidity in London, see Thomas R. Forbes, *Chronicle from Aldgate: Life and Death in Shakespeare's London*.

[7]Margaret Pelling and Charles Webster, "Medical Practitioners," in *Health, Medicine and Mortality*, ed. Webster, p. 235.

[8]Also see Michael MacDonald, "Anthropological Perspectives on the History of Science and Medicine," in *Information Sources in the History of Science and Medicine*, ed. Pietro Corsi and Paul Weindling (London: Butterworths, 1983), pp. 61–80; Leslie F. Newman, "Some Notes on Folk-Medicine in the Eastern Counties," *Folk-Lore* 56 (1945): 349–60; and Edward M. Wilson, "Folk-Lore Survivals in the Southern 'Lake Counties' and in Essex: A Comparison and Contrast," *Folk-Lore* 62 (1951): 259–60.

[9]F. N. L. Poynter, "Patients and Their Ills in Vicary's Time," *Annals of the Royal College of Surgeons* 56 (1975): 142–43; and Alice Clark, *The Working Life of Women in the Seventeenth Century*, pp. 254–59.

[10]Morris Palmer Tilly, *A Dictionary of Proverbs in English in the Sixteenth and Seventeenth Centuries* (Ann Arbor: University of Michigan Press, 1950), P260.

[11]Agnes Arber, "From Medieval Herbalism to the Birth of Modern Botany," in *Science, Medicine, and History*, ed. E. Ashworth Underwood (New York: Oxford University Press, 1953), vol. 1, pp. 317–18; idem, *Herbals, Their Origins and Evolution; A Chapter in the History of Botany, 1470–1670*; Eleanour S. Rohda, *The Old English Herbals* (1922; reprint ed., London: Minerva, 1974).

The symbolic traditions used by many households are especially difficult to document. Notions concerning whooping cough from a later period may illustrate the kind of symbolism used (this was a disease that few learned physicians would treat until the twentieth century, when immunization became available). Donkeys were associated with the disease because of the likeness of their hee-haw to the cough of the sick child. Adults would therefore pass children under the belly of a donkey in the hope that the disease would be transferred to the animal, or children might be fed bread crumbs from a donkey's mouth in an attempt to transfer the donkey's well-being—despite its "cough"—to them. For the same reason, donkey's hair was sometimes tied about a sick child's neck (preferably from a female donkey if the sick child was a boy, from a male donkey if a girl). Adults tried to transfer the cough out of children in other ways, too: a child would be rolled in a sheep's "form" (the dark, dry spot that contrasts with the silvery dewy grass in the early morning) in the hope that as the form disappeared so would the cough; along the coast, a child might be taken to meet the full tide, loosing the cough to the tide as it went out; or a child might cough into a freshly dug hole around midnight, and the hole be quickly filled in, keeping the cough there. "Tommy-tailors," caterpillars of the tiger moth, were sometimes hung around a child's neck to metamorphose the disease.[12] Different communities might well have a host of different cures for common diseases.

Outside of the family and traditional lore, medical help could be obtained from traditional healers known to the community.[13] The traditional healers were people—again, most often women, although not exclusively so—who for one reason or another had acquired a reputation for being particularly skilled at healing.[14] Local midwives, too, practiced the healing arts. The French word *sage-femme* points up the tradition of local healing, for it means both "wise woman" and "midwife."

The world in which most traditional healers acted was not divided into distinct material and spiritual parts. Minds, spirits, appearances,

[12]"Curious Superstition at Lochee," *Folk-Lore Journal* 1 (1883): 30, 195; Frederick Hockin, "Donkey's Hair as a Cure for Cough," *Folk-Lore Record* 5 (1882): 177–78; W. Warde Fowler, "Sheep in Folk-Medicine," *Folk-Lore* 19 (1908): 345; "Shropshire Superstitions," *Folk-Lore Record* 5 (1882): 161; Newman, "Some Notes on Folk-Medicine."

[13]W. G. Black, *Folk Medicine: A Chapter in the History of Culture;* Keith Thomas, *Religion and the Decline of Magic,* chap. titled "Magical Healing," pp. 177–211; Wayland D. Hand, *Magical Medicine: The Folkloric Component of Medicine in the Folk Belief, Custom, and Ritual of the Peoples of Europe and America.*

[14]For more on some ways in which someone might be granted a reputation as a healer, see "The Folk Healer: Calling and Endowment," in Hand, *Magical Medicine,* pp. 43–56.

objects, all mingled with one another in ways that some well-educated contemporaries termed superstitious. Yet even well-educated people entertained at least some of the notions of the world that influenced traditional healing.[15]

In the countryside, the local clergy ministered medically as well as spiritually to their flocks.[16] John Ward, for example, vicar of Stratford-on-Avon from 1662 to 1681, devoted much of his time to medical care, even undertaking minor surgery.[17] Hugh Atwell combined physic (diagnosing and prescribing) with his spiritual ministry in Devon.[18] George Herbert, writing in the 1630s, saw medicine as a regular part of his duties as rector, and many of the Puritan reformers believed that the clergy ought to care for the bodies as well as the souls of their flocks.[19] Gabriel Plattes' *Macaria* (1641) recommended that "the parson of every parish [be] a good physician."[20] Most clergymen, like the gentry, probably dabbled in medicine rather than devoted themselves to it seriously. Yet in May 1672, Robert Wittie of Yorkshire complained to a fellow physician of the large numbers of clergymen, some quite high-ranking, who were practicing medicine, noting that "their pretences not to take fees was but a cheat, for as much as they take plate, webs of cloth, sugar loaves, turkeys, geese, hens, and eggs [instead of money]."[21]

Local healers often practiced charitably if they had a living by other means, or else they exchanged their services for favors from members of the local community: for the right to pasture animals on someone's land, for labor, services, goods, or food. Yet as the market economy spread, some traditional healers supplemented their incomes, or even completely supported themselves, by receiving cash payments for their attentions. As the Elizabethan poor laws were introduced in the late sixteenth and early seventeenth centuries, local parish officers began to pay local wisewomen to look after the sick poor, which

[15]Michael MacDonald, *Mystical Bedlam: Madness, Anxiety, and Healing in Seventeenth-Century England*.

[16]Webster, chap. 4; Pelling and Webster, "Medical Practitioners," p. 199.

[17]Robert G. Frank, Jr., "The John Ward Diaries: Mirror of Seventeenth Century Science and Medicine," *JHM* 29 (1974): 147–79; Arthur Rook, "Medicine at Cambridge, 1660–1760," *MH* 13 (1969): 107–21.

[18]"Devon Medical Worthies," *Devon and Cornwall Notes and Queries*, 2d ser., 13 (1925), p. 145.

[19]Charles Webster, "English Medical Reformers of the Puritan Revolution: A Background to the 'Society of Chymical Physitians,'" *Ambix* 14 (1967): 21–22.

[20]*Macaria* (1641), p. 6.

[21]Letter of R. Wittie to Yarborough, Sloane 1393, fols. 15–16.

indicates that others were probably also paying for these healers' services.[22] Many midwives also began to be paid in coin for their medical services. Some people entered into apprenticeships with skilled midwives to learn the trade.[23] Their training sometimes included anatomy: one Londoner testified that he had learned anatomy from a midwife named Mrs. Nokes, who dissected a "body dead of dropsy."[24] Occasionally even a gentlewoman entered into midwifery as a trade. The best midwives could earn substantial incomes by attending wealthy merchants' wives, gentlewomen, and noblewomen. By 1650 Mrs. Hester Shaw, for example, had accumulated over £3,000 in property—a substantial fortune.[25]

Although women predominated among the ranks of midwives and sometimes entered into general practice in that capacity, few women publicly sold medical drugs or advice.[26] One William Dawson complained loudly against Dr. Robert Savory when he agreed to take Dawson's sister, Hannibal Dawson, as an apprentice in medicine. The 1641 list of members of the London Barber-Surgeons' Company contains no female names.[27]

Traditional exchanges persisted, then, but other medical practices were becoming more common as the monetary economy developed.[28] The market economy grew in the seventeenth century more

[22]Not until well into the eighteenth century did male practitioners begin to predominate in the care of the parish sick poor. See the examples given by R. M. S. McConaghey, "The History of Rural Medical Practice," in *The Evolution of Medical Practice in Britain,* ed. F. N. L. Poynter, pp. 126–29.

[23]Jean Donnison, *Midwives and Medical Men: A History of Inter-Professional Rivalries and Women's Rights,* pp. 8–9. A darker view of midwifery practice is taken by most, based on tracts like Percival Willughby's written for his daughter: *Observations in Midwifery (1640– 70),* ed. Henry Blenkinsop, 1863, with a new intro. by John L. Thornton, pp. 6–7 and passim.

[24]Annals of the Royal College of Physicians (hereafter cited as Annals), vol. 3, fol. 188b.

[25]Donnison, *Midwives and Medical Men,* p. 10. Also see J. H. Aveling, *English Midwives: Their History and Prospects,* pp. 31–34, 47–85; and K. C. Hurd-Mead, *A History of Women in Medicine* (Haddam, Conn.: Haddam Press, 1938), pp. 400–404.

[26]For information on those who did enter the medical marketplace, see Patricia Crawford, "Printed Advertisements for Women Medical Practitioners in London, 1670– 1710," *Bulletin of the Society for the Social History of Medicine,* no. 35 (1984): 66–70.

[27]Annals, 3:211a; T. C. C. Dale, ed., "The Members of the City Companies in 1641 as set forth in the Return for the Poll Tax" (Society of Geneologists, 1935; typescript at the Institute of Historical Research).

[28]See especially F. J. Fisher, ed., *Essays in the Economic and Social History of Tudor and Stuart England: In Honour of R. H. Tawney;* Joan Thirsk, *Economic Policy and Projects: The Development of a Consumer Society in Early Modern England;* Margaret Spufford, *The Great Reclothing of Rural England: Petty Chapmen and Their Wares in the Seventeenth Century;* and for

rapidly than before, if not as rapidly as in the eighteenth century, changing the complexion of local communities.[29] More and more people sold their labor or goods for payments in coin,[30] and they used that money to purchase services, including medical help, from outside the local face-to-face community. Moreover, those who benefited from the growing market economy sometimes also had rising aspirations, and as time passed they more frequently turned their backs on their poor and laboring neighbors.[31] As the more affluent members of local communities accumulated money, they tended to turn away from traditional healers and to purchase medicines or medical advice. Due to the weight of disease, demand for medical services remained high throughout the period; as the market economy spread, people were better able to purchase the services.

Many medical products became commercialized as never before. As English merchants broke into the American and Near Eastern and Far Eastern trade routes, the prices of imported and exotic drugs dropped.[32] In addition, new fashions in medicine caused more and more people to want to purchase remedies compounded from mineral products.[33] The result was the flourishing of an important market in medicinal products, with more people opening shops and traveling the roads to sell drugs. Many of these traders in turn purchased medicinals from "specialists" in the new products rather than purchasing them from local herb-wives or gathering plants on their own.

---

a later period, R. M. Hartwell, "Economic Growth in England before the Industrial Revolution," in *The Industrial Revolution and Economic Growth* (London: Methuen, 1971), pp. 21–41; Neil McKendrick, John Brewer, and J. H. Plumb, *The Birth of a Consumer Society: The Commercialization of Eighteenth-Century England;* and Ralph Davis, *A Commercial Revolution: English Overseas Trade in the Seventeenth and Eighteenth Centuries* (London: Historical Association Pamphlet no. 64, 1967).

[29]See R. H. Tawney, *The Agrarian Problem in the Sixteenth Century;* Peter Laslett, *The World We Have Lost: England before the Industrial Age;* Margaret Spufford, *Contrasting Communities: English Villagers in the Sixteenth and Seventeenth Centuries;* and Keith Wrightson and David Levine, *Poverty and Piety in an English Village: Terling, 1525–1700.*

[30]James C. Riley, "Monetary Growth and Price Stability: France, 1650–1700," *Journal of Interdisciplinary History* 15 (1984): 235–54; D. M. Palliser, *The Age of Elizabeth: England under the Later Tudors, 1547–1603* (London: Longman, 1983), pp. 134–39.

[31]See especially Wrightson and Levine, *Poverty and Piety,* pp. 110–85; Spufford, *Contrasting Communities,* pp. 1–167; and William Hunt, *The Puritan Moment: The Coming of Revolution to an English County,* pp. 1–84.

[32]C. H. H. Wake, "The Changing Pattern of Europe's Pepper and Spice Imports, ca. 1400–1700," *Journal of European Economic History* 8 (1979): 361–403; R. S. Roberts, "The Early History of the Import of Drugs into Britain," in *The Evolution of Pharmacy in Britain,* ed. F. N. L. Poynter, pp. 165–85.

[33]Particularly the introduction of "Paracelsian" remedies, many of which were compounded from metals and other minerals.

London especially pulled people into the market economy—in medicine as in other fields of activity. Like a magnet, the city attracted poor and rich alike: the poor to find work, and the rich to buy luxuries, to take care of business, lawsuits, and politics, and to socialize during the autumn-to-spring "season." The urbanization of the English gentry and aristocracy helped cause what one historian some years ago called "two of the most interesting phenomena of Tudor and Stuart England": the development of the "professions" and the development of a link between the City of London and scholarship.[34]

All over Europe, the urban markets created milieus in which the "professions" flourished; notaries, lawyers, and medical practitioners provided knowledgeable services to middling and well-to-do clients.[35] In England, London was "clearly the breeding ground for the entirely new professions and services that appeared for the first time" in the sixteenth and seventeenth centuries.[36] Medical practitioners who sold their services—from physicians to ordinary practitioners to drug pedlars—gathered in London.

At least two general types of drug pedlars existed, the itinerants and the residents. Itinerant drug sellers usually depended on their face-to-face presence to impress unknown people rather than relying on local word-of-mouth reputations to bring patients to them. They often set up shows or entertainments, attracting crowds to whom they could afterward deliver their patter about their drugs. By the seventeenth century the words *charlatan, mountebank,* and *quacksalver* or *quack,* used to describe such itinerants, had clearly acquired pejorative overtones in many European languages.[37] In 1635, for example, a Frenchman named John Brushye sued Mrs. Jane Maddocks in the court of King's Bench for calling him a mountebank.[38] Physicians and other learned men complained about how drug pedlars cheated the common folk: "It is usual with these men, moving their wandering and uncertain steps from place to place and from town to town,

[34]F. J. Fisher, "The Development of London as a Centre of Conspicuous Consumption in the Sixteenth and Seventeenth Centuries." *Transactions of the Royal Historical Society,* 4th ser., 30 (1948): 50.

[35]Carlo M. Cipolla, "The Professions: The Long View," *Journal of European Economic History* 2 (1973): 37–52.

[36]John Patten, *English Towns, 1500–1700,* pp. 187–89.

[37]Peter Burke, *Popular Culture in Early Modern Europe* (London: Temple Smith, 1978), pp. 94–95. Also see Sandra Billington, *A Social History of the Fool* (Brighton: Harvester Press, 1984), pp. 58–67.

[38]Annals, 3:158b.

by fair deluding promises and policitations, to draw the lives of simple credulous men, for their own gain, into their own hands."[39]

Itinerant drug sellers of all sorts could be found in England. The fairs in and around market towns attracted large numbers of mountebanks, but they might be found anywhere. In August 1667, for example, John Russell, "mountebank, practitioner in physic and surgery," was licensed by the Privy Council "to vend his medicines, prohibiting all strangers not naturalized to practice near him, in such times and such places as he does."[40] At the end of the seventeenth century, Ned Ward mockingly described a London "horse-mountebank" who, coming across a crowd gathered to watch a street fight between two women, "spurred up his foundered Pegasus, and halting in the middle of the crowd, plucked out a packet of universal hodge-podge, and thus began an oration to the listening herd":

> 'Gentlemen, you that have a mind to be mindful of preserving a sound mind in a sound body, that is, as the learned physician, Doctor Honorificicabilitudinitatubusque has it, Manus Sanaque in Cobile Sanaquorum, may here at the expense of sixpence, furnish himself with a parcel, which tho' 'tis but small, yet containeth mighty things of great use, and wonderful operation in the bodies of mankind, against all distempers, whether homogenial or complicated; whether deriv'd from your parents, got by infection, or proceeding from an ill-habit of your own body.'[41]

Ward has the crowd pulling out their purses and buying up all the mountebank's stock.

No doubt few drug pedlars were either as successful or as patently foolish as Ward's caricature. Still, these "quacks" could sometimes make a decent living, even a comfortable one, by moving around and selling their remedies. The itinerant drug pedlars were numerous throughout the seventeenth century; probably their numbers grew as the economy grew.[42]

[39]John Cotta, *A Short Discoverie of the Unobserved dangers of severall sorts of ignorant and unconsiderate Practisers of Physicke in England* (1612), p. 114.

[40]*Calendar of State Papers Domestic, Domestic Correspondence*, vol. 211, fol. 123. For other examples, see Leslie G. Matthews, "Licensed Mountebanks in Britain," *JHM* 19 (1964): 30–45.

[41]Ned Ward, *The London Spy* (1703), ed. Kenneth Fenwick, pp. 101.

[42]See the many examples given in Charles J. S. Thompson, *The Quacks of Old London;* Herbert Silvette, "On Quacks and Quackery in Seventeenth-Century England," *Annals of Medical History*, ser. 3, 1 (1939): 239–51; E. J. Trimmer, "Medical Folklore and Quackery," *Folklore* 76 (1965): 161–75.

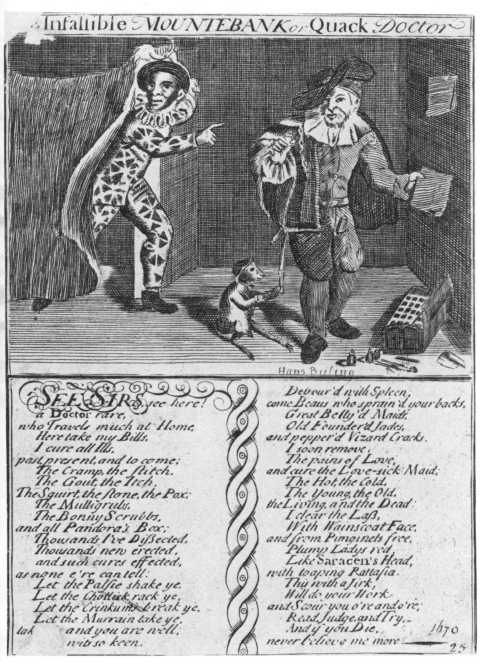

Hans Buling

SEE SIRS, see here!
a Doctor rare,
who Travels much at Home.
Here take my Bills,
I cure all Ills,
past, present, and to come;
The Cramp, the stitch,
The Gout, the Itch.
The Squirt, the stone, the Pox:
The Mulligrubs,
The Bonny Scrubbs,
and all Pandora's Box;
Thousands I've Dissected,
Thousands new erected,
and such cures effected,
as none e're can tell:
Let the Palsie shake ye,
Let the Chollick rack ye,
Let the Crinkums break ye,
Let the Murrain take ye,
and you are well,
with so keen.

Devour'd with Spleen;
come Beaus who sprain'd your backs,
Great Belly'd Maids,
Old Founder'd Jades,
and pepper'd Vizard Cracks.
I soon remove,
The pains of Love,
and cure the Love-sick Maid;
The Hot, the Cold,
The Young, the Old.
the Living, and the Dead:
I clear the Lass,
With Wainscoat Face,
and from Pimginets free,
Plump Ladys red
Like Saracen's Head,
with toaping Rattasia.
This with a Jirk,
Will do your Work,
and Scour you o're and o're,
Read, Judge, and Try,
And if you Die,
never believe me more.

1670

25

Plate 1. "The Infallible Mountebank or Quack Doctor." Engraving by Hans Buling, 1670. Reproduced by courtesy of the Trustees of the British Museum. This satire shows a stage mountebank with his papers and medicines, with his assistant monkey, used to draw crowds.

37

But new advertising techniques based on both the growing economy and the development of widespread literacy and cheap print allowed for rising numbers of another kind of drug seller, one who was resident rather than itinerant. Many drug pedlars no longer had to rely on face-to-face contact with people in order to sell their remedies. They could increase the market for their cures through printed advertisements, which took the form of broadsides tacked up in public places or of printed handbills passed out on the streets or at public gatherings. With advertisements, drug sellers could bring customers to their residences, or to shops, coffeehouses, or other places where their remedies were sold. The one-sheet broadsides and handbills tended to be simple, specifying the usefulness of the medicines, the cost, and where they could be obtained. Some offer proof of the medicine's efficacy, as well, often claiming cures for many diseases.

In the printed advertisements of the drug pedlars, one can almost hear the patter of the seller's voice as he hawks his cures:

A most excellent and rare drink, pleasant and profitable for young and old people, that may be administered at all times, and to women with child without danger, as occasion requireth; and purgeth the body gently, cleanseth the reines and kidneys of the stone and gravel, heat in the back, yard, or secret; freeth the body from itch and scabbedness, chops, or chilblains in the hands or feet, . . . taketh away the morphew, . . . abateth the raging pain of the gout, . . . and is a speedy remedy for the cough, . . . asswageth the raging pains of the teeth, sores or swellings in the throat, mouth, or gums; expelleth wind and torment in the guts, . . . the noise in the head or ears, . . . openeth the sense of hearing, . . . destroyeth worms, . . . and freeth the body from the rickets and scurvy, . . . it is also profitable for women upon all occasions, and encreaseth milk in the breasts of nurses, . . . it helpeth digestion. . . .

This marvelous remedy could be had for two shillings six pence per bottle (one quart), to be taken four mornings in a row, before breakfast, at blood temperature, one half pint at a time. "J. H." also sold "a most precious balsam for man or beast, for diseases and sores inward, and outward" (also for two shillings six pence), and "a most excellent cordial-drink, that restoreth a decayed body, even as seeming near to death, to become healthy, and lusty, and of long life, perfect sight, and fit for all abilities, procreation, and conception" (for almost double the others, at four shillings a quart).[43]

Almanacs, a popular form of cheap literature, often included medical advice, and sometimes they were written with the intention of advertising a medical practice. Most included among their bits of information some utilitarian astrological suggestions for the treatment of medical problems. The buyers of almanacs demanded the presence of the "zodiacal man," a drawing of a man with the veins in the arms and legs illustrated, as well as notes on where and when to bleed someone according to the position of the planets.[44] Many almanacs carried longer sections on medical advice and advertisements for drugs, as did the *Calendarium Astrologium* of 1681 by Thomas Trigge, self-styled "Gent. student in Physic and Astrology." Some medical practitioners published almanacs to help bolster their medical practices, and some astrologers, like the well-known William Lilly, took up the practice of medicine full time when they began to drop astrology.[45]

In addition to broadsides, handbills, and almanacs, the drug pedlars were quick to seize on another advertising device. The newsbooks or "mercuries" (the first newspapers), which were printed during the interregnum, included medical advertisements—and the publishers were criticized for it by some. Samuel Sheppard wrote in 1652 that "there is never a mountebank who either by profession of chemistry

[43]J. H. "A Most excellent and rare Drink . . ." (1650?), in the Thomason Tracts, B.L. 669.f.15(47). Also see the following examples of handbills and broadsides: "Smart's Aurum Purgans" (1664?), B.L. 546.d.44(2); "A Catalogue of Chymical Medicines sold by R. Rotteram at the Golden Bull . . . ," S.P. 29/408/126; Theophilus Buckworth, "Gentlemen, Take Notice . . ." (1680?), B.L. L.R.404.a.4(42); and "Directions for the Sugar Plums . . . ," S.P. 31/1/245.

[44]Bernard Capp, *Astrology and the Popular Press: English Almanacs, 1500–1800* (London: Faber and Faber, 1979), pp. 64–66, 204–6; Allan Chapman, "Astrological Medicine," in *Health, Medicine and Mortality*, ed. Webster, pp. 275–300; Peter W. G. Wright, "Astrology and Science in Seventeenth-Century England," *Social Studies of Science* 5 (1975): 399–422; and idem, "A Study in the Legitimisation of Knowledge: The 'Success' of Medicine and the 'Failure' of Astrology," in *On the Margins of Science*, ed. Roy Wallis, Sociological Review Monograph no. 27 (1979), pp. 85–101. For two examples of advice on how to use astrological lore in medical practice, see John Fage, "student in physicke, and practitioner in Astrologie," *Speculum Aegrotorum: the sicke mens glasse* (1606); and Owen Wood, *An alphabetical book of physicall secrets* (1639), pp. 235–36.

[45]Derek Parker, *Familiar to All: William Lilly and Astrology in the Seventeenth Century* (London: Jonathan Cape, 1975). Lilly's teacher of astrology was the sometime preacher and seller of antimonial cups John Evans, who was prosecuted by the Court of High Commission in 1635 and the College of Physicians in 1640.

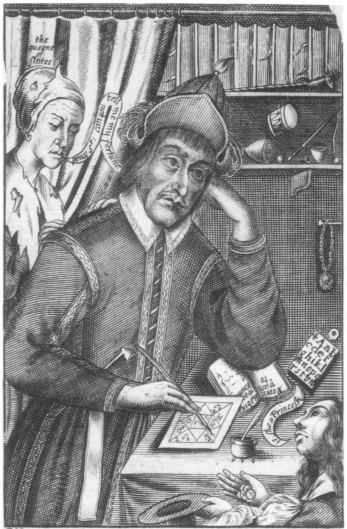

Magnifico Smokentissimo Custardissimo Astrologissimo
Cunningmanissimo Rabbinissimo Viro IACKO ADAMS
de Clarkenwell Greeno hanc lovelissiman sui Picturam

Hobbedeboody pinxit et ✕ ⚲ scratchabat :

Plate 2. "Magnifico . . . Cunningmanissimo . . . Viro Iacko
Adams de Clerkenwell Greeno. . . ." Unattributed engraving of
1663. Reproduced by courtesy of the Trustees of the British
Museum.

The cunningman Jack Adams portrayed as a simpleton. A man is
paying to find out if the "queene of slutes" is a princess while Adams
leans on "Poore Robins" primer as he fills in astrological tables.
Note the alphabet block and toys as well.

or some other art drains money from the people of the nation but these arch-cheats [i.e., printers of newsbooks] have a share in the booty—because the fellow cannot lie sufficiently himself he gets one of these to do it for him." In one 1652 advertisement, coffee, a drink recently introduced from the East, was said to be a sure cure for consumption, dropsy, gout, scurvy, the king's evil, and hypochondriac winds.[46]

Such advertisements might, indeed, be profitable by directing buyers of advertised medicines to the pubs, alehouses, coffeehouses, and assorted shops where the medicines were sold. Ned Ward funned one such coffeehouse from the end of the seventeenth century:

> The walls were hung with gilt frames, as a farrier's shop with horse shoes, which contained abundance of rarities, viz., Nectar and Ambrosia, May Dew, Golden Elixirs, Popular Pills, Liquid Snuff, Beautifying Waters, Dentifrices, Drops, Lozenges, all as infallible as the Pope. "Where," as the famous Saffold has it, "everyone above the rest, Deservedly has gained the name of best"; good in all cases, curing all distempers; every medicine pretends to nothing less than universality. Indeed had not my friend told me 'twas a coffee-house I should have took it for the parlor of some eminent mountebank.[47]

Medical advice could be had from the patrons, too: "They know all that is good, or hurt, / to damn ye, or to save ye" remarked one broadside verse aimed at the coffeehouses.[48]

Beside the drug pedlars pure and simple were those who offered medical counsel as well as remedies. These were the ordinary practitioners or, as the slang of the period had it, "doctors" and "doctresses." They made their livings not only by selling medicines, but by "selling" medical advice, as well.

Evidence for the existence of these ordinary practitioners, most of whom had gotten a practical medical training by apprenticeship, indi-

[46]Both examples are from Ernest S. Turner, *The Shocking History of Advertising* (New York: Dutton, 1953), pp. 22, 24. For some random examples, see *Mercurius Politicus*, Apr. 26–May 3, May 10–17, and July 12–19, 1655; Mar. 10–17 and 17–24, and April 14–21, 1659; *The Intelligencer*, Jan. 25 and 29, 1665.

[47]Ward, *London Spy*, pp. 9–10. The Saffold mentioned here was Thomas Saffold, one of the best-known empirics of London in the seventeenth century; see Thompson, *Quacks*, pp. 41–47.

[48]*News from the Coffee-House . . . A Poem* (1667) B.L. Luttrell Collection, vol. 2. Not just drug pedlars and laymen with medical advice, but physicians the likes of Samuel Garth consulted with patients in coffeehouses. Also see John Keevil, "Coffeehouse Cures," *JHM* 9 (1954): 191–95.

cates that they were not uncommon in the seventeenth century. Robert Wittie, a physician, complained in 1651 that ordinary practitioners, of whom many claimed to be related to or to have learned from "some eminent physician," were multiplying rapidly.[49] George Starkey wrote that Lionel Lockier, whose pills were widely advertised, had learned chemistry from one "Molton of Hogglane."[50] George Thomson noted of himself that he had been taught by a "physician" who had formerly been an apothecary prosecuted by the College of Physicians for making *lac sulphuris*.[51] Mary Trye had learned her trade from her father, Thomas O'Dowde.[52]

The sometimes formal process of medical apprenticeship is well demonstrated in the following letter testimonial:

> [T]he said Robert Le-Neve (as we have [illegible] good information) was educated by his said father [Jeffrey], and by him diligently instructed in that noble science [of medicine], under whom he had practice so long as he lived. But after the death of his said father, he the said Robert betook himself to Doctor John Southwell and practiced with him, and by his own industry and helps aforesaid (being also the inheritor of all his said father's books, notes, and physical observations) . . . hath wrought many excellent cures.[53]

In 1697 Thomas Brown had his stage character "Retorto Spatula d'Ulceroso" (an Italian-born apothecary who believes himself to be a great doctor, surgeon, and chemist) say that he would take an apprentice for £100 and teach him all of medicine.[54]

---

[49]James Primrose, *Popular Errours, or the Errours of the People in Physick*, trans. Robert Wittie (1651), "To the Reader."

[50]George Starkey, *A Smart Scourge for a Silly, Sawcy Fool* (1665), pp. 7–8. See Lionel Lockier, *An Advertisement, Concerning those Most Excellent Pills Called Pillulae Radiis Solis Extractae* (1665). For other remarks on Lockier, see Thompson, *Quacks*, pp. 108–9.

[51]George Thomson, *'Loimotomia'; Or, The Pest Anatomized* (1666), p. 173. Thomson's instructor would appear to have been Job Weale.

[52]Mary Trye, *Medicatrix, Or the Woman-Physician: Vindicating Thomas O'Dowde . . . against . . . Henry Stubbe* (1675), dedication.

[53]Diocese of London, "Certificates and Testimonials," Guildhall MS no. 10,116, box 1, file 1662. A somewhat abbreviated form of the letter is to be found in J. Harvey Bloom and R. Rutson James, *Medical Practitioners in the Diocese of London, Licensed under the Act of 3 Henry VIII, c. 11: An Annotated List, 1529–1725*, p. 59. Doctor John Southwell had an M.D. from Franeker University (R. W. Innes Smith, *English-Speaking Students of Medicine at the University of Leyden*).

[54]He goes on to say that it would cost £1,000 to become a "regular doctor" (by the university route), £1,200 to apprentice with "any surgeon of note," £50 to apprentice with an apothecary, and "perhaps as much" to be put with a chemist: Thomas Brown, *Physick Lies a Bleeding, or the Apothecary turned Doctor* (1697), p. 23.

Some ordinary practitioners, too, advertised their services in print, but often in the form of pamphlets or little books rather than hand-bills and broadsides, so that they would appear to be more respectable than mere hawkers of pills. The technique of using pamphlets to advertise a practice is clearly delineated in *Jones of Hatton-Garden, His Book of Cures,* dated April 18, 1673. Jones began with some seemingly disinterested advice to his readers on choosing a practitioner: "It is not the saying I can or could do great cures, but he that is known to do such cures you must look after, if you intend to have help." Jones was not shy, however, and put forward his little book as proof that he could do great things:

> [I]f you please to read over this little book, you will find that there is but few cures to be named, but what I have cured; the people's names and places where they live, which are your neighbors round about you [whom I have cured, are given], so that you need not go far to know the truth of it; neither need you question, but that I shall do the same cures so long as it pleaseth God to continue the blessing with me; and when He pleases to take it away, I shall do no more.

A list of the people Jones had cured since his coming to London in 1669 followed. He noted that he had printed up other pamphlets before this one and had hired someone to pass them out on the streets, but that "cheats" had been copying his distribution of book-lets and his cures. This book was therefore intended to be a full testimony to Jones's power alone and to the efficacy of his "cordial-pill," balsam, water, and plaster, despite all plagiarizers.

One frequently encounters seventeenth-century books that seem to give medical advice to the public but that, on a second look, are transformed into books intended to advertise a practice. Nicholas Sudell, for example, published *Mulierum Amicus: Or, The Woman's Friend* (1666), which gave directions on compounding medicines for many women's diseases and then noted that if those medicines did not work, he had his own "several secret arcanums and specifical medicines," obtainable at his place in London (the address is provided). William Sermon's *The Ladies Companion, or The English Mid-wife* (1671), dedicated to "the most Accomplish'd Ladies and Gentlewomen of England," was designed "to demonstrate in short, the most facile and easiest directions for women in their gravest extremity, faithfully discovering to them, the sure and true means of help: which secrets by great cure, travel, and long study (through

God's blessing) I have attained to." Sermon went on to note, "I have always had good success in my practice," and to put in a long plug for his "famous cathartique and diuretique pills," but he ended with the respectable disclaimer: "This was published for no private and base end; but as aforesaid, for the sole benefit of my country."

Partially because of the competition among practitioners for patients, then, medical works in the English language proliferated. Increased literacy also played a part in the burgeoning medical book production, by widening the audience. Historians of the early modern period have been familiar for some time with the increase in formal education during the period,[55] and it is clear that literacy spread much further than formal education.[56] Most people therefore had access to the written word through their fellows if not through their own abilities, particularly in London. According to a recent study by Paul Slack, by 1604, had all vernacular medical books been equally distributed among the population, there would have been one book for every twenty people; regimens of health and collections of medical recipes were especially popular.[57]

The rapid growth of a vernacular medical literature provided for the growth of a "middling sort" of medical culture, as well. The books gave basic medical advice so that people could make judgments about medical practices, provided compilations of "home remedies," and gave those who possessed such books a certain amount of power over others, since book owners could proffer "learned" advice to the community. Armed with such books, literate housewives and gentlewomen often advised their poorer neighbors on medical matters, even reading key passages to midwives during labor.[58] These books therefore gave people a certain amount of medi-

---

[55]See especially J. H. Hexter, "The Education of the Aristocracy in the Renaissance," *Journal of Modern History* 22 (1950): 1–20; and Lawrence Stone, "The Educational Revolution in England, 1560–1640," *Past and Present*, no. 28 (1964): 41–80.

[56]Peter Clark, "The Ownership of Books in England, 1540–1640: The Example of Some Kentish Townsfolk," in *Schooling and Society*, ed. Lawrence Stone (Baltimore: Johns Hopkins University Press, 1976), pp. 95–114; R. S. Schofield, "The Measurement of Literacy in Pre-Industrial England," in *Literacy in Traditional Societies*, ed. Jack Goody (Cambridge: Cambridge University Press, 1968), pp. 311–25; Wrightson and Levine, *Poverty and Piety*, pp. 142–54; Spufford, *Contrasting Communities*, pp. 177–218; and idem, *Small Books and Pleasant Histories: Popular Fiction and Its Readership in Seventeenth-Century England* (London: Methuen, 1981), pp. 19–44.

[57]Paul Slack, "Mirrors of Health and Treasures of Poor Men: The Uses of the Vernacular Medical Literature of Tudor England," in *Health, Medicine and Mortality*, ed. Webster, pp. 237–73.

[58]Donnison, *Midwives and Medical Men*, p. 7.

44

cal independence and made them more critical of practitioners in general, while at the same time often introducing them to the advice of certain practitioners in particular.

In addition to writing a medical book or pamphlet, an ordinary practitioner could take other steps to gain increased medical legitimacy in the eyes of the populace: he could try to obtain a medical license. Local bishops, or in their absence their vicars general, were empowered by an act of 1511–12 to examine practitioners in medicine and surgery.[59] If testimonials to the practitioner's correct faith and good art were signed by other medical practitioners and local church officials, the authorities could issue the practitioner a license to practice in the diocese.[60] Additionally, a C.L. (surgical license) or M.L. (medical license) could be obtained from either of the two English universities for a fee after an examination of the practitioner's ability.[61] Finally, the archbishop of Canterbury had the power to issue medical licenses—the so-called "Lambeth degree," from his residence at Lambeth Palace—to whomever he wished. In the middle of the seventeenth century, the fee for a Lambeth degree was thirty shillings, not unbearably expensive.[62] Licenses gave practitioners rights to practice within a diocese or, in the case of the Oxbridge and Lambeth licenses, to practice throughout England. Since the penalties for practicing without a license (from fines to excommunication) were seldom enforced, the licenses seem to have been more important as certificates of ability that could be shown to patients than as remedies against prosecution.[63]

Furthermore, association with a medical guild might give an ordinary practitioner some respectability as well as collective security. For this reason, it is best to view the "surgeons" and "apothecaries" as ordinary medical practitioners who belonged to guilds rather than as medical specialists. Although legally restricted in their practices in London, the surgeons and apothecaries nevertheless frequently engaged in medical practice, gaining their experience by apprenticeship

[59]3 Hen. VIII, c. 11.
[60]See John R. Guy, "The Episcopal Licensing of Physicians, Surgeons and Midwives," *BHM* 56 (1982): 528–42.
[61]Between 1570 and 1658, for example, Cambridge issued 154 M.L.s and 3 C.L.s: Humphrey Davy Rolleston, *The Cambridge Medical School: A Biographical History* (Cambridge: Cambridge University Press, 1932), p. 11.
[62]Frank, "John Ward Diaries," p. 162.
[63]One Mary Buttler gained a practice worth as much as 200s. a case by exhibiting a king's "license" that later turned out to be a "writ under seal out of the Courts at Westminster for attaching one that had not paid her for a cure she pretended to have done" (Annals, 3:171a).

and sometimes a bit of formal education in the same way that most ordinary practitioners did.

The surgeons were sometimes quite learned men, having separated themselves from the medieval barber-surgeons.[64] Thomas Vicary, Thomas Gale, and William Clowes, all sixteenth-century English surgeons, are still praised for their contributions to medical learning. John Gerrard, a surgeon, published both the first English catalogue of a garden and an influential herbal, and established the College of Physicians' physic garden in 1587.[65] The surgeons also seem to have been the first to introduce Paracelsian medicine to England.[66] In 1540, however, the London surgeons were placed with the barber-surgeons in a United Company of Barber-Surgeons.[67] In the Jenkins case of 1602, Sir John Popham, chief justice of the King's Bench, declared that "no surgeon, as a surgeon, might practice physic, no not for any disease, though it were the great pox [syphilis]."[68] In London, then, the surgeons were legally restricted to setting bones, healing outward sores and wounds with topical applications, carrying out bleeding, and undertaking operations such as amputations and cutting for the stone. Many nevertheless knew a great deal of medicine and practiced generally.

The apothecaries grew in number as retail trade spread in early modern England. Originally wholesale merchants and importers of spices, apothecaries constituted one of the fastest growing occupational groups of the period.[69] By the early seventeenth century there were many retail shops in London and growing numbers in the provincial capitals. Physicians and apothecaries worked together to split a new company off from the London Grocers' Company in 1614, and in 1617 the Worshipful Society of Apothecaries was established by royal fiat.[70] De jure, the new guild was a true economic monopoly, since the Crown decreed that no one could practice the

---

[64]Vivian Nutton, "Humanist Surgery," in Andrew Wear, R. K. French, and I. M. Lonie, eds., *The Medical Renaissance in the Sixteenth Century* (Cambridge: Cambridge University Press, 1985), pp. 75–99, 298–303.

[65]For biographical details not otherwise noted, see the *Dictionary of National Biography*.

[66]Paul H. Kocher, "Paracelsian Medicine in England: The First Thirty Years," *JHM* 2 (1947): 451–80; Charles Webster, "Alchemical and Paracelsian Medicine," in *Health, Medicine and Mortality*, ed. Webster, pp. 319, 327.

[67]32 Hen. VIII, c. 42.

[68]*Annals*, 2:155b–157a. On Jenkins case and the conflict between the surgeons and the physicians, see my article "'Against Common Right and Reason': The College of Physicians versus Dr. Thomas Bonham," *American Journal of Legal History* 29 (1985): 301–22.

[69]Patten, *English Towns*, pp. 273, 285.

[70]Underwood, pp. 10–13; Clark, pp. 273–74.

trade of apothecary without belonging to the company, and as such, the new company was resented by the City of London and attacked in the Parliaments of 1621 and 1624.[71] The Society of Apothecaries also de jure restricted the practices of its members to selling medicines prescribed by physicians; the physicians further restrained the activities of the apothecaries by limiting their dispensing to medicines listed in the official *Pharmacopoeia* (published by the physicians), and by retaining the right to inspect the drugs in apothecaries' shops and to examine apprentices who wished to become freemen of the society.[72] Despite these barriers, many apothecaries also engaged in general medical practice.

With the growth of the marketplace and literacy, and the diversification of forms of medical legitimization, private medical practice gained many practitioners a good living, but the golden touch of patronage remained the key to many a practitioner's success. The support of an important local gentlewoman, gentleman, or clergyman, or even better, of an aristocrat or courtier, could cure all a "doctor's" problems. A sure way to secure the interest of patients was to treat successfully someone important.

William Sermon's story is a good example of what could happen to an ordinary practitioner when good fortune in the way of a sick aristocrat came his way. He apparently had attained some medical experience in the armies of the interregnum; even more important to his career, perhaps, was the time he spent shut up in infected houses in Gloucester in 1666 to treat plague victims. Surviving that seems to have earned him a reputation for being able to cure the worst and most difficult diseases. In June 1669, therefore, he was brought to Newhall in Essex to try to cure George Monck, the duke of Albemarle, of a malignant fever—and did. As a result, the king secured a mandated M.D. for Sermon from Cambridge.[73] M.D. in hand, Sermon moved from Bristol to London, where larger opportunities beckoned. He placed an advertisement in the *London Gazette*, informing the public that he "who lately cured the Lord General Albemarle [is in London] and may be seen daily, especially in the forenoon, at his house in West Harding Street, in Goldsmith's rents, near Three-

---

[71]James Larkin and Paul Hughes, eds., *Stuart Royal Proclamations,* vol. 1, pp. 490–93; and "Draft Bill of Proceedings in Court of Star Chamber by the Society of Apothecaries against several persons carrying on apothecaries trade for making and selling defective and inferior medicine, 1621–2," Guildhall MS no. 8285; Clark, pp. 239–46.

[72]Underwood, pp. 13–14.

[73]S.P. 44/31/26.

Legged Alley, between Fetter Lane and Shoe Lane."[74] (This was one of the better neighborhoods in central London, near the present-day Public Record Office.) He went on to gain a good living by selling his "cathartic and diuretic pills" that had cured the duke.[75] His *The Ladies Companion* (1671) and *A Friend to the Sick; or, the Honest English Mans Preservation* (1673) were in large part devices to keep his name before the public.

Sermon's case illustrates the fact that gentlemen such as Monck, and the king himself were opinionated judges of medicine. Among those who had gone to university, the emphasis placed on Greek and Latin letters by medical humanists meant that within the English universities medical teaching was part of the liberal arts, bringing many students into contact with learned medicine.[76] This meant that many university students received some knowledge of ancient and modern medical texts that they could later use in giving medical advice, even claiming some expertise. A gentleman such as John Evelyn treated himself for illnesses, cured the fits of his son, healed a man run down by horses, and discoursed with the duke of York (soon to be James II) on strange cures, to note just a few examples from his life.[77] John Aubrey took a serious interest in medicine, especially in recording various medical remedies.[78] The correspondence of people who were interested in the new science, as well as the correspondence of others, shows the same tendency to record and pass on any medical recipes that might be of use.[79]

The social elite not only dabbled in medical advice themselves, they also employed any ordinary practitioner, apothecary, surgeon, or traditional healer they thought appropriate in cases of sickness.[80] Through this service some of these healers became wealthy. An

---

[74]S.P. 29/265/51.

[75]William Sermon, *An Advertisement Concerning those most Famous and Safe Cathartique and Diuretique Pills* (1672).

[76]Pelling and Webster, "Medical Practitioners," pp. 198, 203. This close association of medicine and arts was common throughout northern Europe: see Pearl Kibre, "Arts and Medicine in the Universities of the Later Middle Ages," in *The Universities in the Late Middle Ages,* ed. Jozef IJsewijn and Jacques Paquet (Louvain: Louvain University Press, 1978), pp. 213–27.

[77]John Evelyn, *The Diary of John Evelyn,* ed. E. S. DeBeer.

[78]Michael Hunter, *John Aubrey and the Realm of Learning,* pp. 43, 96, 107, 109, 139.

[79]See Henry Oldenburg, *The Correspondence of Henry Oldenburg,* ed. A. Rupert and Marie Boas Hall.

[80]Poynter, "Patients and Their Ills," pp. 141–52; also see the case of Anne Conway, in which all sorts of healers were brought in to cure her headaches: *The Conway Letters,* ed. Marjorie Hope Nicolson (New Haven: Yale University Press, 1930).

apothecary who was an immigrant from France, Gideon DeLaune, managed to establish a large medical practice at the English court in the early seventeenth century. He married a son and a daughter into the gentry and left a fortune worth £90,000 on his death. Dr. Radcliffe's apothecary, Dandridge, was worth £50,000 at the time of his death.[81] Of the "principle inhabitants" of London listed by several aldermen in 1640, three surgeons, two medicinal distillers, and five apothecaries are included, in addition to eleven "physicians," several of whom had no known medical degree.[82] The tax list of 1695 notes thirty apothecaries (among other medical practitioners), about half of whom had substantial personal estates worth £600 or more.[83]

Physicians and the Medical Marketplace

But not only drug pedlars and ordinary practitioners depended for their livings on gaining a good reputation among the public; so, too, did the physicians. The only mark clearly distinguishing a physician from an ordinary practitioner was his medical degree (M.B. or M.D.), which he had earned in a university. Ideally this degree certified a physician's mastery of the classical medical texts, but there were wide variations in quality among university degrees as well as among degree holders from any particular university. Moreover, like other practitioners in the days before clinical hospital teaching became a part of English medical education, a physician learned most of his practical skills as everyone else did: on his own or during an apprenticeship.

A small part of the practical knowledge of healing was obtained in the universities, where physic was taught, but more was gained from working under another physician, learning from apothecaries or general practitioners, or trying things out on one's own. A popular proverb therefore had it that "a young physician fattens the churchyard."[84] Practical medical skills were not always closely tied to medi-

---

[81]F. N. L. Poynter, *Gideon DeLaune and His Family Circle* (London: Wellcome Historical Medical Library, 1965), pp. 19, 26; Campbell R. Hone, *The Life of Dr. John Radcliffe, 1652–1714: Benefactor of the University of Oxford* (London: Faber and Faber, 1950), p. 34.

[82]W. J. Harvey, ed., *List of the Principal Inhabitants of London, 1640,* with index by C. F. H. Evans, (Pinhorns, Isle of Wight: Blacksmanbury Offprints, 1969).

[83]David V. Glass, ed., *London Inhabitants within the Walls, 1695* (Chatham, Kent: London Record Society, 1966); "A Supplement to the London Inhabitants List of 1695 compiled by Staff of Guildhall Library," *Guildhall Studies in London History* 2 (1976): 77–104, 136–57.

[84]Tilly, *Dictionary of Proverbs,* P273.

cal theory. Both Oxford and Cambridge as well as most European medical schools therefore required their students to engage in a period of actual practice with an experienced healer before they would grant the M.D. The university-taught medical theory that was the distinguishing mark of the doctors of medicine did not always guide a physician's therapy.

The core of a physician's learning was a Latin (and sometimes Greek) education in the ancient medical texts, supported by the scholastic method of discursive reasoning. This method could derive conclusions from propositions taken from the texts; it was above all a method of "proof" rather than of "discovery," although it could be used to formulate ideas not found in the texts themselves (but thought to be implicit there). As one commentator on the ancient medicine on which the early modern physicians' learning was built put it, "A theory which presents heat and cold, the air, or the four fluids as the causes of diseases can only be proved by dialectics, by logical argumentation. . . . And it is of necessity logical; it is, therefore, accessible only to men educated in philosophy and rhetoric and can only be represented by such men in public demonstration."[85]

Alongside the high medieval traditions of scholastic discourse that remained important in early modern English medical education, philological methods of textual analysis pioneered by the Italians (and brought to England by sixteenth-century humanist physicians such as Thomas Linacre and John Caius) were introducing new intellectual tools for learned medicine. The ancient texts were being read more in the original Greek than ever before, and they were coming under closer critical scrutiny. Problems with the human anatomies of the ancients were pointed out; ancient drug lore was investigated with the help of physic gardens; and clinical training was introduced into several university curricula.

Especially important to the developments in England were the new teachings of the University of Padua.[86] A number of English physicians were trained at Padua in the late sixteenth and early seventeenth

---

[85]Ludwig Edelstein, "The Hippocratic Physician," in his *On Ancient Medicine,* ed. Owsei and C. Lilian Temkin (Baltimore: Johns Hopkins University Press, 1967), p. 105.

[86]On medical humanism, see Charles B. Schmitt, "Thomas Linacre and Italy," in *Essays on the Life and Work of Thomas Linacre, c. 1460–1524,* ed. Francis Maddison, Margaret Pelling, and Charles Webster (Oxford: Clarendon Press, 1977), pp. 36–75; Richard J. Durling, "Linacre and Medical Humanism," in *Essays on the Life and Work of Thomas Linacre,* ed. Maddison, Pelling, and Webster, pp. 76–106; and Jerome J. Bylebyl, "The School of Padua: Humanistic Medicine in the Sixteenth Century," in *Health, Medicine and Mortality,* ed. Webster, pp. 335–70, esp. pp. 339–42.

centuries, and they brought the new currents of medical research back with them. Padua-trained William Harvey, a Lumleian lecturer at the London College of Physicians, put the tradition of humanistic anatomical research to good use in his discovery of the circulation of the blood, published in 1628 in *De motu cordis et sanguinis*.[87] By the 1620s and 1630s, the new humanistic medical endeavors were finding their way into the teaching of medicine at Oxford and Cambridge, too.

Another of the educational revolution's effects on medicine can be seen in the reforms of medical education at the two English universities. The new statutes specified seven years of study beyond the M.A., attendance at medical lectures, and participation in medical disputations.[88] The regularization of medical education allowed the training of more numerous as well as more learned physicians. At Cambridge, for example, between 1500 and 1541 only 1 M.D. and 1 M.B. had been granted. But from the creation of the Elizabethan statutes in 1570 until 1609, 48 M.D.s were granted from Cambridge. From 1610 to 1658, 129 M.D.s were awarded, and from 1659 to 1694, 210 M.D.s.[89]

Yet there were two ways around the long years of textual study. One was to go abroad for a foreign M.D. after having taken a B.A. or an M.A. at Oxford or Cambridge. A physician could then return to England, pay some fees, be examined by the medical faculty of one of the two universities (usually his home university), and then have the degree "incorporated" at that university. This gave the holder all the rights and privileges of an English M.D. Or even more simply, a practitioner might be able to gain the favor of the king or one of his favorites, as William Sermon had done. The king might thereby mandate the granting of a medical degree (or any other degree) from

---

[87]For recent work on Harvey, see Robert G. Frank, Jr., *Harvey and the Oxford Physiologists: A Study of Scientific Ideas and Social Interaction*, chap. 1; and Jerome J. Bylebyl, "The Medical Side of Harvey's Discovery: The Normal and the Abnormal," in *William Harvey and His Age*, ed. Bylebyl, pp. 28–102; Andrew Wear, "William Harvey and the 'Way of the Anatomists,'" *History of Science* 21 (1983): 223–49.

[88]See Phyllis Allen, "Medical Education in Seventeenth-Century England," *JHM* 1 (1946): 115–43; Robert G. Frank, Jr., "Science, Medicine and the Universities of Early Modern England: Background and Sources," *History of Science* 11 (1973): 194–216, 239–69; A. H. T. Robb-Smith, "Medical Education at Oxford and Cambridge Prior to 1850," in *The Evolution of Medical Education in Britain*, ed. F. N. L. Poynter, pp. 19–52; idem, "Cambridge Medicine," in *Medicine in Seventeenth-Century England*, ed. A. G. Debus, pp. 327–69; and H. M. Sinclair, "Oxford Medicine," in *Medicine in Seventeenth-Century England*, ed. Debus, pp. 371–91.

[89]Rolleston, *Cambridge Medical School*, pp. 4–5, 11, 12.

the university; a full one-third of the M.D.s granted by Cambridge between 1659 and 1694 were by royal mandate.[90]

Moreover, more and more English physicians had obtained degrees from foreign universities where an education in the texts did not always take as long as in England. Most French universities, for instance, granted two kinds of M.D.s: the *grand ordinaire,* and the *petit ordinaire* or *per saltum* (meaning "for a fee"). The first was a truly academic doctorate requiring prolonged study; the second was awarded for a fee to those who demonstrated ability and an acquaintance, however slight, with medical theory.[91] The University of Angiers was said by one mid-seventeenth-century Englishman to sell M.D.s for only nine pounds (and spending money to feast the examination committee afterwards was not necessary, as it was at most universities).[92]

More popular still with seventeenth-century Englishmen than the French universities was Leiden. Just across the Channel and Protestant, Leiden attracted many English medical students even though it was somewhat more expensive than places like Angiers. Leiden required its M.D.s to write and publish short theses on medical subjects before defending them orally.[93] This requirement could often be met in a few pages, as the dissertations did not have to be full discussions on medical theory; they might be short exercises on a particular disease or a particular idea, an anatomical study of one organ, or a compilation of various opinions about a medical subject. Usually a residence of several weeks to a few months was a minimum necessity for a Leiden degree, and the degree cost sixteen pounds plus a feast for the professors.[94] A Leiden M.D. represented a much more "clinical" training but a much less rigorous scholastic training than the education in the ancient texts pursued in the two English universities.

The mark of the physician, his M.D., sometimes could help him gain a leg up when it came to assuring potential patients that he was a good practitioner. But a physician's healing skills (as distinct from his

[90]Ibid., p. 12.

[91]Charles Coury, "The Teaching of Medicine in France from the Beginning of the Seventeenth Century," in *The History of Medical Education,* ed. Charles D. O'Malley, p. 127.

[92]Frank, "John Ward Diaries," p. 162.

[93]G. A. Lindeboom, "Medical Education in the Netherlands, 1575–1750," in *History of Medical Education,* ed. O'Malley, pp. 201–16.

[94]Frank, "John Ward Diaries," p. 162.

knowledge) were obtained in the same way as any other practitioner's: by experience. And to acquire a good practice, physicians, like others, had to establish a public reputation for healing. This often was not easy, despite their medical degrees.

The story of how Baldwin Hamey, Jr., established himself is probably typical of how physicians (and others) acquired a practice. His father was a well-known physician and licentiate of the College of Physicians. The younger Hamey was sent to medical school at Leiden, and he incorporated his M.D. at Oxford in February 1630. He soon became a candidate of the College of Physicians, and in 1634 he became a fellow. Nevertheless, his practice foundered and almost failed, until the day Mrs. Mary Peyton came with a sample of her sick daughter's urine. Hamey diagnosed the disease by the symptoms reported by the mother and by inspecting the daughter's urine—a common practice, although the College of Physicians technically prohibited its members from carrying out diagnostic uroscopy when the patient was not present. After Hamey prescribed for the daughter's illness, the girl got well. The cure of the Peytons' daughter brought Hamey a reputation that settled his practice, for Mrs. Peyton's husband was a very wealthy and influential London merchant, and Mrs. Peyton's testimony to Hamey's skills brought the physician many patients.[95]

Hamey's case indicates how important patronage could be in establishing a good practice for physicians. Those who were patronized by the gentry and the aristocracy could do very well. Dr. John Radcliffe, for example, struck it rich when he cured the earl of Albemarle in 1695: he received a diamond ring and £400 from Albemarle, and £1,200 and the offer of a baronetcy from William III (the baronetcy he declined). And John Locke was elevated to importance when Lord Ashley, later the earl of Shaftesbury, took a liking to the young physician.[96]

Physicians, like others, sought to gain a reputation and possibly patronage by publishing works of a more or less learned nature. Publishing knowledgeable works in Latin enhanced a practitioner's reputation among the learned public, while works in English might advance his reputation among the wider public. As the well-placed physician Richard Mead wrote in the early eighteenth century to a young man:

[95]John J. Keevil, *The Stranger's Son*, pp. 48–49.
[96]Hone, *Life of Dr. John Radcliffe*, pp. 58–59; Kenneth Dewhurst, *John Locke (1632–1704): Physician and Philosopher; A Medical Biography* (London: Wellcome Library, 1963).

Should you have an itching to make your name known by writing a book on physic, yet so customary, I will advise you to choose the subject by which you think you will get most money; or that will bring you the most general business, as fevers, smallpox, etc. . . . The method of writing, if in your frontispiece you address not your book to some great man, is to club with some other physicians; and thus by way of letters to commend each other's good practice, and to support and make each other favor. But above all things, take particular care, let the subject be what it will, that the words be well chosen, so to make up an elegant and fervid speech; since you have ten to one that mind the language more than the ideas.[97]

Although Mead suggested writing a book on medicine to help get up a practice, a widely read book on other subjects—science, antiquities, or literature, or an original work of literature—might do as well to establish a physician as a man of learning and parts. Sir Richard Blackmore, for example, gained his knighthood and a position as physician-in-ordinary to King William in February of 1697 after bringing out *King Arthur, An Heroic Poem* (an expansion of his 1695 *Prince Arthur*), which portrayed William as Arthur. Belittled by Pope, Garth, Dryden, and other wits and poets so that his name came to stand for all dull authors, he nevertheless produced other flattering works of poetry and several medical treatises and became, after William's death, physician to Queen Anne.

Physicians developed their own secret remedies to help them gain patients, also like other practitioners. Jonathan Goddard, for instance, was a fellow of the College of Physicians (from 1645), first physician to Cromwell's general staff, warden of Merton College (1651–60), professor of physic at Gresham College (1655–75), and a founding member of the Royal Society—a man of the highest connections. His "Goddard's drops" were well known and widely sold. He is said to have sold the secret recipe for them to Charles II for £6,000. Other physicians' secret nostrums were also widely known, so much so that they could be used in analogies to clarify difficult issues: "The *latitat*," explained one attorney, "is like to Doctor Gifford's water, which serves for all diseases, and so it holds one form in all cases and actions whatsoever."[98]

---

[97]Quoted in Kenneth Dewhurst, "Some Letters of Dr. Thomas Willis (1621–1675)," *MH* 16 (1972), p. 63. Also see the remarks on how publication in natural philosophy could be a route to preferment in Webster, p. 41.

[98]Quoted in J. H. Baker, *An Introduction to English Legal History,* 2d ed. (London: Butterworths, 1979), p. 40.

And like ordinary practitioners who took licenses to certify to patients their worthiness, physicians could gain public legitimacy in ways beyond taking an M.D. They could become licentiates, or, better, candidates and fellows, of the London College of Physicians. They could compete for an academic post at Oxford, Cambridge, or Gresham College. They could try to gain other public posts: to become a royal physician, or to become the physician to one of the five London hospitals (only St. Bartholomew's and St. Thomas's took care of "patients," Bridewell being a workhouse, Bethlehem a lunatic asylum, and Christ's an orphanage, but each employed one physician). Gaining any of these positions testified that other physicians, academics, important merchants, or perhaps even the king himself, thought the physician to be capable, and it introduced him into social and working situations where he would encounter many people. Personal contact was an absolutely necessary prerequisite for physicians, for their views of professional etiquette prohibited them from directly advertising themselves publicly—they had to rely on personal appearance and style, word-of-mouth reputations, and publications to get their names about. Public positions were therefore hotly contested by many physicians.

One other aspect of a physician's practice needs mentioning: consultations with other practitioners. In many instances, patients wanted advice from more than one practitioner and would call in another after consulting with a first. Often the first consulting physician called in others on behalf of the patient. The etiquette of consultations was delicate. "Nothing in the world ought to be carried on with greater gravity and a better decorum than a consultation in physic," notes an anonymous manuscript from about 1700.[99] The College of Physicians specified that the first physician should always speak for the group consensus, that no other physician called in should contradict or embarrass the first, and so on. "A good harmony and understanding among physicians makes their consultations easy to the good of the patient and the honour and advancement of the profession."[100] The College also tried on several occasions to limit consultations to members, but many patients no doubt wished to consult with practitioners not of the College, and so these rules of the College were often honored in the breech. Yet the process of consultation could introduce practitioners to one another, build up bonds of trust

---

[99]"Qualifications of a Physician," Sloane 3216, fols. 42–91; fol. 48.

[100]Ibid., fol. 47b. The rules of the College concerning consultations are given in the 1647 statutes printed in Clark, pp. 414–17.

or create suspicion about other practitioners, lead to a reputation for providing a good second opinion and so bring more consultations, and help physicians without great personal reputations impress patients by calling in colleagues with greater prestige. Even in the personal advice given by physicians to patients, then, the marketplace could intrude.

It should be clear by now that physicians as well as other practitioners entered into the competitive medical marketplace in hopes of securing a good living. The physicians were marked off from all other practitioners by their learning, or apparent learning, certified by their M.D.s. But that was the sole distinguishing mark of the physician, his only clear claim to medical superiority.[101]

Moreover, although the physicians claimed to be medical practitioners of the highest rank, they were not necessarily accepted by all as gentlemen. The notion of a "gentleman" changed over the course of time, and physicians consequently were more likely to be called gentlemen at the end than at the beginning of the century. Some people in early modern England, strongly influenced by the humanist emphasis on learning as a mark of status, did indeed argue that a person should be accorded the rank of gentleman if he studied law, resided in a university, or "professeth physic and the liberal sciences."[102] But when most Englishmen and Englishwomen of the seventeenth century thought of status, other criteria applied, as well, especially the question of how a person lived. Particularly in the early part of the century, the most common opinion was that a gentleman must have an independent income from real property (land). Later in the century, financial investments of other kinds might allow someone to call himself a gentleman. By that period, some physicians carried swords and drove in armigerous coaches, signs of gentility. Yet since many physicians had insecure incomes derived from selling their learned advice, not all were considered gentlemen.[103]

[101]Whether the actual day-to-day therapies of physicians differed significantly from those of other practitioners cannot yet be definitely ascertained, but the differences appear often to have been slight. The rest of this book will show in passing that the most clearly recognized distinction between practitioners was that between M.D.s and non-M.D.s, a difference of certification and training, not necessarily of therapeutics.

[102]William Harrison, 1577, quoted in James L. Axtell, "Education and Status in Stuart England: The London Physician," *History of Education Quarterly* 10 (1970), 141. The difficulties of using Harrison's discussion for a full understanding of late-sixteenth-century English status is pointed out by Palliser, *Age of Elizabeth*, pp. 75–77.

[103]Even in the nineteenth century, physicians were seldom perceived as gentlemen merely because of their medical degrees: see M. Jeanne Peterson, "Gentlemen and Medical Men: The Problem of Professional Recruitment," *BHM* 58 (1984): 457–73. Peterson ascribes the lack of status of the medical "profession" to the physicians' lack of power over others.

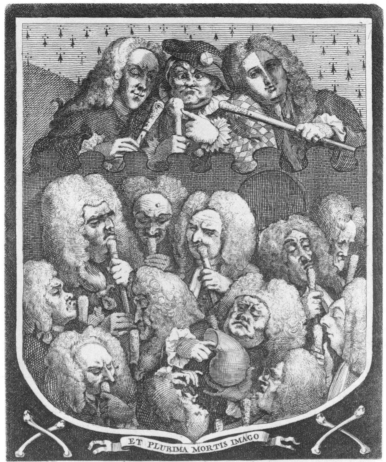

Plate 3. "The Company of Undertakers" or "A Consultation of Physicians." Engraving by William Hogarth, published March 3, 1736. Courtesy of the Wellcome Institute Library, London. The satire takes the form of a coat of arms, explained in the legend. Twelve physicians, with canes and wigs, are shown beneath three well-known empirics of the period: the "Chevalier" Taylor, an oculist (with an eye on his cane); "Crazy Sally" Map, a bone setter (thighbone in her hand); and "Spot" Ward (whose face is half darkened by a birthmark). The legend can be translated as: "And many are the faces of death."

Practicing physicians lived off their practices rather than the land, and no attempt was made to disguise the fact that physicians depended on fees for a living. Physicians, like others, sued patients openly to collect their due. The well-known physician William Harvey used a "secret remedy" in 1621 and 1622 on Sir William Smith in a vain attempt to dissolve a bladder stone in return for a fifty-pound annuity, payable in quarterly installments. When Smith died two months after being cut for the stone, Harvey sued his estate in the court of Chancery for the last quarter's unpaid fee.[104] This fact—that physicians practiced for a profit—removed the profession of physic from the category of a "liberal art" by some definitions, although in the later eighteenth century, as physicians were more likely to be received as gentlemen, the fees became honoraria that could be neither demanded nor recovered by suit.[105]

Like their learned counterparts in the church, physicians competed for a living intellectually; they therefore faced uncertain financial rewards and increasing intellectual demands, making physic, like the church, a profession unattractive to many gentlemen's sons.[106] The educational revolution made it difficult for university-educated men to find decent livings, creating a group of underemployed intellectuals who vied vigorously with one another for any professional position.[107] Undertaking the profession of physic did not therefore guarantee a good income. The normal fee for a physician's visit seems to have been between ten and twenty shillings, which priced physicians out of the reach of many.[108] But these figures are only rough

[104]Geoffrey Keynes, *The Life of William Harvey*, pp. 113 ff. Less well known practitioners also sued: in 1603, for instance, Bartholomew Chapell sued Thomas Lidsam in the Plymouth Borough Court for nonpayment of fees for medical attendance ("Devon Medical Worthies," *Devon and Cornwall Notes and Queries*, 2d ser., no. 13 [1925], pp. 237–38).

[105]Howard Dittrick, "Fees in Medical History," *Annals of Medical History* 10 (1928): 90–101; Fridolf Kudlien, "Medicine as a 'Liberal Art' and the Question of the Physician's Income," *JHM* 31 (1976): 448–59; John W. Willcock, *The Laws Relating to the Medical Profession*, pp. 111–12.

[106]Joan Thirsk, "Younger Sons in the Seventeenth Century," *History* 54 (1969): 366–68. Also see Lawrence Stone, "Social Mobility in England, 1500–1700," *Past and Present*, no. 33 (1966): 16–55; and Richard Grassby, "Social Mobility and Business Enterprise in Seventeenth-Century England," in *Puritans and Revolutionaries: Essays in Seventeenth-Century History Presented to Christopher Hill*, ed. Donald Pennington and Keith Thomas, pp. 355–81.

[107]Mark H. Curtis, "The Alienated Intellectuals of Early Stuart England," *Past and Present*, no. 23 (1962): 25–63.

[108]C. D., *Some Reasons, of the Present Decay of the Practise of Physick in Learned and Approved Doctors . . .* (1675); Edward Chamberlayne, *Angliae Notitia, Or the Present State of England* (14th ed., 1682), pp. 280–81; repeated word-for-word by Thomas DeLaune, *Angliae Metropolis: or, The Present State of London* (1690), p. 156.

guidelines: physicians often treated the poor for less, or even for nothing, while treating the well-to-do in the expectation of far more.

Because nearly all physicians were private practitioners and hence entered the competitive marketplace to earn a living, the diversity of incomes to be gained by practicing physic was great: by one estimate the median estate of physicians who left enough on their deaths to donate money to charity was £1,505, but the average was £2,582 23s. 4d. (figures both remarkably skewed and well below the estates of lawyers and merchants).[109] Many physicians lived well, but all physicians competed in a profession where incomes varied widely. Some even died in destitution. Thomas Grent died in great poverty in 1649; in 1676 John Hale's recent widow had to beg for money because her husband left her nothing on his death; and in 1688 Nathaniel Hodges died in Ludgate Prison where he had been confined for debt, to mention just a few examples from among the fellows of the College of Physicians.

Socially, intellectually, and economically, then, the physicians of seventeenth-century England resembled their learned counterparts in church and university more than the gentry of land, law, or commerce. While the physicians could sometimes achieve social and economic success more readily than other medical practitioners by virtue of their university degrees, they were neither guaranteed such success nor so far elevated socially above other practitioners as to be exempt from their competition.

Of course, some physicians became well-to-do and even gained knighthoods or contracted marriages with the gentry for themselves or their sons and daughters; but this did not make them different in kind from other practitioners.[110] Like other practitioners, by far the majority of physicians never gained entry into the ranks of the gentry.[111] Patronage and riches were no more the monopoly of the physicians than poverty and ignorance were of ordinary practitioners.

Additionally, looking at the practice of physic from the viewpoint of the gentry, one can see that to become a physician by profession would sometimes have been a denigration of a gentleman's status.

[109]W. K. Jordan, *The Charities of London, 1480–1660: The Aspirations and Achievements of the Urban Society*, p. 56.

[110]See the example of an Italian physician marrying into the Devonshire gentry in John Roberts, "A Jacobean Physician," *Devon and Cornwall Notes and Queries* 34 (1978): 80–81.

[111]William J. Birken, "The Fellows of the Royal College of Physicians of London, 1603–1643: A Social Study" (Ph.D. diss., University of North Carolina, Chapel Hill, 1977), pp. 351–57.

This is not to say that English gentlemen could not take an interest in medicine; as noted above, they were likely to acquire some medical ideas at the university. But gentlemen were not to "profess" physic too seriously. Robert Boyle's publisher, for instance, felt compelled to make the following apology for a book of that gentleman's: "[T]hough his method did of necessity lead him to it, yet it might be looked upon as unbecoming of him to meddle with the physicians' art, of which he never did (nor could, by reason of his native honour) make any profession."[112] Since the less than gentlemanly origins and associations of the physicians seem to have been European-wide phenomena,[113] the idea that physicians for the most part were socially far removed from other practitioners ought to be discarded, although by the end of the eighteenth century the profession of physic had acquired a more genteel air.[114]

That physicians were frequently below the rank of gentry had two important consequences for their medical practices. In the first place, it meant that physicians had to enter into the competitive milieu of the medical marketplace to obtain a good practice; indeed, that was a source as well as a consequence of their status. In the second place, the social status of physicians meant that when they were engaged, physicians often had to defer to the medical wishes of their patients. Patients hired whomever they wished, as long as they could afford to do so, and accepted or disagreed with their practitioner's advice as they saw fit.[115] Patients often controlled the medical relationship. While a patient's income and social position frequently affected what kind of medical practitioner he or she sought out, almost everyone had at least occasional access to all kinds of healers, thus being able to

[112]Robert Boyle, *Some Considerations Touching the Usefulnesse of Experimental Naturall Philosophy* (Oxford, 1663), sigs. **r–v.

[113]Luis S. Granjel, *La medicina española del siglo XVII: Historia general de la medicina española,* vol. 3 (Salamanca: Universidad de Salamanca, 1978); Richard L. Kagan, "Universities in Castile, 1500–1810," in *The University in Society,* ed. Lawrence Stone, vol. 2 (Princeton: Princeton University Press, 1974), pp. 367–68, 371–73; Françoise Lehoux, *La Cadre de vie des médecins Parisiens aux XVIe et XVIIe siècles* (Paris: Éditions A. et J. Picard, 1976); and Guido Ruggiero, "The Status of Physicians in Renaissance Venice," *JHM* 36 (1981): 168–84.

[114]In England, indications of the gentlemanly status of the physicians in the later eighteenth century can be found in their changing fees to honoraria (see note 105 to this chapter) and in their occupation of places of political significance: see, for example, the case of the Chamber of Exeter, in which physicians began to appear after 1760 (R. Newton, "The Membership of the Chamber of Exeter, 1688–1835," *Devon and Cornwall Notes and Queries* 33 [1977]: 282–86, 333–36).

[115]Poynter, "Patients and Their Ills," pp. 141–52.

select the practitioner to suit the nature of the appropriate cure.[116] In the end, the physician had to submit to the will of his patients in many cases.[117] Physicians, like other healers, had to offer the kinds of services demanded by their patients and clients, because they competed with one another and with other practitioners for the favor of the public.

One further complication for the physicians must be reiterated: the general knowledge possessed by the public about the basic elements of learned medicine. Despite some changes in the intellectual content of learned medicine, particularly in anatomy and physiology, its analysis of disease—its pathological and therapeutic parts—remained fairly constant. Close attention had to be paid to the six nonnaturals: air, diet, evacuations, exercise, sleep, and mental and emotional stimulation.[118] Disease might be caused when any of the six changed too quickly and the affected person had not taken the proper precautions, or when any of them became "corrupted," or when the patient got too little or too much of something. Then one of the four humors (black bile, yellow bile, phlegm, and blood) might come to a surfeit or decline too much. The trick was to balance the four humors in a harmony with the individual's own unique temperament through attention to the nonnaturals. When the seasons changed, for example, a person's diet and exercise had to be changed, too, slowly, in order to keep the body in balance with the environment. Since all six of the nonnaturals were subject to swift change during travel, Fynes Moryson gave this layman's advice to other layman travelers: "He that feels any change in his body, let him not neglect it, but take physic [here equated with purges], which doing, he may with a small remedy prevent great sickness, and keep his body in health afterwards, not oppressing himself with meat, nor inflaming his blood with violent motion."[119]

---

[116]The case of Dr. John Symcotts illustrates the large variety of people treated by physicians: *A Seventeenth-Century Doctor and His Patients: John Symcotts, 1592?–1662*, ed. F. N. L. Poynter and W. J. Bishop, Publications of the Bedfordshire Historical Record Society, vol. 31 (Streatley, Beds.: 1951).

[117]For a discussion of the effects of patients on medical practice during somewhat later periods, see N. D. Jewson, "Medical Knowledge and the Patronage System in Eighteenth Century England," *Sociology* 8 (1974): 369–85; and Eliot Freidson, "Client Control and Medical Practice," *American Journal of Sociology* 65 (1959–60): 374–82.

[118]Jerome J. Bylebyl, "Galen on the Non-Natural Causes of Variation in the Pulse," *BHM* 45 (1971): 482–85; P. H. Neibyl, "The Non-Naturals," *BHM* 45 (1971): 486–92.

[119]Fynes Moryson, *An Itinerary* (1617; reprint ed., New York: MacMillan, 1908), p. 393. Also see James Hart, *'Klinike,' Or, the Diet of the Diseased* (1633), and Jane O'Hara-May, *Elizabethan Dyetary of Health*.

What was a commonplace for the laity was the expertise of the physicians. Physicians conceived of the practice of physic not as an art of therapy alone but as a philosophy of health. The physician's training gave him access to a learned knowledge of nature and man. He knew a great deal about the secrets of nature and the ways in which man and nature fit together; the very word *physician,* or *physicus,* was derived from the Greek *phusis,* or *nature.*[120] Concerned first with health, ideally a physician was not called on merely in cases of illness. Advising on a diet proper to an individual's temperament provided the foundation for a physician's medical counsel. Appropriate exercise would be suggested, too. Mild herbal drugs and other treatments (such as purging, sweating, vomiting, and bleeding) could be prescribed in more pressing situations to expel any humors that had become excessive. An understanding of the natural processes of the body and mind, an understanding of the workings of nature as they applied to the whole human being, could be had by studying the texts. Theoretical medicine could also help to guide a physician's therapies in pressing situations. In addition, empirical therapies that did not necessarily arise from an understanding of the natural processes might prove useful.[121]

Perhaps an analogy with the learned physicians' counterpart, the lawyers, can better make the point. A person retained a lawyer to get advice on how best to run his or her affairs. A knowledge of the normal course of law, obtained from a bookish education, is essential to giving that kind of advice. Generally, when the advice is followed, few if any problems arise. But sometimes the client runs into trouble—in medical terms, becomes ill. Then the lawyer's consultations become concerned not with the regular operation of things, but with overcoming the irregularity. General advice proposing a mild remedy is usually enough. But if matters continue to deteriorate, a more drastic intervention of some kind may be called for, and the lawyer has to take action of some kind. Here, if it concerns a case going to trial, for example, a knowledge of the law still guides his actions, but the lawyer's practical knowledge of the opposition, the judge, the jury, the court system, the influences of money, power, and prestige,

---

[120]This view of the essential nature of the practice of physic remained widely accepted in the seventeenth century. See, for example, [Christopher Merrett?], *The character of a compleat physician, or naturalist* (1680?), pp. 2–3.

[121]As an example of medical therapies prescribed by learned physicians which often had no necessary relationship to Galenic theory, see the assessment of William Brockbank, "Sovereign Remedies: A Critical Depreciation of the Seventeenth-Century London Pharmacopoeia," *MH* 8 (1964): 1–14.

and so forth may play an equal or even greater role in helping his client than a bookish knowledge of the law. The lawyer may decide to supervise the actions of a private detective, or he may interview people on his own or call in expert advice or other lawyers for consultations on various matters. But in all this activity, practical, worldly experience not gained in law school, or only touched on there, is crucial.

Just so, the learned physician preferred to give counsel to a client on how to remain healthy. This required theoretical skill, for each individual's temperament was understood to be unique. Theory led the physician to an appreciation of what course was best for each client's health. Written counsels could be composed without an examination of the client—messages, the testimony of servants or relatives, an examination of the patient's urine, and other bits of evidence could set the physician on the path to the right texts for composing his advice on a client's well-being. When illness occurred, the physician aided nature in its fight to restore order. Mild correctives could bring things back to normal in most cases: more rest and more exercise, altering one's habits, changing one's residence or companions, changing one's diet, and so on. If a disease became serious, practical measures could be taken in which theory might be a rough guide but in which a worldly knowledge and experienced judgment might yield success where theory failed. Practical results, not learning alone, counted in cases of illness.

Thus, the learning of the physicians helped them cure patients, but it also, and more importantly to many physicians, enabled them to counsel clients on health. When it came to mere healing, eclectic practices were the rule, as the case of Richard Napier so clearly demonstrates.[122] The physician might also call in other physicians for consultations, get expert advice from apothecaries, surgeons, or other practiced empirics on specific details, and possibly supervise the ministrations of others. Behind all, however, learned physic and counsel were the physician's stock in trade. Hence, the renowned physician Sir Thomas Browne could write in 1646 to Henry Power, a medical student at Christ's College, Cambridge: "*Materia medicamentorum,* surgery and chemistry, may be your diversions and recreations; physic [i.e., studying nature] is your business."[123]

[122]Napier's medical practice is partially described in MacDonald, *Mystical Bedlam;* it will be more extensively described in a forthcoming University of Wisconsin Ph.D. dissertation by Ronald Sawyer.

[123]Quoted in Pelling and Webster, "Medical Practitioners," p. 205.

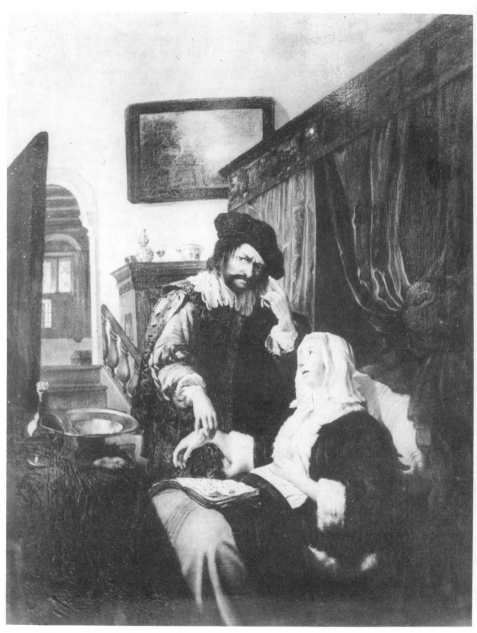

Plate 4. Untitled portrayal of the consultation of a Dutch physician and a patient. Oil by or after Frans van Mieris I. Courtesy of the Wellcome Institute Library, London. In this painting, the physician points to his temple to indicate his theoretical wisdom after taking the pulse and (by the implication of her open mouth) hearing the report of his patient.

Browne's advice was almost a commonplace: physic constituted learning, while mere medicine consisted of experience in therapy alone. One anonymous manuscript giving "Advise to a Young Physician" puts matters this way: first, "every morning seek a blessing from God Almighty"; second, be expert at Latin, and study Greek and Arabic well for an understanding of the ancient texts; third, "learn thy philosophy exacto, wherein consists the knowledge of man, the prime subject of medicine"; and fourth, "observe that if thou attempt to be a physician without those former qualifications, thou shall never become famous nor in respect." To study medicine itself, a further but secondary requisite for becoming a physician, one ought, the manuscript instructs, to begin with a solid author such as Daniel Sennert, beginning with his anatomy and working through his *Institutes*. "And for thy recreation, learn to know the [herbal] simples," first from the gardens and fields, then, together with compound medicines, from an apothecary's shop, "and frequent his shop civilly." One should also know some surgery, "so that, being in the country, thou do not be ashamed for want of a surgeon" to open the veins quickly and easily. When it comes to practice, the manuscript counsels again begin with prayer. "Then give advice deliberately, and that only for the present condition, remitting thy second advice, to a second visit." Before giving advice, the physician should examine the patient for his or her constitution and age. The season of the year and the disease itself were both to be considered, too. "Be sparing to prognosticate. And begin always with the most safe medicine."[124] Such remarks seem sensible enough, but the author clearly stresses the knowledge of languages and philosophy and the reading of good medical authors. Physicians need only a smattering of "recreational" knowledge of herbs and surgery. The main weight of practice is to be in *advice*.

We have seen, however, that physicians had to get up a practice in competition with one another and with other practitioners. The medical marketplace, controlled by informed patients, could directly threaten the ideal of a learned practice of medical counsel. Many nonphysicians, for example, claimed that learned advice based on a theory of health as balance among the humors, with bleeding, purging, and diet as its main therapies, promoted incompetence. They

---

[124]"Advyse to a young physitian. to one who intends to studie medicine and live thereby," Sloane 163, fols. 1–5. The manuscript bears a date of 1647 in another hand, but it may be of slightly earlier provenance.

drew on a popular suspicion here: "The physician is more dangerous than the disease."[125]

Most of the ordinary practitioners and empirics practiced medicine rather than physic. When it came to medicine, they often argued, experience, not bookish learning, was the important criterion for choosing a practitioner; therefore, with their practical experience in medicine, they were better practitioners than the learned and logic-chopping physicians—or so they claimed. Apparently many patients believed them, too.

As a result, complaints about patients were common among physicians. In 1637 Thomas Brian wrote that few physicians believed in being able to diagnose a disease from a distant inspection of the urine alone. They were constantly saying that the urine was a harlot or a liar, and that one visit to a patient was worth twenty inspections of the patient's urine. Yet, Brian wrote, "the vulgar sort are so strongly prepossest (by reason of their ignorance) that physicians can discern (by the urine) the disease, the conception, the sex, the party's age, with many other absurdities, that I fear it will be an hard matter to dispossess them of that opinion."[126]

Dr. C. T. (probably Timothy Clarke) wrote that practitioners who loudly advertise themselves and their virtues impress the populace, but "a learned and rational physician, especially if he have the misfortune of being modest, is looked upon at the best but as a weak, and a timorous man." He also declared that patients did not pay their bills unless they thought some great difficulty was had in rendering a cure (whereas to him the true art of physic consisted in making difficult matters look easy). Thus to increase his reputation and insure payment, one physician who was called to treat a great lady in the country (who was despaired of by her family but who the physician could see would soon get well) made up four little pills of bread and, putting them in a fine box, presented them to the lady, dissolved them in water with a flourish, and gave the concoction to her to drink. Just as he thought, she went into a sweat and recovered. People ever after importuned him for his secret pills.[127]

Because the medical marketplace did not function ideally, the anonymous author of a seventeenth-century manuscript treatise entitled "A Just and Necessarie Complaint concerning Physicke" at-

[125]Tilly, *Dictionary of Proverbs*, P267a.
[126]Thomas Brian, *The Pisse-Prophet or, Certaine pisse-pot Lectures* (1637), sigs. A2r-v, and p. 1.
[127]Dr. C. T., *Some Papers writ in the Year 1664 . . .* (1670), pp. 3, 39, 21–22.

tacked physicians, "unlawful intruders into the art and faculty of physic," "visitants and attendants . . . belonging to the patients" (i.e., their friends and servants), and the patients themselves. The physicians, he declared, had "prostituted the most noble and excellent art of physic" by "aiming more at their own particular ends and profit than the public good." The next group the author accused of damaging medicine had received "no true education, qualification, authority, or accommodation, [and were] intemperate and such as make not conscience of their actions, whose ends are not the good of the people, but their own private lucre and profit." Those who attended the sick gave "sinister commendations of physicians either as they are allied, or have some other relation to them."

Moreover, this author thought that the patients themselves had much to answer for. First, they did not complain "in due time" but delayed calling a physician until they had "tried their own blind experiments and conclusions, thereby often laying such ill foundations that no good building can be wrought thereon." Second, "if he presently finds not cure or ease as soon as he expects then forthwith he changeth his physician and applies himself to another, and commonly lays the fault on his former physician whereas the truth is seldom but his own either in not following and not conforming to the counsels and directions of his physician." Third, the patients expected "cure and satisfaction from [the inspection of] urines." Fourth, patients took "offense at the physician his refusal to visit them when they are visited with the pestilence." And fifth, the author condemned patients "for their disrespective demeanor and ingratitude to their physician." The author concluded with a quotation from Laurent Joubert's *Erreurs populaires et propos vulgaires* (1579): "And thus they deal many times with their physicians during their sickness, promising them golden mountains, peaks, and precious stones or some yearly pension at least. But being once recovered they are of a far other mind."[128] Who, besides the patients and medical entrepreneurs, could have loved such a state of affairs?

Because the medical marketplace often assigned to physicians the status of medical servants to their patients, it not only bred social and economic insecurities, but also posed a deep threat to the physicians' ability to maintain themselves as a learned group. Patients often

[128]Sloane 2563, fols. 1–19. The manuscript appears to be the unfinished draft of a book for publication. It is written in a mid-seventeenth-century hand and may be from the interregnum, since it begins "in this hopeful time of Reformacōn."

wanted quick and immediate cures rather than a reasoned discourse on illness. As a result, vociferous conflicts arose between practitioners over medical services. Since all were competing for a practice, every practitioner had to make public claims to expertise and might try to support those claims with his or her own scholastic or nonscholastic reasoning. This bred public quarrels over medical therapies and philosophies.

In addition, the rather abstract and distant relationship between patient and healer that existed when medical help was purchased from a stranger may have contributed to the promotion of an "ontological" notion of disease. The flexibility of the monetary economy and its stimulation of demands for new goods and services made some of those who lived off of it eager to make medical innovations. The medical marketplace became an important force for change in medical practice, for when practitioners sold their advice to the sick rather than to the healthy, as the medical marketplace more and more demanded that they do, there was less and less justification for studying long years in the ancient texts. The medical marketplace increasingly focused the attention of practitioners on therapy rather than on "wellness," on the disease rather than on the patient.[129] The implications for the status of physicians, which was derived from an ability to master medical theory, were enormous, and were so because the patients often had strong opinions on medical practice and a large variety of practitioners from whom to choose. It was a buyers' market, so medical practitioners were forced to modify their behavior.

The learned physicians and their allies, who frequently had high ideals of what medicine ought to be, often took a rather jaundiced view of the medical marketplace. Yet many physicians did have two common bonds that gave them an important advantage in their struggles with rival practitioners and unruly patients: they had the status of learned men and a common view of the medical milieu, both of which were shaped by their university educations. As a self-conscious group, the learned physicians had an important weapon in their arsenal: they could organize themselves institutionally in order to set collective standards and to govern others. Political means could help the physicians secure their sought-after place at the head of the medical hierarchy by granting them powers both to maintain high

---

[129]For a quite different view of these changes in medicine, their implications, and causes, see Michel Foucault, *The Birth of the Clinic: An Archaeology of Medical Perception*, trans. A. M. Sheridan Smith.

standards of learning in physic and to coerce their rivals into obedience to their direction.

Given the state of the medical marketplace, any group would have encountered difficulties in attempting to govern medical practice. But as we shall see, the growth of the public power of the English Crown in the early modern period offered an opportunity for the physicians to so govern. The physicians found that the English monarchy was willing and able to intervene in the affairs of its subjects from a certain vision of the "public good." The Crown provided opportunities for the learned physicians by supporting their powers to supervise the medical community, thus protecting the physicians' social and intellectual position. The ways in which the Crown helped the physicians determined the powers that the physicians could bring to bear against their rivals.

2

Knowledge and Power:
The London College of Physicians

Singular, communed the guest with himself, the wonderfully un-
equal faculty of metempsychosis possessed by them, that the puer-
peral dormitory and the dissecting theatre should be the seminaries
of such frivolity, that the mere acquisition of academic titles should
suffice to transform in a pinch of time these votaries of levity into
exemplary practitioners of an art which most men anywise eminent
have esteemed the noblest.

James Joyce, *Ulysses*

The physicians of early modern London were engaged in a sometimes precarious profession. Socially, intellectually, and medically,
troubles abounded, particularly for younger physicians. But if the old
formula that "a physician was a gentleman, while apothecaries and
surgeons were mere craftsmen" can no longer be accepted, the formula does express an ideal that existed in the minds of the London
physicians.[1] They would have liked medical practice to have been
limited to the members of the three City medical corporations, with
the Society of Apothecaries and the Barber-Surgeons' Company subordinate and obedient to the College of Physicians; and they would
have liked to have been respected as gentlemen, confining the others
to the status of shopkeepers.

The physicians' wishes may not have been entirely granted by
London society, but through the agency of the College of Physicians

[1]Bernice Hamilton, "The Medical Professions in the Eighteenth Century," *Economic History Review* 4 (1951): 141. For just one example of how Hamilton's views have been repeated, see W. A. Speck, *Stability and Strife: England, 1714–1760* (Cambridge: Harvard University Press, 1979), p. 50.

the physicians had a mechanism to strive for their goals. The College encouraged and protected the learning of the academic physicians, their one clear claim to the status of a gentleman; it also had juridical powers to make that learning the standard by which all other practitioners might be judged, thus establishing barriers against the medical competition of others.

The College of Physicians as a Learned Society

The London College of Physicians was in large part a learned society, at least internally. The new medical humanism of Thomas Linacre and his learned colleagues had originally provided the impetus to found a medical corporation in London that would rival some of the Continental ones.[2] In order to encourage medical learning Henry VIII granted a royal charter to this small group of academic and largely court physicians in September 1518. In its early years, the College met at Linacre's home, apparently most commonly to discuss medical ideas.

The Crown seems to have viewed the encouragement of medical learning as a good thing for the larger "common weal." Thus the immediate cause for the chartering of the College was an outbreak of epidemic plague in 1518, an epidemic during which the Crown issued the first set of plague orders ever by an English government.[3] The humanist idea of governing for the larger public good rather than simply for the purpose of carrying out justice allowed Henry VIII's government to extend its authority in new ways, including into the sphere of acting for the public health. The College therefore provided a reservoir of knowledge that could help the monarchy temper the effects of plague—again, as other corporations of physicians did on the Continent.[4]

[2]On Continental precedents for the College of Physicians, see Gweneth Whitteridge, "Some Italian Precursors of the Royal College of Physicians," *Journal of the Royal College of Physicians, London* 12 (1977): 67–80; and Charles Webster, "Thomas Linacre and the Foundation of the College of Physicians," in *Essays on the Life and Work of Thomas Linacre, c. 1460–1524,* ed. Francis Maddison, Margaret Pelling, and Charles Webster (Oxford: Clarendon Press, 1977), pp. 198–222.

[3]Webster, "Thomas Linacre"; *Letters and Papers, Foreign and Domestic, of the Reign of Henry VIII* (London: HMSO, 1864), vol. 2, pt. 2, p. 1276.

[4]See Carlo M. Cipolla, *Public Health and the Medical Profession in the Renaissance;* Richard Palmer, "Physicians and the State in Post-Medieval Italy," in *The Town and State Physician in Europe from the Middle Ages to the Enlightenment,* ed. Andrew W. Russell, pp. 47–61; and José Mária López-Piñero, "The Medical Profession in Sixteenth-Century Spain," in *Town and State Physician,* ed. Russell, pp. 85–98.

The College was chartered, then, to encourage medical learning and to make that learning available to the Crown in moments of public emergency. Two other matters complicated the purposes of the College, however: the charter created a system of patronage for the court physicians by granting them, the first officers of the College, the right to be sole practitioners in physic in London and within seven miles; and it granted them juridical powers to hand down penalties against those infringing on this right. By giving humanistically trained physicians the right to regulate other medical practitioners, Henry VIII made their learned medicine the standard by which the practices of all others might be judged. As a body of learned physicians at the pinnacle of a Crown-sponsored medical hierarchy, the College encouraged medical learning both by emulation and by simply not allowing uneducated physicians to practice. A parliamentary act in 1523 both extended the licensing power of the College throughout the whole of England (a provision later ignored) and, more importantly, gave the royal charter of the College statutory authority.[5]

The notion that the College was a society of learned men remained very much in evidence in the seventeenth century. Admission to full membership in the College—that is, to the rank of fellow—was limited in the sixteenth century to Englishmen with medical doctorates (of any university). After the arrival of a new monarch in England in 1603, however, the College opened its doors to "British" M.D.s (in 1606) to allow James I's Scottish royal physician, John Craige, to become a fellow. At the same time, however, it set a new limitation on new fellows: all of them had to have studied for seven years past the M.A. for the M.D., the same length of study specified by the two English universities.[6]

Further changes came in 1621, as the College sought the help of various members of Parliament in obtaining ratification for a new charter. The two M.P.s representing Cambridge University complained that there were more fellows of the College who had obtained their M.D.s abroad than ones who had earned them in England, thus causing the College to consider for the first time limiting membership to medical doctors of one of the two English universities. The idea was discussed again in 1624 (another year of debate over medicine due to the sitting of a Parliament), and it was adopted in 1626,

[5]14 and 15 Hen. VIII, c. 5.
[6]Annals, 2:189b.

thus afterward forcing prospective fellows who had earned M.D.s abroad to "incorporate" their degrees at Oxford or Cambridge. In 1642 those with non-Oxbridge M.D.s were admitted but forced to pay a double entry fee and to give a bond on their promise to incorporate the degree at Oxford or Cambridge within two years. But sometime during the 1650s the rules about not being admitted without an incorporated Oxbridge doctorate were reestablished, only lapsing in the years shortly after 1687, when the number of fellows was doubled.[7]

In addition to requirements clearly establishing long academic preparation for entry, a further barrier to the unlearned was presented by requiring the candidates for the fellowship to undergo a three-part examination in physiology, pathology, and therapeutics. The examinations were given orally, normally on three separate occasions and, naturally, in Latin. The examinations were rooted in the texts. For instance, the revised statutes of the College in 1647 specified that questions could be put from the following texts: in physiology, from the *Elements of Hippocrates, On Temperaments, On the Uses of the Parts, On Anatomical Procedures, On the Natural Faculties* (all texts by Galen), "and on other natural parts of medicine"; in pathology, from *On the Art of Medicine, On the Affected Parts, On Differences of Sicknesses, On Fevers, On the Pulse,* and *The Book of Prognostics,* all also by Galen; in therapeutics, from *On Hygiene* and *On Method in Medicine* by Galen, and *Regimen in Acute Diseases, On Ancient Medicine, On Crises,* and the *Aphorisms,* Hippocratic works.[8]

Once the potential fellow had exhibited his degree and agreed to undergo his examination, he was allowed to visit each of the fellows individually at their homes so that they could weigh his character as well as his knowledge and judgment. At a meeting of the whole College, the fellows would vote on admissions by dropping black or white markers into an urn. If elected to a fellowship only to find the statutory number of fellows complete, the newcomer would be made a candidate, being allowed to attend meetings but not to vote, until a fellowship became vacant and he was the most senior candidate, whereupon he would normally be raised to the empty seat.

The College of Physicians also allowed M.D.s and non-M.D.s to practice under its aegis through the granting of licentiate status to men with some knowledge of medicine, or some ability to treat

[7]Annals, 3:43b, 67b, 217a.
[8]Clark, p. 410. The Latin statutes of 1647 are printed on pp. 393–417.

illnesses. They, too, were subject to an examination, usually in Latin, although exceptions could be made for English interviews. Approved licentiates could practice within the College's jurisdiction, that is, within a seven-mile radius of London, including within the City itself. Usually the licentiates could not be fellows because they did not have M.D.s or did not have their medical doctorates incorporated at the English universities. The quality of such practitioners could range from that of Thomas Sydenham, renowned throughout Europe for his expertise in curing fevers; to Caleb Coatesworth (made licentiate in 1688) or Sir John Colbatch (1696), a disenfranchised apothecary called a quack by many and a great man by some; to many practitioners who are known only by name, some of whom no doubt would have been hard to differentiate from good ordinary practitioners. In fact, when the physicians of the College wished to refute publicly the charge that they were a "monopoly," they pointed to their licentiates, a category of practitioners that, they claimed, showed that virtually any worthy practitioner might gain admission to the College.[9] Thus, the College of Physicians was a body whose full members, the fellows, were highly educated physicians otherwise engaged in private practice, and whose licentiates were only somewhat less academic in their training.

The members of the College ordinarily met together on at least four annual occasions: the day after Michaelmas (September 30); the morrow of St. Thomas the Apostle's Day (December 22); the day after the Annunciation of the Virgin Mary (March 26) or, as Catholic feast days fell into disrepute, on the morrow of Palm Sunday; and on the day following St. John the Baptist's nativity (June 25). At three of these annual meetings, all the statutes governing the behavior of the members were to be read. Other meetings could be called as occasion warranted. At these annual meetings the College also voted on corporate matters and elected new members. The fellows undoubtedly renewed acquaintances and discussed private, professional, and academic business at regular meetings, as well.

The learned nature of the group was emphasized by the required attendance at the annual lectures (the Lumleian lecture in surgery and

[9]The revised statutes of 1647, for example, are clear on this point: "Aequum autem censemus, ut censores, et socii, examinatos omnes, quotquot tam doctrina quam moribus idoneos repererint, ad medicinae praxin admittant: ne Collegium nostrum monopolii accusetur: modo tamen statutis Collegii morem gesserint." (We are nevertheless of the opinion that it is just that the censors and fellows admit to medical practice all those having been examined and found sufficient in learning and conduct, as many so ever there are, so that our College may not be accused of a monopoly; but only as long as they uphold the statutes of the College faithfully. My translation.) Clark, p. 410.

the Gulstonian in anatomy); later the Harveian Oration was added.[10] These occasions allowed the lecturers to demonstrate their knowledge and to point out new facts and ideas to intellectual colleagues (rather than to medical students, who needed to learn elemental things), thus giving the lecturers a chance to do original work if they wished to do so. The most important result was William Harvey's discovery of the circulation of the blood, made while he was a Lumleian lecturer, although other College lecturers also furthered medical theory in the course of their preparation for the talks. (Many appointed lecturers, however, considered the talks an onerous duty to be avoided if possible, or performed perfunctorily if necessary.)

But not all was intellectual business, for the College also observed an annual feast, although the fellow chosen to organize and supply the feast often preferred to pay a fine rather than undertake the exertions and expenses of such an event.

In addition to the social and intellectual fruits of membership, a College fellow gained tangible legal privileges, as well. Members of the College were exempt from serving on assizes, juries, inquests, attaints, or any other "recognition"; they were exempt from lower City offices such as watch and ward or constablewick; and they were exempt from bearing or providing arms (a form of taxation), although they had to go to court on a number of occasions to maintain this privilege in the face of monarchical and municipal actions.[11] Such exemptions were not negligible in a period when minor City offices, jury duty, and war taxes frequently imposed daily burdens on the citizens of London. All in all, the College of Physicians must have seemed to its members to be something like an occasional university college for regular but not burdensome academic exchange and conviviality.

Although the College membership was small, the number of members grew over the course of the seventeenth century at the same pace that the City of London grew. In 1605 the three royal physicians were to be made "supernumerary" to the twenty-four fellows, making a total of twenty-seven full members. By 1614 the number of royal physicians had grown to six, making for thirty fellows, and the number of royal servants was further increased by one in 1616. In 1618, therefore, the statutes were revised to allow for thirty-four

[10]On the Lumleian Lectureship (1582), see F. W. Steer, "Lord Lumley's Benefaction to the College of Physicians," *MH* 2 (1958): 298–305; on the Gulstonian Lectureship (1632), see Clark, pp. 251–52. The Harveian Oration was added in 1656.

[11]John W. Willcock, *The Laws Relating to the Medical Profession*, pp. 137–41. Willcock maintains that the physicians were not exempt from the last duty, but the College was able to maintain the exemption in the seventeenth century.

fellows, with four supernumerary royal physicians. The new charter of 1664 expanded the number of fellows to forty, and in the same year the category of "honorary fellow" was created; nevertheless, the College often went over its statutory limitation on the number of actual fellows. Another charter, in 1687, set the number of fellows at eighty.

Counting the number of fellows alone, one finds that the increase in their statutory number from twenty-four in 1605 to eighty in 1687 (a 333 percent increase) was faster than the growth of the population of London (from c. 200,000 in 1603 to c. 575,000 in 1695, or a 287 percent rise); the actual increase in fellows from twenty-four to seventy matched the rate of London's population growth of the same years almost exactly (291 percent). (For the total numbers of members of the College, see appendix 1, table 6.) In the end, then, although never as large a body as the Royal Society (which had social as much as intellectual requirements for entry), the College of Physicians was a sizeable learned society that adapted well (in terms of numbers, at least) to its changing urban environment.

Watching over the members and the fortunes of their institution were the officers of the College. A group of eight "elects" existed, a group that itself chose fellows to replace deceased or resigned elects in a self-selecting oligarchical fashion (much like that of other corporations of the day). From among the elects were annually chosen the president and two elders, or *consiliarii,* the chief College officers.

The election of officers occurred at the regular Michaelmas meeting of the College. After all the members had gathered together in the main meeting room at the College's building, the former president made a speech and placed the mace of office in the hands of the senior of the *consiliarii.* All the members but the elects were excused; the senior *consiliarius* then nominated an elect as the new president, a nomination voted on by the other elects. The other fellows and candidates of the College were then invited to return to the room, and they helped to choose the other officers: a registrar, a treasurer, and four censors, nominated by the new president but voted on by all the fellows. Ordinarily the elects did not hold these lesser and more burdensome offices, except that one elect was usually chosen to be one of the censors. Committees to look into specific matters or to make recommendations for action could be appointed by the president when the need arose.[12]

The officers received some compensation from the fees of new

[12]For a list of the officers of the College from 1630 to 1710, see appendix 1, table 1.

members. In 1681, for instance, after he was accepted, an M.D. had to pay the College £4 to become a candidate—but in addition, he had to pay 10s. to the president, 6s. 8d. to the treasurer, 6s. 8d. to the registrar (plus an additional 5s. to him to enter his name in the Annals), and 3s. 6d. to the beadle, for a total of £5 1s. 6d. Three years later, the entry fee for candidates and licentiates was raised to £20 in addition to the other "subscriptions."

The most active officers were those who sat on the *comitia censorum* (also sometimes called the *comitia minora* or *comitia menstrua*): the president and four censors, with the registrar attending to keep a record. This committee met frequently, ordinarily on the first Friday of every month (after late 1640, on the first Thursday of every month; then again on the first Friday later in the century)—although frequently the *comitia* met more often during the October to June "season," when all the fellows were in London. The *comitia censorum* carried out the regulatory functions of the College: inspecting the apothecaries' shops and examining their apprentices, examining prospective fellows, disciplining members, and hearing cases against illicit or bad practitioners. How actively this committee pursued its business might vary a good deal depending on whether the elects had chosen a president who cared about enforcing the privileges of the College, and whether he in turn had chosen energetic and activist censors to serve on this important regular committee.[13] The College's private face might be seen in its academic and social functions, but its public face was seen in the activities of the *comitia censorum*.

The College's Public Face

The committee of censors was empowered to sit as a court to judge medical practice in either of two ways.[14] They had the right to impose a fine of five pounds for each month someone practiced without their license, and they could also imprison those they found guilty. After a complaint was made to the president and censors, the accused and witnesses would be brought before the committee by the College's beadle, or occasionally by a constable or marshall's servant,

[13]For an account of the number of meetings of the *comitia censorum* and other College meetings, see appendix 1, table 3; the average attendance is given in table 4.

[14]The College's court of censors was explicitly recognized by the court of King's Bench in 1699 as a court of record (but implicitly so viewed much earlier): "Dr. Groenevelt v. Dr. Burwell et al'," 1 Ld. Raym., 454, *English Reports* 91.

since an act of Parliament required all law officers to do as the officers of the College bid them.[15]

Seated gravely on elevated seats at the front of the main meeting room in their long crimson gowns and speaking to one another in Latin, the formidable *comitia* took testimony. In most cases the president and censors attempted to overawe the offenders, seeking confessions of illegal behavior and promises not to break the medical statutes again. In cases in which they believed a practitioner had acted particularly badly, to have repeated her or his offenses, or to have been contemptuous of their authority, the officers might impose a fine, sometimes imprisoning the offender until the fine was paid or until the guilty party had humbled herself or himself and begged forgiveness.[16] In particularly recalcitrant cases, the College officers might sue an offender in a higher court—ordinarily in Exchequer to recover a fine, or in King's Bench to imprison someone who had influential friends, or even in Star Chamber if the case concerned institutional disputes. The juridical authority of the College of Physicians, then, could cause difficulties for those who were in contempt of the College's medical statutes.

Yet, as in many other instances in which administrative bodies had great juridical authority in early modern England, the actual strength of the College was far less than the law would indicate. A close examination of the medical milieu reveals that the physicians of the College could not even compel all physicians in London to join their ranks. Many physicians practicing in London failed to join the College, more often because they refused to do so than because there were no places for them. For example, the aldermen's list of the wealthiest inhabitants of London in 1640 listed two known physicians who were not of the College in addition to six who were.[17] A look at the tax assessment made at the end of the century yields a similar impression: of the inhabitants within the walls of the City, forty were physicians and "doctors." Some of the "doctors" were doctors of divinity and some were ordinary practitioners, but most seem to have been physicians. Only twenty of the forty "doctors" were members of the College.[18] By the end of the century, many well-to-do people

[15] 1 Mariae, St. 2. c. 9.

[16] The statute of 1 Mariae also ordered the keepers of prisons to lock up those charged by the officers of the College and to hold them at the officers' will.

[17] W. J. Harvey, ed., *List of the Principal Inhabitants of London, 1640*, with index by C. F. H. Evans (Pinhorns, Isle of Wight: Blacksmanbury Offprints, 1969).

[18] David V. Glass, ed., *London Inhabitants within the Walls, 1695* (Chatham, Kent: London Record Society, 1966); "A Supplement to the London Inhabitants List of 1695 compiled by Staff of Guildhall Library," *Guildhall Studies in London History* 2 (1976): 77–104; 136–57.

and their physicians had moved beyond the walls of the city to the western suburbs. But it seems that throughout the seventeenth century, a large proportion—perhaps as many as one-third—of the practicing physicians in London were not members of the College of Physicians.

Part of the reason that the College could not compel the membership of all physicians in London is that university degrees and licenses in medicine and surgery specified that their holders had the right to practice throughout England; the exception of not being able to practice in London without the permission of the College seemed unjust to university graduates. Many university graduates in medicine therefore felt entitled to practice in London by virtue of their degrees, without the license of the College. The case of Dr. Thomas Bonham is an example: in the first decade of the century Bonham pleaded the right to practice in London by virtue of his university degree alone.[19] Such problems continued for the College throughout the seventeenth century: in June of 1676 three men who presented themselves as physicians with degrees from Cambridge demanded the right to practice in London,[20] and in February of 1702 a number of junior M.D.s of Oxford practicing in London tried to get the universities to petition Parliament on their behalf so that all graduates in physic would be allowed to practice in London without undergoing examination by the College.[21]

In addition to not being completely successful in monopolizing the right to grant M.D.s permission to practice in London, the College could not always keep other practitioners from practicing within the City. Beside the M.D. and M.B. degrees, the universities also granted licenses to practice medicine and surgery after applicants passed an examination and paid a fee of forty shillings.[22] Moreover, the Act of 1512, which empowered bishops to grant licenses for medical practice within their dioceses and explicitly granted the bishop of London jurisdiction over London and seven miles around—the same territory

---

[19]See my article, "'Against Common Right and Reason': The College of Physicians versus Dr. Thomas Bonham," *American Journal of Legal History* 29 (1985): 301–22.

[20]Annals, 4:116a–116b. Perhaps the Annals are not exact on this point, or perhaps the three were disingenuous: neither "Dr." Hallwood nor "Dr." Swale is listed as having obtained a medical degree from Cambridge, Oxford, or Leiden, although John Master obtained his M.D. from Oxford in 1672: Joseph Foster, *Alumni Oxonienses, 1500–1714*, 4 vols.; R. W. Innes Smith, *English-Speaking Students of Medicine at the University of Leyden*; John and J. A. Venn, *Alumni Cantabrigienses*, 2 vols.

[21]Annals 6:183.

[22]John H. Raach, "English Medical Licensing in the Early Seventeenth Century," *Yale Journal of Biology and Medicine* 16 (1944): 283–88.

that the College regulated—was never legally rescinded or super-seded. Certainly not all of these licentiates were university graduates, although from 1635 to 1640 Archbishop Laud denied practice to anyone within his jurisdiction who did not have a university degree in order to insure that all licentiates were proper Anglicans.[23]

Even activist fellows of the College helped others gain medical legitimacy through the bishops' license by signing letters testimonial. The officers of the College, however, sometimes tried to prohibit College members from signing testimonial letters, conceiving that the College alone had the power to license London practitioners. For instance, in 1635 it was "propounded and agreed, that no man shall give testimony for the sufficiency of any practitioners but according to the statute."[24] But this attempt, like others, ultimately failed. Both Richard Morton and Charles Goodall, candidates of the College, signed John Firmin's letter testimonial of 1676, for example.[25] Goodall was one of the major upholders of the authority of the College in the same year he signed the letters.[26] Even strong supporters of the College's licensing powers, then, sometimes helped others to get licenses to practice through the agency of the bishops rather than through the College. The alternative routes to medical licensing served to weaken the College's legal monopoly on medical practice in London.[27]

Nevertheless, when the College officers chose to act, and when their authority to do so was recognized and encouraged by the monarchy, the College did constitute something like a monopoly in the terms of the day. The quid pro quo between College and Crown, and so the views of the court toward the incorporated physicians, varied over the century, and cannot be easily generalized. But it is possible to establish the attitudes toward the College's juridical power held by

[23]Robert S. Roberts, "The London Apothecaries and Medical Practice in Tudor and Stuart England" (Ph.D. diss., University of London, 1964), p. 148; Christopher Hill, *Intellectual Origins of the English Revolution*, p. 83.

[24]Annals, 3:156a–156b.

[25]Diocese of London, "Certificates and Testimonials," Guildhall MS no. 10,116, box 4, file 1675–76; also in J. Harvey Bloom and R. Rutson James, *Medical Practitioners in the Diocese of London, Licensed under the Act of 3 Henry VIII, c. 11: An Annotated List, 1529–1725*, p. 49.

[26]In that year, Charles Goodall published *The College of Physicians Vindicated* (1676), written against an illict practitioner, Adrian Huyberts; he later wrote the very influential *The Royal College of Physicians of London, Founded and Established by Law*, 2 vols. (1684).

[27]It should be noted that the vast majority of the bishops' licenses for practice did not limit the practitioners to any local area; some of the licenses, however, specified a right to practice only outside the area of the College's jurisdiction.

both the public and the officers of the College itself if we look at some of the activities of the *comitia censorum*.

The behavior of the censors during the "College year" (that is, from one autumn election to the next) 1639–40 can be taken to be as representative of their actions during periods when the College was modestly active. The officers were elected on September 20, 1639, and served until October 1, 1640. Continuing as president was the seventy-one-year-old Simeon Fox, the son of the martyrologist John Fox. Raised among the nobility, educated at Padua, candidate of the College in 1605 and fellow since 1608, Fox, who resided in St. Martin's Ludgate, had become an elect in 1630 and president in the autumn of 1634 (he served in that capacity until the autumn of 1641).

Sitting as most senior censor was fifty-four-year-old Othowell Meverall, who had been made an elect the previous year. Of a modest family, living in St. Lawrence Jewry parish, he had been a censor since the autumn of 1637 and had also been registrar since 1638; his 1613 M.D. from Leiden had been incorporated at his alma mater, Cambridge, in 1616, just before he became a candidate of the College. He had been made a fellow two years later. The next most senior censor was forty-two-year-old Edmund Smith, who was elected to his second year in that office in 1639. Son of a London minister of modest means, he had gone to Caius College after attending Merchant Taylor's school and had stayed on as a fellow there until 1627, when he took an M.D. and moved to London, becoming a licentiate of the College in 1627, a candidate in 1628, and a fellow in 1632.

The two new censors were Francis Prujean and John Clarke. Like Smith, Prujean was forty-two years old, the son of a cleric of modest means, and a Caius man. Four years after earning his M.A., he applied for an M.D. by "grace" (1621) and went to London, where he became a licentiate of the College and, in the next year, a candidate. The M.D. was finally conferred on him in 1625, and in 1626 he became a fellow. The fifty-six-year-old John Clarke, living in St. Martin-within-Ludgate, was yet another Cambridge man. Born of a minor gentry father in Essex, he matriculated at Caius College, but his B.A. and M.A. were from Christ's. Two years after he had taken his M.D. he became a candidate of the College (1617), and after five more years he was raised to the fellowship.[28]

---

[28]Fox died in 1641; Meverall and Clarke were senior officers during the College's parliamentary career in the 1640s; Prujean played an important role in the College's return to conservatism in the 1650s and was knighted by Charles II in 1661; Smith served as one of Charles I's physicians-in-ordinary during the wars.

While the College as a whole met six times during 1639–40, the *comitia censorum* met fourteen times on their own. They negotiated with the Society of Apothecaries (which was being threatened with the revocation of its charter by quo warranto in the Privy Council for not obeying the College), examined the apprentices of apothecaries who had been proposed as freemen of the society, visited the apothecaries' shops and destroyed the drugs they thought bad, solicited the nominations for two physicians to go north with the army in the Bishops' Wars, gave the three examinations to two licentiates and one candidate, and heard twenty-nine complaints against twenty-three individuals for disobedience to the medical statutes.

Of the twenty-three people accused of breaking the medical statutes, two were apothecaries, two were surgeons, two "doctors," one a minister, and sixteen (two of them women) unidentified by "profession," most probably ordinary practitioners. Fifteen of these offenders appeared before the censors to be questioned, and in ten cases a verdict was recorded. At least eight of the ten were severely warned and let go on a promise not to practice again (and probably thirteen of the fifteen were admonished not to practice again, but no record of a verdict exists in the other five cases). One person was fined and imprisoned, and one was to be indicted in another court.[29]

The eight accused who did not appear included Aron Streater, a minister accused of "setting up bills," or advertising for patients. Elizabeth Story, of Robin-Hood Court in Shoe-Lane, was complained of by Jane Bentley for taking in her husband for a week or ten days in order to cure him of the "renes." (Story was said to have treated him with isingeglasse and milk, to have fluxed him with an ointment, and then to have purged him.) Then there was the complaint against William Pigot made by Francis Eland, an apothecary; several witnesses who claimed that a patient had died under Benjamin Turner's care; Mary Berdwell, speaking against Giles Barton; William Kempson, against one Hooper, a barber in King's Street next to the Blackamoore's Head; several witnesses complaining about Peter Lorayne, alias DuChamboure (including Mr. Jackson, who said Lorayne had undertaken to cure him but had abandoned him when he was in a great extremity); and Robert Smith, who brought the name of James Trikley to the censors for illicitly practicing on his wife.

It is not clear why the censors did not move against these eight more energetically, but probably the accused had moved from London or had not clearly charged money for their services or had not

[29]Annals, 3:202b–207b.

been accused by creditable witnesses. All these were reasons the censors had not undertaken more vigorous investigations of practitioners in other instances.

Of the fifteen who voluntarily came to the College when summoned or who were compelled to come by the beadle, probably thirteen, but certainly eight were let off with a sharp reprimand. So Peter Francis, of Amsterdam, who said he only practiced on cases of gout by using external applications and a few simples compounded together (which he said he would name, but the compositions of which he refused to divulge), was let go. So, too, was John Hunt of Boomyard in Herefordshire, with a warning and his promise never to practice again after being presented for "setting up bills for [the] cure of many diseases."[30]

Roger Starlinge was accused of trying to cure John Yardley's wife of the pox for forty shillings but of only making her worse, being compelled to call in the help of Dr. Moore (probably the Catholic licentiate of the College, John Moore). Starlinge's defense was that he was a freeman of a surgeons' company (although not of the London Barber-Surgeons' Company) and that he had first consulted with Dr. "Frear" (Dr. John Fryer, an M.D. of Padua and a candidate of the College, although not a fellow because of his Catholicism), who had received ten shillings for the consultation. (Starlinge had diagnosed the disease as the pox because the woman had a headache and her husband had gonorrhea.) The censors decided to check on the wife's condition and to speak with Fryer. On a later occasion, therefore, they brought Starlinge before them again and let him go, since Fryer vouched that he did sometimes consult with Starlinge.

Robert Twige, of St. Saviour's parish, was let go with a warning after being accused by William Barrat of practicing physic because "the accusation seemed to be malicious." Josiah Wotton, of St. Alphage's parish, was accused by John Usher of Oldstreet for poorly trying to cure him of the ague by using a vomit and a plaster and giving him bread to eat "which had certain syllables written upon it," and of doing the same for a child for a fee of five shillings. Wotton in turn put the blame on an apothecary in Aldermanbury, Mr. Wheatley. Wheatley later appeared before the College and confessed all. John Bird, of Merton College, Oxford, was admonished not to practice again. A "doctor" Eyres, accused of setting up bills, had his wife come to plead his case and to beg off.

Also, Dr. Alexander Read, a fellow of the College closely associ-

[30]Hunt's case is one of those given in Goodall, *Royal College of Physicians*, p. 470.

ated with the Barber-Surgeons' Company, complained of a surgeon, Mr. Downinge, who later appeared before the College. On that occasion Anna Wall, the widow of John Grove, testified that Downinge had treated Grove, but that Grove had died under his hands; Downinge claimed that the prescription had come from Dr. Read. The censors called Downinge before them on another occasion and proved to their satisfaction that Wall's charges were true and that there were other instances of death at his hands; yet they felt that since the matter had occurred two years earlier, the current complaint was motivated by "discontent," and so they let Downinge go with a strong admonition not to practice again.

Richard Gilbert, a maker of small knives who also set bones, and Matthew Lucatello were let go with warnings and their promises not to practice. Mrs. Lander, a medical associate of George Butler's (an empiric who caused the College trouble for many years), had fluxed at least two patients with mercury pills for six pounds or more per treatment—but she, too, was let go on her promise not to practice again. Finally, Mr. Phige, an apothecary, appeared before the censors on charges of practicing on Mrs. Ganocke, but he claimed he had done so at the direction of Dr. William Staines (a new M.D. and candidate of the College), Dr. Aaron Gurden (who was later tried by the censors for illicit practice), and Mr. Hill (an empiric who was protected by Lord Holland), and so he was let go, probably with a warning, although no declaration is written down.

Of one individual who was brought before the College in 1639–40, there is no detailed record. Mr. Barton is merely mentioned as someone to be indicted—that is, sued in another court. Any records of the case were probably in the possession of the College's lawyer.[31]

The only case in which the censors imposed a fine in 1639–40 was that of Francis Roe, alias Vintner, of St. Botolph's parish. He was accused by William Clarke, of White Chapel, of having undertaken to cure his wife of a "tympany." He had obtained four pounds already (three for the expenses said to be incurred in the treatment), and three more pounds were to be paid for his advice. Vintner declared that he had been at Trinity College, Cambridge, for a year or two, and had learned medicine from his father ("Mr. Vintner the empiric"). After hearing the charges and Vintner's reply on the first occasion, the censors ordered him to return at their next regular meeting. At that next meeting, further evidence of Vintner's practice

[31]In 1635 the College employed one Mr. Jenkins of Grays Inn to draw up a document, and also one Mr. Keling, a solicitor. In December 1640, Mr. Leightfoot was hired as their lawyer. Whether any of these three men handled Barton's case is unknown.

was taken. The registrar of the College entered the story as follows: Clarke's wife had come to Vintner's study, where he diagnosed her illness (the diagnosis is not recorded). His prescription was elaterium (a purgative made from precipitate from the juice of the "squirting cucumber"), "a medicine he had not," and so he sent her "into the open streets home, and said it was a cordial." The censors thought this ignorant or dangerous (and they probably thought the charge exhorbitant), and so they sentenced him to a ten-pound fine and imprisonment.

It was probably the same Vintner against whom more complaints were heard two months later. This time Ellen Tomson and Anne Clarke (probably his former patient) declared that he had earlier undertaken to cure John Clarke (Anne's son?) of a "surfeit and the jaundice," giving him physic every three days for five weeks and receiving over twenty pounds for his treatment. Probably this earlier practice was successful enough to cause John's mother, Anne, to return to Vintner when she was ill herself, resulting in an unhappy outcome and thus ending in her complaint to the College. The censors were probably trying to find out more about Vintner's practice on this second occasion in the event that he tried to pursue his medical activities in London.

Why the censors singled out Vintner for a fine and imprisonment while letting others go with a warning is not entirely clear from the record. Perhaps his accuser, Clarke, was an important person whom the censors wanted to cultivate. Probably they periodically made an example of someone to intimidate the others. He was also a man with Latin and thus could easily be confused with regular physicians. The amount of money Vintner was charging also seems extraordinarily large, and it is clear that when the censors fined and imprisoned someone, they sought clear and unambiguous evidence of illicit practice or malpractice *for money* from creditable witnesses.

It is also clear that the activities of the College censors were well enough known to the public to result in citizens bringing to them complaints in cases in which they felt themselves wronged by a practitioner. Patients or their friends and relatives would sometimes have had difficulty in bringing a bad practitioner to justice in a common law court, for those practitioners who had taken a license could not be sued for malpractice, even if death occurred.[32] Moreover, the so-called "Quacks Charter" of 1543 implied that even unlicensed practi-

[32]Christopher Merrett, *A Collection of Acts of Parliament, Charters, Trials at Law, and Judges Opinions Concerning Those Grants to the Colledge of Physicians London* (1660), p. 66. Merrett quotes Fitz Herbert tit. Cor. p. 311. Briton fol. 14 to this effect.

tioners could be exempted from suit if they possessed traditional knowledge of healing.[33] One physician complained that all these factors meant that malice had to be proven in cases of malpractice. Proving malice was undoubtedly difficult to do, and therefore few legal remedies seem to have been open to relatives of someone who died of "quackery."[34] Many patients or their relatives who believed that harm had been caused to them or theirs by a medical practitioner therefore looked to the College as a court of recourse.

In addition to when they believed that they had actually been harmed by a practitioner, members of the public complained in two other instances: when a patient had paid large fees for no results, or when a practitioner was suing a patient for fees and the patient thought the practitioner had done no good. For example, in January 1633, the censors heard a complaint against Mary Butler, who had charged twenty pounds for treating a woman suffering from a "dead palsy"; Butler was trying to recover the second ten pounds by suit. Later in the century, and in the early eighteenth century, the censors spent much of their time adjudicating what patients thought were unreasonable bills. In November 1702, Mrs. Gillian thought that Henry Barnaby's bill of nineteen pounds, five shillings was extravagant, for instance; when the censors summoned the apothecary Barnaby to appear before them at their next meeting, he reduced the bill considerably.[35]

The censors of the College might be alerted to the illicit practice of someone through means other than patient complaints, however. Members of the College might also hear of a practitioner in the course of their work or leisure. They might be called in to treat someone after another practitioner had failed, and so have an opportunity to bring that practitioner to the attention of the censors. They

[33]34 and 35 Hen. VIII, c. 8. The words of the act make it clear that the act was intended to protect traditional healers, those giving ointments and plasters, from the depredations of the surgeons.

[34]Willcock, *Laws Relating to the Medical Profession*, p. 86, notes three kinds of malpractice other than "wilful malpractice": "avaricious malpractice," "negligent malpractice," and "ignorant malpractice." I suspect that these last three actions grew out of eighteenth-century interpretations of the law, but until an investigation of common law cases is undertaken from the sixteenth to the nineteenth centuries, the issue of the common law and malpractice will remain unclear.

[35]It should be pointed out here that the commonly held belief that apothecaries were allowed to charge for their medicines but not for their advice after the Rose case of 1703–04 was not one the censors adhered to. For instance, when Mrs. Temple complained of overcharging by the apothecary Mr. Jackson in 1718–19, the College suggested to her that she owed him £30 for the drugs *plus* £5 for his attendance.

might notice public advertisements or medical pamphlets and books by the unlicensed. The College's beadle was empowered to search out illegal practice. Also, the prescriptions kept on file in the apothecaries' shops would be inspected during visitations by the censors, revealing the names of illicit practitioners of physic who sent their patients to the shops to buy drugs.

The Crown also brought people to the College's attention on the few occasions when it sought the College's help in legal matters. In one case it used the College as an expert committee to help with the prosecution of one Cromwell, accused of poisoning his master.[36] In another case the Star Chamber referred to the College and its censors the case that William Clowes, Jr., the king's serjeant-surgeon, was pursuing against James Leverett, an old gardener who cured by his touch, something Clowes thought demeaned the king's own royal touch. The College undertook an experiment in Leverett's case, making him touch various patients selected by College members over a one-month period. They seemed to be inclining in Leverett's favor until Clowes came to the College, bringing a seven-count accusation against Leverett as an "impostor and couzener of the King's people," whereupon the College agreed to declare in Star Chamber that Leverett "adds scorn and contempt towards those whom the sacred hand of His Majesty hath touched for the evil."[37]

It must also be said that the censors found some particularly resourceful individuals very difficult, if not impossible, to bring to heel, despite many attempts. The case of John Buggs occupied the College for over eight years and shows the limits of the College's powers as well as the College's persistence. He was first complained of on July 3, 1630. Living in Warwick Lane near the College's own building, Buggs, as an apothecary, had practiced medicine on the son of Mr. Murray in Foster Lane, and the son had died the same day. When questioned by the College, he refused to incriminate himself by answering. The servant of Dr. Thomas Grent, a fellow, accused him, but Buggs continued to refuse to answer. After an interruption of some months due to an epidemic of plague, Buggs's case was taken up on November 12. The boy's father (this time recorded as Mr. Nicholas Marrin of Fetter Lane) said Buggs had boasted of being a physician and had treated his son for several days, leading Marrin to

---

[36]This was the Lane case of 1632: Annals, 3:119b–123a; the details are given in Underwood, pp. 256–61.

[37]Annals, 3:175a–183a; the details are given in Geoffrey Keynes, *The Life of William Harvey*, pp. 263–69.

hope for his son's recovery. When he saw that the son was going to die, however, Buggs summoned Marrin to a wine-seller's shop and presented him with a bill for services rendered. Marrin and Isabella Wersley also said that Buggs had given one Mr. Pinkurne a vomitory made from Spanish wine which only made the sick man worse.[38]

The officers of the College wanted to take action against Buggs, but they could not, since he had friends at court, and members of the king's household were exempt from prosecution. In February 1631, therefore, the College wrote a letter to Philip, earl of Pembroke and Montgomery, the Lord Chamberlain, asking that he give the College "leave to take the ordinary course of law for suppressing of the unlawful practice" of Buggs and several other named "empirics, and all others that shall assume the like colors" of being "His Majesty's servants." The Lord Chamberlain replied that none of the persons mentioned "nor any others are admitted to His Majesty's service to entitle them to the practice of physic against the charter of the College," and therefore the College could "freely take the benefit of His Majesty's laws for their relief."[39]

The College let matters rest until September 1631, when they took testimony about Buggs's practicing medicine again. Not until May 11, 1632, however, was more testimony taken, apparently after the censors had searched his shop for bad medicines and Buggs had in turn sued the censors. The College then locked Buggs up in the Fleet prison until he paid a fifty-pound fine for his offenses. At the end of June, Lord Heath, lord chief justice of the Common Pleas, wrote the College that Buggs wanted to be freed on a writ of habeas corpus, but that Heath would not release him unless the College wished him to. The College returned grateful thanks to the chief justice, but called Buggs "a dangerous empiric. And against whom there are many complaints in our Register, and never any man behaved himself with that insolency and contempt against our College as he hath done." They ended: "Sir, the trust that the King and state hath placed upon us, bends us in all duty and conscience to prosecute such dangerous abusers for the preservation of the lives of His Majesty's people." Therefore they wanted Buggs to be kept in prison until he had paid his fine.[40]

After a plea by the Society of Apothecaries, on October 12, 1632, the College finally agreed to release Buggs from prison (after a five-

[38] Annals, 3:101a, 102a.
[39] Annals, 3:107a.
[40] Annals, 3:113a, 118a–119a, 124b–125a.

month incarceration) on condition that ten pounds of his fine be paid immediately, twenty pounds in the next six months, and twenty pounds more by the next October; additionally, he would have to "seal a release of errors" admitting his mistakes. But a complaint that Buggs was practicing again came to the College in December, and another in March of 1633. By July 1, Buggs's first twenty-pound installment not having been paid, his bond was considered forfeit, and he and the men who stood surety for him were sued.[41]

In the meantime, Buggs had matriculated at Leiden on May 11, 1633, and took his M.D. there on July 15, with a thesis "De pleuritude vera et exquisita" dedicated to Sir Kenelm Digby.[42] When the College continued to accuse Buggs of illicit practice in 1634,[43] he presented his Leiden M.D. to Cambridge and obtained its license to practice medicine.[44] The College protested this to Dr. Collins, the Regius Professor of Physic there, urging him to reexamine Buggs and to find him unfit. But Collins replied that Buggs had gotten around him since any two doctors of the university could submit a recommendation to the whole university senate of regents and nonregents, who in turn put names forward to the vice-chancellor, who granted the degrees and licenses. The College ordered Buggs sued in the Court of Exchequer for the recovery of the fine.[45] But in May 1635 Buggs incorporated his M.D. at Oxford, as well.[46]

In June and again in December the College took testimony against Buggs for malpractice. But Buggs had important patrons—so influential were they, that when the position of physician to Christ's Hospital fell vacant in May 1636, the College feared that he or some other "irregular man would by the favor he had with the officers of that place to the prejudice and dishonor of this society" gain the position, and so they petitioned the Lord Mayor. Throughout 1636, 1637, and 1638, the College pursued Buggs, but despite their harassment of him, it seems he was never fined again.[47] The other courts were no doubt reluctant to declare someone with an M.D. incorporated at Oxford who had influential friends to be an illict practitioner, and the College could not get evidence of clear malpractice. By the time of his death in 1640 (at thirty-seven years of age), Buggs was

---

[41]Annals, 3:126b, 128a, 131a–131b.
[42]Innes Smith, *English-Speaking Students,* "John Buggs."
[43]Annals, 3:135b, 136b.
[44]Venn, *Alumni Cantabrigienses,* "John Buggs."
[45]Annals, 3:146a–147a.
[46]Foster, *Alumni Oxonienses,* "John Buggs."
[47]Annals, 3:155b–156a, 161b, 164b–165a, 168a, 169b, 189a, 195b.

living in St. Andrews Holborn and was one of the most wealthy inhabitants of Billingsgate Ward.[48] Buggs's case illustrates the problems the College censors had in excluding successful practitioners from London and their persistence in trying to do so.

The College's Regulatory Activity

The censors handled cases brought by patients, the Crown, and members of the College. How the College of Physicians used its powers in the seventeenth century can be seen by examining a breakdown of hearings in *comitia* against other practitioners, taken from the College's Annals from 1630 to 1705.

The jagged ups and downs of the College's actions over the years (appendix 2, table 1) are notable, and are remarked on later.[49] The number of individuals complained of was lower than the total number of complaints heard, due to the fact that often two or more hearings were necessary before the *comitia* determined the outcome of a particular case. Fewer individuals actually appeared before the College than were complained of. Of these cases, few resulted in a recorded verdict, as not all cases were considered serious enough by the censors to be pursued to a final decision. Of all the judgments rendered by the *comitia* (appendix 2, table 2), few resulted in the greatest punishment of imprisonment or fine—or both.

A different analysis shows what kinds of cases the censors most often considered worth pursuing to a final judgment and indicates how the College viewed its legal responsibilities. Comparing the total number of malpractice cases with the number of individual complaints (appendix 2, table 3) makes clear that the number of malpractice cases was normally only a small fraction of the total individual cases heard. That is, the College more often heard other kinds of cases—cases of illicit practice—than it heard malpractice cases. In other words, a few people pursued their complaints against bad practitioners by bringing them before the College, but normally the censors preferred not to intervene in cases of malpractice.

The public and the College thus seem to have perceived the function of a regulatory body in quite different ways. The College preferred to enforce its authority by pursuing rival practitioners so as to

[48]Harvey, ed., *List of the Principle Inhabitants of London.*

[49]Table 1 begins in 1630 because Charles Webster (or one of his associates) will be publishing data from before 1640 at some time in the future.

frighten them from practice or to make those who were physicians take up membership or quit London: the College was primarily concerned with illicit practice. It could not force every practitioner to conform to the College, but it could make occasional examples of those who did not.

The interests of the College are more clearly revealed through the "professions" of the practitioners brought before the College (appendix 2, table 4). Only four ministers appeared before the College, and these only before the civil war, in the period of the "alienated intellectuals" in which educated men had difficulties finding a living.[50] The major category of practitioners with which the College was concerned was unspecified. In most cases they can be assumed to have been ordinary practitioners. Next in number came "doctors," the physicians' immediate rivals. Many apothecaries were also investigated.

The evidence of the Annals is not consistent enough to tell us with certainty whether most of the practitioners of an unspecified occupation—those who were most likely ordinary practitioners and drug pedlars—were brought before the censors more commonly by the public than by members of the College, but the scattered records suggest that such was the case. The censors themselves, then, seem to have been most worried about physicians, apothecaries, surgeons, and educated ordinary practitioners—other learned "professionals"—infringing on the College's jurisdiction illicitly.

When the censors took action against an outsider, it usually amounted to trying to impress and overawe the offender. In an age when public law was administered rather arbitrarily, and often with the intention of causing public humiliation and gaining confessions of wrong and promises to reform rather than imprisonment, the College had some success in warning off rivals.[51] If the healer did not stop practicing after such a warning, the College did not press matters unless that person appeared before it again on another charge. When the College did seek to fine and imprison someone, it needed clear testimony to show that the defendant had practiced physic, and that he or she had been paid for those services; if something untoward had

[50]Mark H. Curtis, "The Alienated Intellectuals of Early Stuart England," *Past and Present*, no. 23 (1962): 25–63.

[51]See J. A. Sharpe, "The History of Crime in Late Medieval and Early Modern England: A Review of the Field," *Social History* 7 (1982): 187–203; Cynthia Herrup, "New Shoes and Mutton Pies: Investigative Responses to Theft in Seventeenth-Century East Sussex," *History Journal* 27 (1984): 811–30; and idem, "Law and Morality in Seventeenth-Century England," *Past and Present*, no. 106 (1985): 102–23.

happened to a patient as the result of bad practice, so much the better for the College's case. The College seldom tried to eliminate from practice the many traditional healers who sought payment in kind or even practiced charitably (unless, as in Leverett's case, a complaint was brought by an important person or body). The College was more worried about its learned "professional" rivals, all of whom made their livings by charging monetary fees for their services. In fact, the physicians of the College were to a degree exercising a monopoly by trying to use their legal powers to prohibit the practices of their medical rivals.[52]

The political nature of this activity is demonstrated by the College's dependence on the support of the Crown. The midcentury civil war changed the College's behavior. The College could not rely on the Crown for support after 1641, and so the number of cases over which it presided dropped between 1641 and 1657, with some years seeing no activity at all (appendix 2, table 1). The censors entertained complaints against only four individuals from 1658 to 1681. With the resurgence of monarchical authority in England after the Exclusion Crisis of 1679, the College began to revive its monopolistic activity, having a peak of activity after the new charter of James II in 1687. Changes followed the revolution of 1688, with a brief lull and then a resurgence under the Whig Junto. With the period of intense political confusion after the end of the Nine Years' War, however, the College lost the test of the Rose case in the House of Lords, and apothecaries were allowed the right to practice physic. After 1704 the censors increasingly became merely arbiters of fees.

The political correlation of College strength with monarchical strength is seen in the average number of complaints the censors heard per meeting of the *comitia* over the years (appendix 1, table 5). Again, the relationship between the activities of the censors against other practitioners and the strength of the English Crown seems clear. Showing how and why the College and Crown worked together (or, on rarer occasions, at cross-purposes) is part of the task of the chapters that follow.

---

[52]Charles Webster has portrayed the juridical powers of the College as "weak" in the first half of the seventeenth century, meaning that it could not dominate all others as it might have wished: Webster, "William Harvey and the Crisis of Medicine in Jacobean England," in *William Harvey and His Age*, ed. Jerome J. Bylebyl, pp. 1–27. I do not think that the College of Physicians was necessarily weaker than any other corporate body of the period; it was probably stronger than some, and it certainly harassed (if not more) a great many people.

The claims of the learned physicians to moral and intellectual excellence in medicine may not have impressed everyone in early modern England, but those claims did have institutional authority. The physicians wished to present their art as the most "noble" of all, and so further their desires for high status and intellectual respectability. They won their argument not in the medical marketplace, but in the councils of the Crown.

For many of the early modern English monarchs, increasing their own powers to regulate the lives of their subjects for the "common good" was a self-conscious goal. To achieve these ends, they chartered or further strengthened various bodies and gave them power to sit in judgment of those who engaged in various enterprises. In the first part of the century at least, the Privy Council, with its court of Star Chamber, was the ultimate judge of the activities of these new and revived institutions.[53]

Crown "innovations" such as these regulatory bodies, however, raised the hackles of those who saw in their activities methods of government that served the interests of the few while undermining the rights of others. The physicians found that they could institutionally ally themselves with the Crown in order to exercise public authority in medical matters. But in the process they became identified by many as servants of the monarchy.

Most members of the College of Physicians seem to have supported their links to the Crown in order to encourage and sustain a respect for academic medicine and to gain juridical superiority over all medical practitioners. Yet, as servants of the king (at least abstractly), they found themselves dependent on the policies and authority of the monarchy. In the early seventeenth century the members of the College of Physicians saw their fortunes rising rapidly. They were being pulled up out of the competitive mire of the medical marketplace by the growth of monarchical government under James I and his son.

[53]See, for example, J. P. Dawson, "The Privy Council and Private Law in the Tudor and Stuart Periods," *Michigan Law Review* 48 (1950): 393–428; 627–56; and Derek Hirst, "The Privy Council and Problems of Enforcement in the 1620s," *Journal of British Studies* 18 (1978): 46–66.

3

Revolution and Reform: Changing the Enterprise of Physic, 1630–1660

> Because a knowledge of letters is entirely indispensable to a country, it is certain that they should not be indiscriminately taught to everyone. . . . If learning were profaned by extending it to all kinds of people one would see far more men capable of raising doubts than of resolving them, and many would be better able to oppose the truth than to defend it.
>
> Cardinal Richelieu,
> *Testament politique*

The College of Physicians built up a close relationship with the monarchy during the reigns of James I and Charles I, but it abandoned the relationship as early as the autumn of 1641, when what became known as the Long Parliament began to assemble. What had appeared to be an institution closely linked to the Crown soon became a staunchly Parliamentarian group, in part because the College was situated in London, but also in part because of the political sympathies of the officers elected in 1641.

During the civil wars and the Protectorate, the members of the College took note of each new shift of the winds, reorienting their affairs in order to preserve or rebuild as much of their authority as possible. Officers came and went, depending on who had the most influence with the changing governments. Policies were made and reversed, depending on which might gain the best advantage. During the 1640s, when parliamentary or army committees ran affairs, the College ducked its head and prosecuted few rivals. As its public, regulatory behavior was slowly abandoned, the corporation's more private role as a learned body grew in importance to its members, and many physicians began to study seriously the new philosophy. During the 1650s the College established good relations with the Protectorate governments and briefly began to prosecute more people, only to have its statutory power broken in a judicial decision in 1656.

Through it all, the College maintained its existence in English law, although its statutory authority to regulate other practitioners was, finally, taken away. A corporation closely identified with the policies of the early Stuarts survived the Revolution as a learned society rather than as a public authority. Yet the College of Physicians as an institution survived the storms of a dangerous era because of the keen political instincts of its members.

The College and the Early Stuarts

Under James I and his son, the royal physicians and, through them, the College of Physicians, came to exercise considerable political influence. The relationship between the College and the physician who was undoubtedly the most important in the land, the French Huguenot Sir Theodore de Mayerne, was thus particularly important. A royal physician of the French king, Mayerne was protected by Henri IV from the attacks of the Faculté de médecine in 1603 when Mayerne published an apology for chemical remedies. Having first visited the English court in 1606, Mayerne moved permanently to the court of James I in 1610, after Henri IV's assassination, and became the first physician to the English king and queen.

While at first naturally suspicious of the London College of Physicians after his experiences in Paris, he began to find it a useful body, and in 1616 he accepted the offer of a fellowship, although he declined the offer of becoming an elect in 1627, saying that his busy schedule at court would not allow him to attend College business—in fact, he rarely came to meetings. Knighted in 1624, he remained first physician to Charles I and his queen and was the first physician in name to Charles II, as well, although Mayerne mostly remained in the vicinity of London during the civil wars until his death in 1655. During the latter part of James I's reign, and during his son's until 1641, the College's fortunes were strongly affected by the College's relationships with Mayerne and, through him, with the court.

What bound the College's fortunes closely to Mayerne's and the king's was the separation of the apothecaries from one of the twelve great livery companies of London, the Grocers' Company. On his

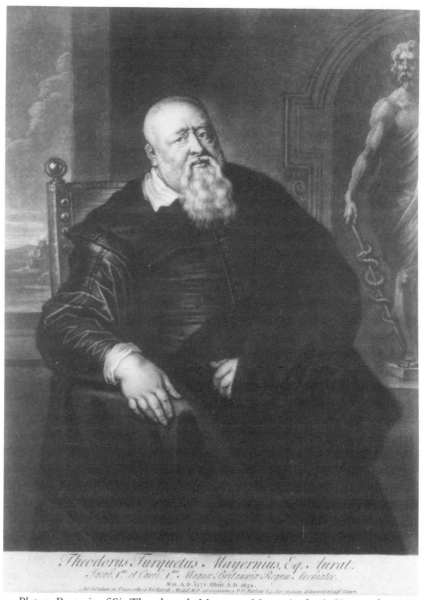

Plate 5. Portrait of Sir Theodore de Mayerne. Mezzotint by J. Simon after P. P. Rubens. Courtesy of the Wellcome Institute Library, London.

arrival in 1610, Mayerne allied himself with Gideon DeLaune, another French Huguenot and the apothecary to Anne of Denmark, a man who had been denied admission to the Grocers' Company because he was foreign-born. Mayerne and DeLaune used their influence to try to split off the apothecaries into a separate guild, as they commonly were in France. The first attempts to get a bill passed in Parliament to this effect were defeated in 1610 by an angry Grocers' Company and the City of London. But stimulated by the calling of a new Parliament in 1614, Mayerne, DeLaune, Henry Atkins (another royal physician and a fellow of the College), and the renegade apothecaries petitioned the Crown in April. By mid-May the law officers, Sir Francis Bacon and Sir Henry Yelverton, recommended the formation of a new apothecaries' company, and a charter was ready in what must have been an unprecedented three days.[1]

The Grocers' Company and the City of London were threatened by this action (the city government was very closely associated with the great livery companies),[2] but Atkins got the College of Physicians to support the separation. The College had obtained the right to inspect the wares of apothecaries in an act of 1553, and in 1588 it had seriously considered issuing an official pharmacopoeia that would specify the drugs the apothecaries would be allowed to dispense (the idea was dropped in 1594).[3] The proposed new company, however, would be even more subordinate to the College.[4]

The "Addled Parliament" was soon dissolved, but by June the College had firmly committed itself to an association with the Crown by supporting the new company over the strong opposition of the City of London. The College then sent a flattering letter to the king seeking his support in the College's attempts to control empirics. By 1618 the king had created the new apothecaries' company by royal fiat, and the College had published its *Pharmacopoeia*. The *Pharmacopoeia*, together with the new privileges of the College, seemed to place the direction of the apothecaries in the hands of the physicians.[5] From the middle of the reign of James I, then, a mutually beneficial association began to develop between the College and the Crown by

[1] Underwood, pp. 9–12.

[2] See Robert Ashton, *The City and the Court, 1603–1643*, pp. 5–82.

[3] 1 Mariae, St. 2, c. 9; Annals, 2:75b–76a; Clark, pp. 160–61.

[4] Annals, 3:16b; Clark, pp. 221–23; Underwood, pp. 13–14.

[5] Annals, 3:17a; James Larkin and Paul Hughes, eds., *Stuart Royal Proclamations*, vol. 1, pp. 389–91; also see George Urdang, "The Mystery about the First English (London) Pharmacopoeia (1618)," *BHM* 12 (1942): 304–13; and idem, "How Chemicals Entered the Official Pharmacopoeias," *Arch. Int. d'Hist. des Sciences* 7 (1954): 314.

way of the royal physicians, an association which only became closer under Charles I.

The Crown defended the College and the new Society of Apothecaries from attacks in the Parliaments of 1621 and 1624, and from attempts by the Barber-Surgeons' Company to obtain the right to administer internal remedies. In turn, the College gave advice to the Privy Council on fighting the plague in 1625, provided physicians to oversee the vast numbers of sick and wounded brought back to Plymouth, Portsmouth, and Southampton after Buckingham's dismal expedition to Rhé in 1627, and in the same year advised the council on a matter of public health when the citizens of St. Botolph-without-Aldgate complained about pollution from an alum works run by patentees of the king.[6]

During the first year of Charles's "Personal Rule," when plague again threatened the city, the links between the College and the Crown became even stronger. The Privy Council placed the College at the head of the government's attempts to limit the epidemic's effects and had the College write part of the first of what became the three "Books of Orders."[7] In 1631 Mayerne proposed to the council that the royal physicians and the College be brought together with a few privy counselors and aldermen in a board of health that would police London.[8] And when the Society of Apothecaries in the 1630s began to cause trouble for the College, the Privy Council and the Star Chamber fully supported the Colleges' steps to discipline and subordinate the Society.[9] Mayerne and Sir Thomas Cadyman (a Catholic physician to Queen Henrietta Maria and a member of the College) obtained a patent for a Company of Distillers in 1638 as part of the attack on the recalcitrant Society of Apothecaries.[10] In sum, partially

[6]Annals, 3:63b, 72a–72b; Acts of the Privy Council, p. 182. The alum works were ordered stopped by the Privy Council and were eventually moved to Newcastle: J. W. Gough, The Rise of the Entrepreneur (New York: Schocken Books, 1969), pp. 176–96.

[7]Acts of the Privy Council, pp. 313–14; see Paul Slack, "Books of Orders: The Making of English Social Policy, 1577–1631," Transactions of the Royal Historical Society, 5th ser., 30 (1980): 1–22.

[8]S.P. 16/187/60; the English translation by Martin Lister is S.P. 16/533/17. Mayerne's overall emphasis on government by a learned elite fits well with his father's political beliefs: Louis Turquet de Mayerne published Monarchie Aristo-Democratique (1611), dedicated to the States General of the United Netherlands, urging that merchants and liberal professionals run the government, that the old nobility merely carry out their orders. See R. Mousnier, "The Exponents and Critics of Absolutism," in The New Cambridge Modern History (Cambridge: Cambridge University Press, 1970), vol. 4, pp. 120–21, 131.

[9]Underwood, pp. 41–57, 243–316.

[10]Distillers' Company, "Charter and Statutes, 15 Charles I, 1639," Guildhall MS no. 6228. Also see Ashton, City and the Court, pp. 76–79.

through the activities of Mayerne, the College of Physicians and the Privy Council established a quid pro quo under the first two Stuarts, especially during Charles I's "Personal Rule," in the interests of more effective government for the public good.[11]

But late 1639 saw the outbreak of war with Scotland, placing the political status quo in jeopardy. During the "Short Parliament" that met in the spring of 1640, the Society of Apothecaries entered a petition against the College (and, by implication, the medical policies of the Crown). The Parliamentary Grand Committee for Grievances ordered the medical institutions to bring in their books for examination, and the College prepared counterpetitions. By May, however, the Parliament and the king had deadlocked on a number of issues, and the Parliament was dissolved, allowing the College once again to counterattack the apothecaries in the councils of the Crown.[12] Yet the political climate of England was undergoing swift changes, and the College's alliance with the Crown was about to be broken.

By the end of the summer, the Bishops' Wars against the Scots had turned badly against the king, and he was forced to call another Parliament. In the uncertain atmosphere on the eve of the meeting of the new Parliament,[13] the College sensed a shift of political winds, and it tried to place the burden of institutional innovation on the apothecaries' company. In doing so, it began to distance itself from the monarchy, an indication that many members of the College anticipated that this Parliament would be different.

The College itself entered a petition in the new Parliament, claiming that the physicians of the College were "sole and primary judges of physicians and physic and medicines and makers and compounders thereof in and near to the City of London" by virtue of certain charters and acts. But recently the apothecaries had "procured themselves to be severed from the Company of Grocers" and had obtained a charter of incorporation, "which hath been condemned in Parliament." (This much is disingenuous, for the College had clearly

[11]For more details, see my article "The Medical Politics of London under the First Two Stuarts."

[12]"Information on the College of Physicians," Sloane MS no. 3914, fols. 90–90b (hereafter cited as Sloane 3914); "Petition of the Apothecaries [with] the Answere of the Doctors thereunto, 1640," R.C.P. 340/25; "A Brief of the Apothecaries Cause against the Colledge of Physitians and new Patent of Distillers and the College Answer, 1640," R.C.P. box 4, env. 33; "A Deduction of the Apothecaries Behavior Toward the College," R.C.P. box 4, env. 31.

[13]For important insights into the political mood of that autumn, see Conrad Russell, "Why Did Charles I Call the Long Parliament?" History 69 (1984): 375–83.

wished to separate the apothecaries from the Grocers' Company; the "condemnation" referred to an action in the 1624 Parliament, in which a grievance against the new company was entered by the City of London and opposed by the College of Physicians.) The apothecaries, the College claimed, "suppose they have gained thereby" so that they "are now become so bold as to condemn your petitioners and their government." Therefore, the physicians concluded, "unless some strict and speedy course be taken, the general damage thereby arising will be insupportable."[14]

In setting out the charges in this petition, the College of Physicians clearly bent the facts to portray itself as the defender of the Parliament. Perhaps few M.P.s remembered the controversies over the Society of Apothecaries in the early 1620s, in which the College and the Crown acted to force the separation of the apothecaries from the grocers over the objections of the City and the Parliament. But while the Grand Committee of the Parliament ordered the Society of Apothecaries to bring in its books and to testify on the physicians' charges, the College was asked to bring in its books, too.[15] The College had given the Parliament a fine opportunity to settle the differences between the medical corporations in the way that it, rather than the Crown, saw fit, although it was an opportunity in which the College took the lead.

Because the College moved to have its disputes settled in the Parliament, it had to do other things that the Crown must not have welcomed. Most particularly, it restored John Bastwick in a special session on December 18. Bastwick, one of the "Puritan triumvirate," had been expelled from the College in 1635 after being prosecuted by the ecclesiastical Court of High Commission. He had been condemned by that court in 1637, suffering heavy fines, the loss of his ears, public exhibition in the stocks and, finally, imprisonment. But he and his fellows were released from their prisons in one of the first acts of the new Parliament, and they were welcomed back to London at the beginning of December by large throngs and joyful celebrations. Clearly, the College could not oppose the restoration of Bastwick to his fellowship and still hope to gain the favor of the Parliament.[16]

[14]Annals, 3:208b; Sloane 3914, fols. 91–91b.

[15]Sloane 3914, fol. 91b.

[16]Annals, 3:209a; on Bastwick, see Stephen Foster, *Notes from the Caroline Underground: Alexander Leighton, the Puritan Triumvirate, and the Laudian Reaction to Nonconformity* (Hamden, Conn.: Archon Books, 1978); and Brian Manning, *The English People and the English Revolution* (London: Heinemann, 1976), pp. 14–16.

Other compromises, too, became necessary soon enough. During the tumultuous days of December, January, and February, a preoccupied Parliament had more important matters than questions of medical regulation on its mind. The case was being prepared against Strafford; attacks on the lieutenancy and regional councils were begun; the courts of High Commission and Star Chamber, even the Privy Council itself, were being investigated by parliamentary committees; and the Triennial Bill was readied: all were attacks on the Crown's recent policies. But by mid-March, Parliament took up the petition of the College and began investigating the London medical corporations. The College set up a permanent committee to oversee its business in Parliament. Before it did so, however, a meeting of sixteen of the most important members of the College was held to discuss whether the College should add to or alter its statutes, which would be read by Parliament.[17] Presumably they debated whether to alter the statutes before they presented all the College books to Parliament, in order to place the College in the most favorable light possible.

But then, in late May or early June, the College shifted tactics, entering a petition in the House of Lords. By June, as some of the reformers in the House of Commons began to push for more radical changes, the Crown's influence in the House of Lords increased. The College of Physicians saw a better opportunity to get its will done in the upper house in the spring of 1641.

The petition of the College to the House of Lords outlined the acts and charters giving the College authority over ignorant practitioners of physic, and then complained that "many illiterate and unskillful, ignorant, and inexperienced persons have taken upon them" the practice of physic, "contrary to the said charters and Acts of Parliament to the great peril and danger of many of His Majesty's subjects, and to the disgrace of the necessary and useful science and faculty of physic." The College's bill was entered in the House of Lords by the second week in June, but so was a petition of the Barber-Surgeons' Company against it requesting the right to administer internal remedies, a right they had claimed unsuccessfully since the sixteenth century.[18] The Lords, however, decided to pursue medical matters

[17]Annals, 3:210a–210b. The physicians on the permanent committee were Othowell Meverall, John Clarke, and Edmund Smith, all officers of the College.

[18]Sloane 3914, fols. 94–97b; Clark, pp. 273–74; *House of Lords Journals,* vol. 4, p. 270; "Exceptions by the Chirurgeons to the Bill preferred by the College, 1641," R.C.P. box 4, env. 40. The Barber-Surgeons' Company complained that it wanted the Commons to act on its petitions but that the Commons had been too busy with other matters.

themselves and turned the issue over to a committee after a second reading of the College's bill on June 19. During June and July the Lords considered the College's requests and the exceptions of others.[19] But then the Parliament recessed for a time, and the College's business could not be taken up until Parliament reconvened in the autumn.

A New Era

By the time autumn came, political changes of great moment had occurred, and the College was forced to choose between Parliament and king. Rooted in London, it would change its policies and side with the Parliament.

The second session of the Long Parliament opened on October 20, 1641, against the background of an England full of not completely unfounded rumors of plots and conspiracies on the part of Catholics and Royalists against the Parliament and its supporters.[20] As a result, the Parliament swung back toward the side of Pym and other reformers in the House of Commons. On the same day that Parliament reconvened, the College of Physicians elected a new group of leaders. When the College had met for its regular elections on the morrow of Michaelmas, it had had to postpone its business because too many of its fellows had been absent.[21] This may indicate a boycott of the College's election by fellows who were sympathetic to the members of Parliament in favor of wide-ranging reform. For whatever reason, the College convened a quorum for the election on October 20, and the results reflected the new fears of a Royalist and papist plot in England.

The leadership of the College of Physicians was transformed that

---

[19]The Barber-Surgeons' exceptions were put before the committee in writing before July 12, whereupon the College directed its solicitor to "inquire for the surgeons' charter; . . . [to] procure a copy of the condemnation of the surgeons' bill, which was rejected 30 March, 1607; [and] to procure a copy of the condemnation of the apothecaries' charter." The College also drew up a reply to the Barber-Surgeons' objections, which was put before the committee of the Lords on July 28 (*House of Lords Journals,* vol. 4, p. 280; Sloane 3914, fols. 96–99; Annals, 3:211a; "An Answer to the Exceptions of the Surgeons, 1641," R.C.P. box 4, env. 40).

[20]Caroline M. Hibbard, *Charles I and the Popish Plot.*

[21]Annals, 3:211a.

October, taking on the character of a moderately Parliamentarian group. The aging Simeon Fox (he was seventy-three and died the next year), who had held the president's office for the preceding six years, during which the College had cultivated its connections with the Crown, was replaced by fifty-six-year-old Othowell Meverall, a graduate of Puritan-influenced Christ's Church, Cambridge, a second son of a gentry family of Staffordshire.[22] Thomas Ridgley, about sixty years of age, also from a distinguished Staffordshire family that supported the Parliament,[23] was elevated to the position of elect, replacing the recently deceased sixty-five-year-old Sir Simon Baskerville "the rich," who had been a physician to James I and Charles I. Both Meverall and Ridgley seem to have been sympathetic to the goals of the Parliament in late 1641. John Clarke, Meverall's friend and approximate age, a fellow graduate of Christ's Church, and a fellow Parliamentarian, also became an elect. He seems to have been voted into a nonvacant spot. As a result, for a time there were nine elects of the College (whereas the statutes provided for only eight); the new elections suggest the office was packed. The College as a whole shifted its view of the political world to a position it had slowly been moving toward since late 1640.

The crisis between king and Parliament continued to grow. The Great Remonstrance of the Commons in November was followed by Charles's bungled attempt to arrest by force the five leaders of the Commons in January. By the spring of 1642, as the king raised his banner to rally his forces, civil war was clearly in the offing. The effect of the situation on the College of Physicians gradually became apparent. In 1642 John Clarke became a *consiliarius* as well as the College's treasurer. Thomas Winston, age sixty-five, an elect and a royalist, left England for the Continent. Other elects, such as William Harvey, sixty-two, left London to follow the king. They were replaced by Laurence Wright, fifty-two, a Parliamentarian and later physician-in-ordinary to Oliver Cromwell, and Paul DeLaune, about the same age, who in 1643 was sent by the Parliament to the New Model Army.[24] The College fell into the hands of a group of younger

---

[22]William J. Birken, "The Fellows of the Royal College of Physicians of London, 1603–1643: A Social Study" (Ph.D. diss., University of North Carolina, Chapel Hill, 1977), pp. 170–73.

[23]Ibid., pp. 173–79.

[24]Neil Cantlie, *A History of the Army Medical Department,* 2 vols. (London: Churchill Livingstone, 1974), p. 24.

physicians who were sympathetic to the Parliament and to current notions of the reform of the professions.[25]

The behavior of the College therefore changed abruptly in 1642. The new men in charge decided that prosecuting others for malpractice or illicit practice, something that the College had done consistently since the end of the reign of Elizabeth, caused them more harm than good in public opinion. In addition, many Parliamentarians were beginning to urge a reform of the three professions (law, church, and physic). They charged that the physicians regulated medical practice not for the good of society but for their own selfish interests alone. An apothecary, Edward Cooke, who had earlier been disciplined by the College, complained to Parliament that the College tyrannically infringed on the liberties of citizens, and he received a serious hearing (he is said to have left more than £14,000 to Parliament on his death in 1644). With the king and Parliament at war, the College had to find support in the Parliament or else stand in danger of being undermined, perhaps even disbanded. Members who were secretly sympathetic to the Royalist cause were at risk: Baldwin Hamey, Jr., was shot at through his window in 1643, the ball passing so close to his ear that he was ever after hard of hearing.[26]

The new officers of the College needed all their diplomatic skills and social authority to carry the College through such difficult days. As supporters of Parliament, they discontinued the College's regulatory activities against others. The only sentence they handed down in 1642 was to warn Mrs. Isabella Larimore not to practice medicine.[27] By allowing apothecaries, surgeons, and other ordinary practitioners to go about their business without interference, the College hoped that it would not be vigorously attacked by its rivals in the Parliament.

But not only did the College drop some activities, it also undertook others in an attempt to gain new friends. In June 1642 the House of Commons borrowed money from physicians of the College. President Othowell Meverall, in his speech of September 30, 1642, condemned certain "bad" members of the College, possibly Royalists.

---

[25]Only about twenty fellows remained active in the College: Meverall (age 56), Clarke (c. 55), DeLaune (c. 50), Wright, Sr. (c. 50), Grent (c. 45), Prujean (c. 45), Alston (c. 45), Hamey, Jr. (40), Goddard (23), Rant (36), Catcher (c. 40), Glisson (43), Sheaf (33), Salmon (c. 35), Ent (35), Bates (c. 28), Staines (c. 30), Micklethwaite (c. 30), Regimorter (c. 30), and Wright, Jr. (c. 24). (Compiled from the lists of attendance at the College meetings in 1643 and 1644.)

[26]John Keevil, *The Stranger's Son*, pp. 73–76.

[27]Annals, 3:218a.

The College officers also administered on behalf of Parliament the Oath of the National Covenant to all "physicians, practitioners in physic, and apothecaries" in that year. A year later, it also tendered the oath to the members of the Barber-Surgeons' Company. The College did resolve to defend its members against having to be part of the watch and ward of the City in 1643. But it also offered advice to the mayor and the Court of Aldermen on a new imported drug called "ramatroe"; at the same time, it got back from the City its quill of water, which had been cut off during disputes between the College and the City ten years earlier.[28]

Because the College was not policing the medical community in the charged political climate, other practitioners did not feel that they had to be licensed by the College or by any other body. There were even proposals in the College to open the fellowship to any M.D., not just to those whose degrees were from Oxford and Cambridge. The consequences of the College's laxness quickly became apparent. Ralph Bishop (of Exeter College, the vice-chancellor of Cambridge) wrote to President Meverall in 1644 to complain that some students in physic had withdrawn from his university before incorporating their degrees. He feared that "(if some timely course prevent it not) we shall be utterly deprived of any students or inceptors in that learned faculty." This, he feared, was due to the College opening its doors to men without Oxbridge degrees. Meverall reassured Bishop that every member of the College still had an M.D. of Cambridge or Oxford; he stood behind his alma mater. But this seems to have been a somewhat disingenuous reply, for in 1642 it had been Meverall himself who had proposed opening the fellowship to M.D.s not of one of the two English universities.[29] Although as it turned out no one seems to have been admitted without an English M.D., the College was defining itself as a much more open institution. This, coupled with the lack of action against others, signaled other practitioners that some kind of fundamental change in the policy of the College had taken place.

The proliferation of ordinary practitioners in the new environment did not please all members of the College, however. In the meeting of September 30, 1645, another shakeup in the College leadership occurred when the strongly Parliamentarian Clarke became president and Meverall was moved to *consiliarius* and treasurer. Clarke took a

---

[28]*Commons Journals,* vol. 2, pp. 409, 542, 601, 610; Annals, 3:217a, 218a–219a.
[29]Annals, 3:223a–223b; Clark, pp. 277–78.

more active role in exerting the regulatory influence of the College. Once again cases were heard against people practicing without the College's license and engaging in malpractice. The members of the College themselves acted to bring in these cases. At the beginning of December 1645, "a proposition was made by Mr. President to go to the sheriffs of London to desire their warrant for the convention of empirics before us." A committee made up of President Clarke, Francis Prujean, and William Rant was given the task of approaching the sheriffs.[30]

But political events conspired to stop this revival of regulatory activity. The king's forces were defeated at Naseby in June, and the period between late summer 1645 and late winter 1646 was a period of new expectations of normality in England.[31] The College began to move back toward its strict policies during this interlude, but in the winter of 1646 there were renewed fears of a papist foreign intervention on behalf of Charles I, and after Charles surrendered to the Scots in May, the Parliamentarians were split by bitter arguments over how to restore order in the country. After February 1646, therefore, the number of cases taken up by the College dwindled. The renewal of political confusion brought the College up sharply; it stopped trying to regulate others and took stock of the situation.

Its inability to prosecute actively its professional rivals undercut a basic justification of the College. The College of Physicians therefore entered a period of decline in both public importance and internal strength. Clearly a turning point was reached in December of 1646, when a statute was proposed "for preventing the absence of fellows, which frustrateth many of our meetings." For that meeting, however, only fifteen fellows could be mustered—too few to make up a quorum to pass the statute, even if all fifteen had agreed to it. The problem was referred to the censors for their advice on how to proceed. The following March, the College debated whether to change its "oaths" (*juramenti*) to "faiths" (*fidei*)—this would have identified it more clearly with those Puritans who refused to swear oaths—but this measure was voted down in April. Both meetings on the subject of the oaths were poorly attended. That same April's meeting found the registrar absent and concern for the College's treasury expressed: little money was coming in from fines or dues. New statutes were

[30]Annals, 3:228a.
[31]Robert Ashton, *The English Civil War: Conservatism and Revolution, 1603–1649*, pp. 278–79.

proposed in May (unfortunately, no details are given).[32] Apparently the College of Physicians lost much of its internal strength when its members were politically divided and its juridical reason for being, its regulatory power, was in abeyance. Something had to be done if the College was not to expire altogether.

These years of crisis for the College pointed clearly to the institutional need of its members to find a new set of reasons that would support its existence, encourage new members to join, and bind members together in a way that would protect their claims to being the best practitioners. Yet the difficult years proved creative institutionally and intellectually, and they gave the College a direction of lasting consequence: it reverted to the simpler status of a learned society.

New approaches to the medical milieu were stimulated in large part by the intellectual activities of some physicians. A group of young Londoners, most of whom were trained in medicine, began meeting semiformally in London in order to discuss the "new philosophy." They found themselves confined largely to the metropolis and the surrounding Parliamentarian areas and lacking, no doubt, some of their gentry clientele. With time on their hands and with little public business, these younger physicians began to have a heightened interest in the new ideas being put forward in Europe. They began to meet in the so-called "1645 group," a group that continued to meet from that year until the late 1650s.

Members usually gathered at Dr. Jonathan Goddard's rooms in Wood Street or at his rooms in Gresham College, after he became professor of physic there in 1655. Twenty-eight years old in 1645, he had previously been a tutee of John Wilkins's at Magdalen Hall, Oxford, where he had been introduced to the new humanistic medicine before going on to study under Dr. Francis Glisson at Cambridge, where he took his M.B. in 1638 and his M.D. in 1643. The other prominent original members of the 1645 group included Theodore Haak, age forty, an émigré to England from the Palatinate, and Father Marin Mersenne's most important English correspondent; John Wilkins, thirty-one, a mathematician who had previously tutored, in addition to Goddard, Doctors Walter Charleton and William Denton in medicine and philosophy at Oxford; John Wallis, twenty-nine, who had studied medicine under Glisson at Cambridge and who had been the first to defend the Harveian circulation in a disputation there;

---

[32]Annals, 3:233a–234b.

George Ent, forty-one, an M.D. who had studied at Cambridge and Padua, and a good friend of William Harvey's; Charles Scarburgh, thirty-one, an M.D. of Oxford (1646) who had studied under Glisson at Cambridge before fleeing with the Royalists during the civil wars to Oxford, where he became Harvey's protégé; and Christopher Merrett, thirty-one, also a friend of Harvey's, an M.B. (1638) and M.D. (1643) of Oxford under Dr. Thomas Clayton. These men scrutinized the new natural philosophy, in which anatomy and physic played a major role.[33] Some of the physicians and other members of the 1645 group moved to Oxford in 1648 and became instrumental in inaugurating a group there known as the Oxford Philosophical Club, which pursued anatomical and medical questions.[34]

A spinoff of the 1645 group was a group of nine physicians, including the four M.D.s of the 1645 group, who began to meet at the College of Physicians to investigate rickets. One of the investigators, Daniel Whistler, had completed his M.D. at Leiden in 1645, undertaking a disputation on rickets there for his degree.[35] Rickets was considered to be a new disease in the seventeenth century, and so not necessarily amenable to the therapies of the academic physicians.[36] But the English physicians who looked into rickets investigated its anatomical and pathological signs and then formulated therapies consistent with academic medicine to counter the disease. The cooperative study resulted in a monograph coauthored by Francis Glisson, George Bate, and Aussuerus Regimorter in 1650 that showed how the new medical research could be used to develop empirical evidence in order to support traditional systems of academic therapy.[37] In other words, the new medical studies being developed by these men might be based on empirical evidence as much as on Galenic ra-

---

[33]The major sources of information on the 1645 group are two letters from Wallis, often reprinted in the literature on the early Royal Society, of which the 1645 group is considered a precursor. For a good account, see Robert G. Frank, Jr., "The Physician as Virtuoso in Seventeenth-Century England," in *English Virtuosi in the Sixteenth and Seventeenth Centuries*, pp. 80–84.

[34]The program of the "Oxford Physiologists" is detailed by Robert G. Frank, Jr., in "Physician as Virtuoso"; and idem, *Harvey and the Oxford Physiologists: A Study of Scientific Ideas and Social Interaction*.

[35]Daniel Whistler, *Disputatio . . . de morbo puerili Anglorum, quem patio idiomate indigenae vocant The Rickets* (Leiden, 1645; reprint ed. London, 1684). Also see his "De Rachitide," Sloane 1263, fols. 329–35.

[36]See Lloyd G. Stevenson, "'New Diseases' in the Seventeenth Century," *BHM* 39 (1965): 1–21.

[37]Published under the title *Tractatus de rachitide*. Also see Edwin Clarke, "Whistler and Glisson on Rickets," *BHM* 36 (1962): 45–61.

tionalizations, yet they could be used to support the therapies of academic medicine.

As the work on rickets shows, the enterprises undertaken by physicians after the mid-1640s continued the academic tradition of discursive reasoning, but at the same time modified it so as to link theory to research in things. Some of the more old-fashioned physicians, to be sure, remained aloof from the new endeavors as trusting too much in physical evidence and as undermining firmly held tenets of Galenic and rationalistic medicine. Yet for a time many London physicians took up the new science, which had both English and Continental sources, and furthered it as nowhere else.

The reasons for this flowering of science among the physicians during the interregnum and early Restoration—the outward institutional weakness of the College of Physicians and the persuasiveness and attractiveness of the new ideas—are both negative and positive. The physicians were using new ideas and techniques to create a reformed medicine based on a revised system of anatomical Galenism, modeling their endeavors both on the previous work of anatomists such as William Harvey and on that of academic chemists and natural philosophers, the men of the new philosophy. In the process, they promoted a new kind of "scientific" medical learning that incidentally maintained their place at the top of the medical hierarchy as learned men, something the College of Physicians could now do only as a learned society, not as a regulatory body.

The new medical researches in mid-seventeenth-century England owed much to the intellectual ferment on the Continent. One influence flowed to England from the critical humanism of the northern Italian universities, beginning at Ferrara but flourishing at Padua in the middle of the sixteenth century.[38] A second influence on the English physicians came from Leiden, where important scientific and medical developments were also underway, partially in imitation of the Paduan developments in botanic and anatomical research and clinical teaching in the hospital. Franciscus de la Böe Sylvius had been teaching clinical medicine in the Leiden city hospital since 1636. He also taught chemistry in his medical courses at the university, although doing so in the discursive textbook style rather than in the more mystical Paracelsian manner. Additionally, Sylvius was the first teacher of medicine in Holland to demonstrate the truth of the Har-

[38]See especially Jerome J. Bylebyl, "The School of Padua: Humanistic Medicine in the Sixteenth Century," in *Health, Medicine and Mortality in the Sixteenth Century*, ed. Charles Webster, pp. 335–70.

veian circulation. His colleague Jan de Wale had his best English pupil, Roger Drake, defend Harvey's ideas in a public disputation in 1639.[39]

In addition to the research- and practice-oriented humanistic medicine imported from Italy and the Netherlands, English physicians were in touch with French philosophical developments of the late 1630s and early 1640s. The circle of scholars corresponding with Father Marin Mersenne were taking up the approach of Galileo to the world: they were trying to use Christianized ancient philosophies, mathematics, empirical observations, and occasional demonstrations to uncover the hidden reality of things. Members of the Mersenne circle, particularly René Descartes and Pierre Gassendi, were working out new philosophies that were to place corpuscularianism at the root of all physical phenomena. They also took an interest in how their principles could explain physiology: in 1637, for example, Descartes had accepted the theory of the circulation in his *Discourse de la méthode*. Mersenne corresponded with Theodore Haak and, during the 1640s, when many English Royalists resided in Paris, Kenelm Digby, Thomas Hobbes, and other members of the circle around William Cavendish, duke of Newcastle, were personally working with the Mersenne circle, finding the new philosophy to be persuasive.[40]

The effect of the developments at Padua, Leiden, and Paris on the formulation of programs for medical research in England in the 1640s can be seen in the proposals of William Petty. His *Advice of W. P. to Mr. Samuel Hartlib for the Advancement of Some Particular Parts of Learning* was drawn up after his return to England in 1646 and published in 1648—during the same period that young physicians in England were meeting to discuss the new developments.[41] After serving a

[39]G. A. Lindeboom, "Medical Education in the Netherlands, 1575–1750," in *The History of Medical Education,* ed. Charles D. O'Malley, pp. 201–16; and idem, "The Reception in Holland of Harvey's Theory of the Circulation of the Blood," *Janus* 46 (1957): 183–200. Also see Owen Hannaway, *The Chemists and the Word: The Didactic Origins of Chemistry,* p. 154.

[40]See Robert H. Kargon, *Atomism in England from Hariot to Newton,* pp. 63–84; also Harcourt Brown, *Scientific Organizations in Seventeenth Century France (1620–1680),* chap. 3, "Mersenne and England."

[41]It might be suggested that this book was, as the title says, advice *to* Hartlib, suggesting ways in which Hartlib could use new developments on the Continent to help his reform program. In 1646 and 1647, Robert Boyle, who had also been on the Continent in the early 1640s, was supplying Hartlib "with appraisals of the work of contemporary natural philosophers," especially the work of Descartes, Mersenne, and Gassendi (James R. Jacob, *Robert Boyle and the English Revolution: A Study in Social and Intellectual Change,* p. 28).

stint in the navy, Petty had gone to the Low Countries in 1643, at age twenty, to learn medicine. He studied at Leiden, Utrecht, and Amsterdam, and he seems to have been especially impressed with the clinical teaching in the hospital at Leiden. In 1645 he was introduced to the Newcastle circle in Paris through his mathematician friend John Pell (who had also been in the Netherlands), and through that group learned of the new corpuscularianism.[42] On his return to England in 1646, Petty joined the loose association of reformers around Samuel Hartlib and brought together a number of new ideas in a proposal to improve medicine.

Petty advocated the establishment of a hospital (or hospitals) as a research center for reforming medicine. Medical theory could be developed along experimental and mathematical lines and brought into a close relation with practice in such an institution. The steward of the hospital would be a mathematician—that is, a representative of the new science. A physician, a surgeon, and an apothecary would jointly supervise the medical care given in the hospital and keep careful track of the success of various treatments. A younger vice-physician and a student of physic of five or six years' standing in a university would assist the physician, while a surgeon's mate and an apothecary's mate would help their respective superiors, and an apprentice (learned in Latin) would be given to each. Widows could be employed as nurses. The purpose of such a hospital would be two-fold: the recovery of the patients and the improvement of knowledge.[43]

Petty's foresighted vision of the possibilities of using the hospital as a research and teaching institution was not to be realized in England for another one hundred years, except for the brief lives of the parliamentary military hospitals of the Savoy and Ely House.[44] But while Petty did not, as some radicals did during the interregnum, advocate the dismantling of the old institutional structure of physic, he clearly believed that the physicians would have to reform their medical ideas and therapies by working in a research environment under someone else's supervision and in conjunction with surgeons and apothecaries.

[42]On Petty's involvement with the Newcastle circle in France, see Kargon, *Atomism,* pp. 68–69.

[43]William Petty, *The Advice of W. P. to Mr. Samuel Hartlib for the Advancement of Some Particular Parts of Learning* (1648), pp. 9–17. Also see the description of this work in Richard F. Jones, *Ancients and Moderns: A Study of the Rise of the Scientific Movement in Seventeenth-Century England,* pp. 89–92.

[44]Webster, pp. 293–98.

The central idea of the proposal was to advance knowledge for the good of all, despite the prerogatives of existing institutions and despite the claims of the physicians to medical superiority based on a knowledge of the texts. Petty represents the hopes of many younger men who were interested in the new medicine and the new philosophy and who had little patience with the older academic medicine.

Petty was not, then, a member of the College of Physicians, but his hopes for an improved system of medical science and medical practice were seen in some of the younger fellows of the College. These physicians had already begun to respond to the same challenges as Petty by meeting to discuss new ideas and by undertaking new researches. The new ideas were promoted by other groups, too, some of them close to the centers of power in revolutionary England. No doubt this helped the physicians interested in the new learning to convince others of the importance of their activities. Most importantly, as the Independents in the army and the House of Commons gained control during and after 1647, the circle around Samuel Hartlib, who had important Independent supporters, became influential in promoting intellectual and social reforms.[45] Part of this group's program was to transform medicine, and many of the reformers wished to develop a new medical philosophy based on chemical processes. Whether or not someone sought a new chemical medicine, however, the basic goal of all the reformers was to revive the hidden potentials of nature for the better health of mankind.

The physicians who had begun to meet to discuss advancing medical knowledge in light of the new researches exerted their combined influence to move the College of Physicians toward becoming an up-to-date learned body. Although the College had begun to fall apart in the winter of 1646–47, measures were undertaken to revive it in the spring of 1647. The medical researchers got the College to discuss amending the official *Pharmacopoeia* in July and September of 1647. A committee was set up to redo the book, and some of the most important and active members of the new group participated.[46] At the end of June 1648, President Clarke suggested that the College erect "a laboratory," and his idea was "assented to by every ones' suffrage." In October an anatomy lecture was delivered after a lapse of some

[45]This has been described in detail in Webster.
[46]Annals, 3:235a; 4:10a. The committee members were the four censors (in 1647–48, Prujean, Rant, Ent, and Micklethwaite), the president (Clarke), and Meverall, Hamey, Catcher, and Bates.

years. A proposal to have William Johnson build a chemical laboratory in a room in the gateway to the College was voted down for the moment, but soon Johnson's laboratory became an important part of the College's intellectual program.[47] In the moment of the College's greatest outward weakness, then, a quiet revolution took place, reorienting much of the College's energy toward making it into a learned society that would pursue research, or at least provide the facilities and encouragement for some of its members to do so.

In the spring of 1647, the College reformed itself institutionally, as well. Clarke got lesser criteria for membership accepted and began to increase the number of fellows and licentiates. This could not have happened if old-fashioned academic knowledge had been as valued by the members as it had been before. And despite the fact that new statutes governing the behavior of the members and other practitioners were proposed and passed,[48] the College concentrated on carrying out its obligation to the public to prosecute dangerous practitioners rather than illicit competitors. Yet even in malpractice cases it undertook few prosecutions. Very probably these changes were due to the strong Independent and reformist views of Clarke and some other influential members of the College in the years from 1646 to 1649. They were more interested in reforming the profession along new intellectual and institutional lines than their predecessors had been.[49]

Yet even as the College of Physicians was being reformed, it came under attack from radicals, who found their voices in the late 1640s. Some people did not or would not see the College moving toward becoming a learned body that only prosecuted others for malpractice. The institution's previous monopolistic behavior formed many people's image of the College. No doubt this attitude came in part from suspicions about the motives of the more conservative members of the College: were they just letting things change due to the exigencies of the moment while really hoping to restore their old ways when the king returned to power? The institutional authority of the College posed a threat to the liberties of Englishmen, a number of radicals argued, even if the institution was not being obnoxious at the moment. With the gradual disappearance of censorship in the mid-1640s, the College came in for a certain amount of public abuse.

[47]Annals, 4:13a, 17a, 18a.
[48]Clark has a discussion of the statutes on pp. 278–81.
[49]Also see Birken's remarks in "Fellows of the Royal College," pp. 307–8, 318–22.

The critics of the physicians of the College were outspoken during the interregnum. Many reformers and radicals in the 1640s tried to promote visions of a new society in which there would be true justice for all. In such a society, corporations such as the College of Physicians would have to be abolished. One radical, John Cooke, a solicitor who would present the army's case against Charles I in January of 1649 and sign the verdict of death, published a book in which he took up the plight of the poor. He castigated hoarders of grain who drove up the price of bread, and he urged magistrates to shut down all alehouses and to provide free bread for the needy. He advocated twelve other steps for the relief of the poor, including, in number eleven, having the learned physicians, "whereof God increase the number," give free advice to the indigent. The physicians, he noted, generally charged ten shillings for a visit, which was "as grievous many times as the disease itself" to the poor. (The exorbitant fees also applied to apothecaries and surgeons, who should give free advice, too, Cooke noted.) "But if you cannot be at leisure to prescribe to the poor gratis," Cooke went on, addressing the physicians, "pray do not hinder any man that would be the poor man's doctor." He cited the case of William Trigge, whom he had defended from the College of Physicians in 1640, as an example of what was wrong with the medical corporations. The common law, Cooke insisted, provided that any person with skill could not be stopped from offering his or her medical services. Yet the College had sued Trigge and many others for illicit practice. The implication was clear: the College of Physicians was a monopolistic innovation of government that had no place in the common law; it should therefore be treated as an instrument of absolutism, and the revolution ought to strike it down along with the king.[50]

Others familiar with the injustices of the corporate control of medical practice were also publishing tracts in the late 1640s that criticized the pattern of medical regulation. Peter Chamberlen, a fellow of the College of Physicians but obviously no longer a supporter of the institution, loudly claimed to speak for the women and children of England. The College, he wrote in 1647, plotted against him and persecuted him. (The College did oppose his attempts to gain a patent

[50]John Cooke, *Unum Necessarium: Or, the Poore Mans Case: Being an Expedient to Make Provision for all poore People in the Kingdome* (1648), pp. 41–63 (pagination skips from 41 to 62).

for setting up public baths in the following year.)[51] There could be no cause for this unless, he darkly noted, it was "covetousness" supported by legal powers that is "the true cause that fills their hearts with malice, and their mouths with slanders."[52]

Chamberlen, Cooke, and others in the late 1640s still viewed the College of Physicians as a group of conservative, haughty M.D.s who acted to drive out of London all rivals so that they could keep their fees high. The situation benefited very few people in the city, these critics charged, and they wanted the public to be better served. The reformers of the College could not quiet the more radical opponents of their institution. But both the institutional and the intellectual character of the College had begun to change, nevertheless.

Partial Retrenchment

After Charles I was executed in January 1649, the College of Physicians began to move in a more conservative direction, as did most of the political nation. First, it began to take more actions against empirics. The members voted on June 1, 1649, that "all are to be cited that set up bills" (advertisements), and on June 28 a new solicitor, Thomas Ellis, was appointed to pursue cases against "such as practice without the license of the College." Second, more and more men of formerly Royalist political views were admitted to the fellowship. Even a man like Walter Charleton, who had been a physician extraordinary (that is, without regular salary) to King Charles I, sensed the changed views of the College and applied for membership in November. A debate raged over his admission on the point of whether he ought to be subjected to an examination or whether he should be allowed in without examination because he had been in the king's employ.[53]

Third, members of the College who had become radicalized were expelled. Two members of the College who had criticized it openly,

---

[51]Annals, 4:15a–17b; Peter Chamberlen, *To the Honourable House of Commons Assembled in Parliament, the Humble Petition of Peter Chamberlen, Doctor in Physick* (1648); *A Paper Delivered in by Dr. Alston, Dr. Bates, Dr. Hamens, Dr. Micklethwait . . . to the Honourable Committee for Bathes and Bath-Stoves . . . together with an Answer thereunto by Peter Chamberlen* (1648); and Webster, p. 298.

[52]Peter Chamberlen, *A Voice in Rhama: or, The Crie of Women and Children* (1647).

[53]Annals, 4:20b, 22a–22b, 24b. In February it was decided to examine Charleton (fol. 26b), and he was made a candidate.

Peter Chamberlen and William Goddard, were ejected three weeks after Charleton became a candidate for membership. Chamberlen had publicly criticized the College, had been involved in many schemes to support the Long Parliament and the army, and had written sectarian religious tracts.[54] William Goddard (not to be confused with Jonathan Goddard, one of Cromwell's physicians and a member of the Council of State) had refused to come to any College meetings and had been publicly unruly.[55] The fears of John Cooke were on the verge of being confirmed: the institutional liberalization of the College, if not its intellectual invigoration, had been forced on it by political events, and now that the political atmosphere was changing again, so too was the College's behavior.

The shift to a more conservative position continued into 1650, when Francis Prujean supplanted Clarke as president. The elections of this period have the aspect of a counterrevolution within the College. The new president had been accused of popery in 1643 and afterward, although he was probably a high Anglican rather than a Catholic. Also in 1650, Sir Thomas Cadyman and Edmund Smith were made elects. Both had been Royalists. Cadyman had been physician to the queen and had cofounded the Distillers' Company with Sir Theodore de Mayerne. During the civil wars, he had been physician general to the Royalist army. Smith had been physician-in-ordinary to Charles I during the wars. On the death of Cadyman in 1651, Sir Maurice Williams replaced him as an elect. Williams had also been a Royalist, having been physician to Lord Thomas Strafford during Strafford's tenure as viceroy of Ireland. In 1653 Thomas Winston, a Royalist physician who had fled to France in 1642, was reinstated in his position as elect. And in 1654 William Harvey, who had been the personal physician to Charles I during the wars, was elected president, although he declined the honor.[56]

Yet Cooke's fears would not be confirmed all at once. At the end of

[54]On Chamberlen's criticisms of the College, see *A Voice in Rhama;* also see the many tracts listed under his name in the British Library. His pamphlet of 1650, *To My Beloved Friends and Neighbors of the Black-Fryers,* speaks of his conversion by the spirit of God ("A most strong impulsion of the Spirit") which he wished to promulgate ("to come and publicly declare amongst you, what the Lord hath done for my soul").

[55]William Goddard may at this time have become a chemical physician, as well, since he later joined the proposed "Society of Chymical Physitians": see the list printed in Henry Thomas, "The Society of Chymical Physitians," in *Science, Medicine, and History,* ed. E. Ashworth Underwood, vol. 2, p. 63.

[56]Annals, 4:28a, 53b–54a; *Calendar of State Papers Domestic,* 1660, vol. 16, p. 103; *Calendar of the Committee for Compounding, Domestic,* 1643–1660, July 21, 1648. Also see Birken, "Fellows of the Royal College," pp. 110–12, 203–9, 222–27, 324–27.

October 1650, the College tried to coerce fourteen physicians practicing in London into joining the College; but since it could not legally enforce its privileges given the current state of affairs, it settled for hearing only one or two cases of malpractice per year (brought to the censors by the relatives of harmed patients), only to recommend these cases to common law courts. After 1650, meetings of *comitia censorum* continued to be few.[57] During the confused and unstable next several years under the Barebones Parliament and the Protectorate, the College became more conservative internally while at the same time keeping itself clear of direct legal and political conflicts.

Yet even though the College was becoming more conservative in its membership and, probably, in its hopes of regaining powers of medical regulation, plans to make it a truly up-to-date learned society continued. In January 1651 an outlay of twenty pounds was voted for anatomical and surgical instruments that the College needed for dissections, and at the beginning of April in that year, the College's chemist, Johnson, was ordered to prepare certain chemical medicines each month and to bring them out for inspection and discussion.[58]

Especially important to the continuing revival of the College as a learned society was the generosity of some of the Royalist members of the College. Baldwin Hamey, Jr., purchased the College building from Parliament (after it had been confiscated from the landlord, the dean and chapter of St. Paul's, in 1649), and rented it back to the College at a nominal five pounds per year in 1651.[59] And in July the new president, Francis Prujean, asked: "If I can procure one, that will build us a library, and a repository for simples and rarities, such a one as shall be suitable and honorable to the College, will you assent to have it done, or no, and give me leave, and such others, as I shall desire, to be the designers and overlookers of the work, both for conveniency and ornament?" The fellows voted yes. It turned out that William Harvey, seventy-three years old but still active in research, had approached his friend Prujean and offered to donate his library and other materials to the now securely established College. Money was also appropriated from the College's treasury for the new library, which opened as the Harveian Museum and Library in 1654.[60] Donations of important and valuable books from other peo-

[57]See appendix 1, table 3.
[58]Annals, 4:32b, 33b. Johnson is recorded as having acted as instructed in June and December (4:34b–35a, 38a).
[59]Keevil, *Stranger's Son,* p. 116.
[60]Annals, 4:35a, 37b. Also see Clark, pp. 285–86.

ple soon began to expand its size.[61] Both Harvey's generosity and the model of his previous research made him one of the heroes of the College from this time on.[62]

Harvey's reasons for donating materials to the College were shared by other physicians in the period who pursued research in lieu of regulation. According to Sir Charles Scarburgh (writing at a later date), Harvey first thought of donating his things to Cambridge. But, in conversation with Scarburgh, Harvey declared: "I see plainly that, were I to dedicate my fortune, as I had intended, to the promoting of the knowledge of truth and the public weal [by giving it to the now Puritan-dominated Cambridge], I should do nothing other than make Anabaptists, fanatics, and all manner of thieves and parricides my heirs."[63] The College of Physicians had become a more conservative institution than Cambridge while yet having many members interested in taking up new medical investigations.

Yet in promoting the "public weal" through learning, Harvey was advocating a program of quiet research that avoided political issues. According to George Ent, he, like other physicians perhaps, replied to the question of "Are all affairs well, and right?" with:

> How can they [be], . . . when the Commonwealth is surrounded by intestine troubles; and I my self [as a former physician to Charles I] as yet far from land, tossed in that tempestuous ocean? And, unfeignedly (added he) if the comfort of my studies, and the remembrance of many things, long since fallen under my observation, were not some refreshment to my mind, I know not what could prevail upon me to survive the present.[64]

In other words, the pursuit of learning and research was an escape from the present for Harvey, a present full of difficulties and political turmoil. Admittedly Harvey was suicidal in his old age. But others have remarked on how science can sometimes become "a mental shelter for intolerable pressures" of a political or ideological nature.[65]

---

[61]Sir Richard Napier, for example, gave the College a thirteen-volume edition of Greek commentators on Aristotle, valued at £25, on September 30, 1652 (Annals, 4:43b–44a). Also see *Collegii Medicorum Londinensium Fundatores et Benefactores* (1662).

[62]Robert G. Frank, Jr., "The Image of Harvey in Commonwealth and Restoration England," in *William Harvey and His Age,* ed. Jerome J. Bylebyl, pp. 117–19.

[63]Quoted in Gweneth Whitteridge, "William Harvey: A Royalist and No Parliamentarian," *Past and Present,* no. 30 (1965), reprinted in *The Intellectual Revolution of the Seventeenth Century,* ed. Charles Webster (London: Routledge and Kegan Paul, 1974), p. 188.

[64]Quoted in Whitteridge, "William Harvey," p. 188.

[65]The phrase is Mark Kuchment's in his review of Mark Ya. Azbel's *Refusenik* in *Isis* 44 (1983): 453.

The quiet pursuits of the mind could help satisfy Harvey's own troubles while at the same time benefiting the profession and the public. Other physicians seem to have felt similarly.

The College of Physicians was steadily made into an organization that promoted learned research in physic. The Harveian Museum and Library became a meeting place for the physicians and others who wished to explore both new and old learning in the 1650s. Collaborative researches were even undertaken with apothecaries and noncollegiate physicians. In 1657 Walter Charleton published an introduction to his *Immortality of the Human Soul* that described the College of Physicians as a Solomon's House: the ideal scientific academy outlined by Sir Francis Bacon.[66] Shortly before, in June of 1656, the Harveian Museum had been given statutes governing its operation; and in July, the first Harveian oration was given by Thomas Emily.[67] In 1658 a former and future member of the royal governments, Henry Pierrepoint, lord marquis of Dorchester, earl of Kingston-upon-Hull, and viscount Newark, who had retired from public life during the Protectorate, became an honorary fellow of the College of Physicians.[68] By 1659 and 1660 the library of the College was being used by noncollegiate scholars, such as Castle and his friend Thomas Murrey, Arabic scholars who were allowed to take the Arabic editions of Avicenna home with them to use in compiling a dictionary.[69] The intellectual character of the College of Physicians continued to be reshaped after the mid-1640s.

Many physicians devoted their efforts toward collectively establishing their prestige as learned men by engaging in research, and their efforts paid off. Walter Charleton became a leading spokesman for corpuscularianism. Several other physicians published on physiological subjects.[70] Whereas virtually no anatomical or physiological works had originated in England before 1640 (with the great excep-

[66]See Charles Webster's "The College of Physicians: 'Solomon's House' in Commonwealth England," *BHM* 41 (1967): 393–412, which reprints Charleton's introduction.

[67]Annals, 4:62a–63a, 64a.

[68]Pierrepoint had been a Privy Counselor to Charles I at Oxford and would become a Privy Counselor to Charles II from 1660 to 1673. He had taken up the study of physic after moving to London in 1649 and being treated by Harvey, Scarburgh, and others. Some of his medical manuscripts are in the Sloane Collection at the British Library.

[69]Annals, 4:72a, 74b, 74b–75a, 75a–75b. Christopher Merrett brought out a catalogue of the College library in 1660: *Catalogus librorum, instrumentorum chirurgicorum, rerum curiosarum, exoticarumque Coll. Med. Lond. quae habentur in Musaeo Harveano.*

[70]Charleton's most important tracts promoting atomism in the 1650s were his *Darkness of Atheism Refuted by the Light of Nature* (1652) and *Physiologia Epicuro-Gassendo-Charletoniana* (1654). For indications of the increase in anatomical publications by English physicians during the 1640s and 1650s, see the tables in Frank, "Image of Harvey," pp. 106, 109.

tion of Harvey's *De motu cordis et sanguinis,* published at Frankfurt in 1628), the mid-1640s to the mid-1650s ushered in a few decades of important English medical research. As Charles Webster recently remarked, "on intellectual matters, the Fellows [of the College] were strikingly successful in capturing an up-to-date image" during the interregnum.[71]

A great many of the most influential Englishmen, whether Royalist or Parliamentarian, took an interest in the new science, part of which concerned medicine. No doubt many of the physicians were encouraged to pursue their researches by generalized intellectual support from the social and professional elite. Men like William Sprigg, a close associate of Cromwell's, promoted "experimental science" as part of the social reform that would usher in a new age of peace, prosperity, and liberty; chemistry, anatomy, and medicine composed a very substantial part of his view of what the new science was.[72] Charles Webster has aptly described how the belief in the benefits of the new science could fit into the hopes of some people, particularly members of the Hartlib circle, for the millennium.[73]

Royalists, too, were interested in the new science and medicine. After all, the Newcastle circle, a group of Royalist émigrés in France, was significant for bringing corpuscularian ideas to the attention of people in England. William Harvey and some of his associates were Royalists. And Charles Stuart himself took a deep interest in chemistry while in exile in France, and on his restoration brought back with him Nicaise Le Febvre (who taught chemistry at the Jardin du Roi from 1651 to 1660) to become his royal chemist.[74]

Yet a number of more radical thinkers continued to see the work of the College as a mere continuation of its former elitist activities. The College physicians continued to publish most of their works in Latin, and as their work on rickets showed, they also used their new experimental and anatomical findings to bolster their academic therapies. They were, in other words, modifying but not fundamentally changing their view that an academic elite ought to remain the most important and prestigious group of practitioners. However up-to-date

---

[71]Webster, p. 308.

[72]R. L. Greaves, "William Sprigg and the Cromwellian Revolution," *Huntington Library Quarterly* 34 (1971): 109–17.

[73]Webster, esp. chap. 1.

[74]On the importance of chemistry at the Jardin du Roi in Paris, see Jean-Paul Contant, *L'Enseignement de la chimie au Jardin Royal des Plantes de Paris* (Cahors: A. Covelant, 1952); and Rio Howard, *La Bibliothèque et le laboratoire de Guy de la Brosse au Jardin des Plantes à Paris* (Geneva: Droz, 1983).

many of their activities may have been, however they may have changed the content of learned medicine, the physicians could not convince all people that they had the larger public interest at heart.

Some men led an attack on the College of Physicians by translating Latin medical works into English. Latin, in their eyes, was a holdover from the days in which the Catholic church lorded it over honest men by keeping them in ignorance through the use of an esoteric language. If Latin medical works were translated into English, all men could learn medicine themselves and not be enslaved by an elite profession.

Nicholas Culpeper became the best known of these antiauthoritarian translators. He entered the lists in 1649 with a translation of the College's *Pharmacopoeia,* entitled the *Physical Directory,* which contained a strong assault on the College, and in 1653 he issued a translation and augmentation of the 1650 revised *Pharmacopoeia* that contained a preface on astrological medicine as well as an attack on the College. He wished to overthrow the physicians, but Culpeper also believed that the liberties of the subject would best be preserved by ending the professions of law and church, as well. In one of his almanacs, Culpeper predicted struggles between lawyers and clergy, commenting that "when thieves fall out, honest men come by their goods again." His antimonarchical tenets and semisectarian religious opinions are clear. Culpeper's works were welcomed by the parliamentary press and caused the College much embarrassment.[75]

Still other attacks on the College of Physicians came from practitioners who were trying to reform physic along chemical lines. This reform was to unlock the secrets of nature through a combination of spiritual and empirical pursuits. One brand of chemistry derived from Paracelsianism and Hermeticism fit in well with the heightened religious sensibilities of the period. An understanding of God's book of nature, proponents believed, could be aided by a knowledge of scripture; the key lay with a hands-on knowledge of chemistry. The semi-anti-intellectualism of this attitude—the emphasis on inspiration and intuition over scholastic learning—undermined the claims of the physicians to superiority due to their academic educations. Paracelsus himself had been no friend of academic physic. On one occasion he declared: "The physician comes from nature, from nature he is born; only he who receives his experiences from nature is a physi-

[75]Bernard Capp, *Astrology and the Popular Press: English Almanacs, 1500–1800* (London: Faber and Faber, 1979), pp. 107, 79, 107–108; Webster, pp. 267–72; also see F. N. L. Poynter, "Nicholas Culpeper and His Books," *JHM* 17 (1962): 152–67.

cian, and not he who writes, speaks, and acts with his head and with ratiocinations aimed against nature and her ways."[76]

By the mid-seventeenth century, many empirics and ordinary practitioners, and some noncollegiate physicians, followed the teachings of Jean Baptista Van Helmont, who had modified Paracelsian teachings in significant ways.[77] Several of these "spagirical" philosophers and physicians and their ideas to reform natural philosophy, education, and medicine found sympathetic ears in many Paracelsian and Puritan circles during the 1640s and 1650s.[78]

One outspoken chemical reformer was Noah Biggs, who followed Van Helmont in attacking both the Galenic program and the Paracelsian program while advocating a new approach to medicine based on Helmontian principles.[79] He also aimed a scathing attack at the College of Physicians, which he saw as a conservative and ignorant group of monopolists. Biggs's book, 'Mataeotechnia medicinae praxeos.' The Vanity of the Craft of Physick (1651), was addressed to the Parliament, which, Biggs said, had been directed by Cromwell to undertake the reform of all the professions. As for the academic physicians, Biggs had nothing but contempt: they "have nothing in their mouths but ars longa, vita brevis; and true enough: for they cure either late, or never, which makes their art long; but they kill enough, which makes life short." "The whole method and body of physic, as it is now prescribed and practiced, with the desires of good men," he

[76]Quoted from Paracelsus: Selected Writings, ed. Jolande Jacobi, p. 49. The best work on Paracelsus himself remains that of Walter Pagel, Paracelsus: An Introduction to Philosophical Medicine in the Era of the Renaissance.

[77]Walter Pagel, Jean Baptista Van Helmont: Reformer of Science and Medicine; idem, "Religious Motives in the Medical Biology of the Seventeenth Century," BHM 3 (1935): 97–128, 213–31, 265–312. Also see Allen G. Debus, The Chemical Philosophy: Paracelsian Science and Medicine in the Sixteenth and Seventeenth Centuries, vol. 2; see pp. 357–59 for Debus's description of Van Helmont's idea of the divine office of the physician.

[78]P. M. Rattansi, "Paracelsus and the Puritan Revolution," Ambix 11 (1963): 24–33; Webster, esp. pp. 273–82; and idem, "Alchemical and Paracelsian Medicine," in Health, Medicine and Mortality, ed. Webster, pp. 301–34.

[79]For a brief review of Biggs's medical ideas, see Debus, Chemical Philosophy, vol. 2, pp. 502–7; Webster, pp. 263–64; Jones, Ancients and Moderns, pp. 99–101, 132–33, 303–4. Debus sees Biggs as typical of the "Paracelsian" reformers in the period despite Biggs's avowed Helmontianism: see "Paracelsian Medicine: Noah Biggs and the Problem of Medical Reform," in Medicine in Seventeenth Century England, ed. Debus, pp. 34–38.

The identity of Biggs has never been established, but I like to think that he was either Thomas Biggs, brother-in-law of Rear Admiral Richard Badiley, or his son, Henry Biggs, both of whom were surgeons employed at the dockyards of Deptford and Woolwich between 1649 and 1657, the pseudonym "Noah" stemming from their work environment (Calendar of State Papers, Domestic, 1649–50, p. 532, and 1652–53, pp. 351, 352).

wrote, "groans for a reformation."[80] As the learned physicians were at that time practicing their "craft," it was "vanity."

Much of the problem, Biggs said, came from the spiritual corruption of the physicians. The mistake of the academics was to rely on ancient doctrines, derived from pagan sources, which failed to see God's creation in the proper terms:

> An evil spirit has gone out, to seduce them [the physicians] to lie unto themselves, and to the truth of God. For these things they see, hear, taste, and handle, they known not what they are, neither without nor within themselves. He is too inward in the private cells and recesses of His creatures, for their shallow and unhallowed eyes to penetrate; and none of them all can see Him without fire: not the chemists' kitchen-fire, but the true philosophical fire.

The academicians, Biggs claimed, pursued "studies, books, orations, councils, conversations, chairs, and practices" through nothing but "trifles and anxious disput[ation]s," and so advanced learning in medicine hardly at all. Anatomical investigations—the basis of the claim by many of the new research-oriented physicians to a knowledge of the human body and hence to a knowledge of diseases and their cures—had never actually helped the physicians cure, Biggs claimed. The true philosophical fire, the spiritual philosopher's alchemical operation, Biggs said he himself possessed, and so he claimed to be able to cure a great many people. Thus, as part of his reform of medicine, Biggs advanced the view that spiritual adepts such as himself, not the academically trained physicians, should be free to pursue their own studies and cures without interference from the College of Physicians, the universities, or other bodies.[81]

Biggs was a radical in his ideas about the content of learned medicine, but his program was aimed at demolishing the academics, not at ending the domination of the learned over other practitioners. He would substitute his own men for the academic physicians. The vulgar people, as he put it, held the medical profession in contempt. The herbal medicines administered by most physicians were ineffectual, and therefore the art of "pyrotechny"—that which involved the purification of substances by fire, or chemistry—ought to take the place

[80]Biggs, 'Mataeotechnia medicinae praxeos.' *The Vanity of the Craft of Physick* (1651), sig. b2v, p. 16.

[81]Ibid., sig. b3, pp. 6, 9.

of herbal medicines. As it was, "any knave, whore, bawd, old woman, or any that have the impudence, dares boldly rush into a Galenical way of physic, without control." They "dare play with and dandle the lives of men and women in their hands; and unto so high a pitch of impudence have they flown, that they dare build their nests in the College's turrets, and use [the College's] highest medicines, and plead prescription, custom, and present practice of the most eminent physicians." For their own good, then, the learned physicians of the College should end their attempts to control others whose practices could hardly be distinguished from their own, and pursue instead the truly learned medicine of chemistry that Biggs advocated be pursued within his proposed "Academy of Philosophic Freedom."[82]

Other men, too, promoted chemical medicine as the kind of medicine that ought to replace the older Galenic and academic medicine. Men such as John Webster, George Starkey, and John Heydon published works advocating chemical medicine and its underlying philosophy,[83] while translations of Paracelsus, Van Helmont, and many other Continental chemical physicians emerged in the 1650s.[84] Many people associated with the Hartlib circle viewed chemistry as the key to unlocking nature's secrets, and a "chemical council" was established near Hartlib's house in Charing Cross in 1654.[85] A book published in 1655 entitled *Chymical, Medicinal, and Chyrurgical Addresses: Made to Samuel Hartlib, Esquire* that contained nine essays had a strongly alchemical bent. The last essay (translated from a German theological treatise) predicted that soon a universal medicine would make everyone healthy, end death, and so eliminate the medical profession.

As far as the physicians of the College were concerned, the chemists and some of the empirics would not have posed as great a problem as they did had they simply been mountebanks and hawkers of wares through newspaper advertisements and broadsides: such men would be easily distinguished from the learned physicians. But many books and pamphlets were being published that offered medical ad-

[82]Ibid., pp. 18, 225–28, sig. b3.

[83]John Webster, *Academiarum Examen* (1654); George Starkey, *Nature's Explication and Helmont's Vindication* (1657); John Heydon, *A New Method of Rosie Crucian Physick* (1658). Also see Jones, *Ancients and Moderns,* pp. 108–14, 104–38.

[84]See Debus, *Chemical Philosophy,* pp. 509–10; Rattansi, "Paracelsus and the Puritan Revolution"; and Charles Webster, "English Medical Reformers of the Puritan Revolution: A Background to the 'Society of Chymical Physitians,'" *Ambix* 14 (1967): 16–41.

[85]Webster, esp. pp. 384–402; also see Barbara Kaplan, "The Medical Writings of Robert Boyle: Medical Philosophy in Mid-Seventeenth-Century England" (Ph.D. diss., University of Maryland, 1979), pp. 35–40.

vice and seemingly learned medical disquisitions on various subjects. Chemists and empirics also often claimed the title of physician or "medicus" on the title pages of their tracts.

A problem therefore existed for the academic physicians of the College: how to get the public to recognize the learned physicians as the only legitimate ones when the College's juridical power could not be used against the interlopers. A struggle for public opinion ensued. As the physician James Primrose put it in a book translated from Latin in 1651: "The greater danger hangs over the sick by those practitioners in physic, which have but little knowledge therein, than from [those] that know nothing at all." "Therefore," he continued,

> let the people from henceforth think him a learned physician, not who knows a little Greek and Latin, or some other science besides physic [such as chemistry], but who being well instructed in the rules of physic, and well read in Galen and Hippocrates, understands thoroughly the diagnostic, prognostic, and therapeutic parts of physic; for he that is either wholly ignorant of these things, or understands them but meanly and in part, can scarcely be accounted a good physician.[86]

Only a university education and a proper medical degree could guarantee that a physician would fit the qualifications proposed by Primrose. But how were the physicians to prove publicly that they alone truly understood the "rules of physic"? Part of the answer lay in the "scientific" research program that had already been undertaken by members of the College of Physicians.

The engagement of the physicians in anatomical and "scientific" research gave the members of the College an opportunity to mount a public counterattack against their rivals. Soon after Noah Biggs's *The Vanity of the Craft of Physic,* which in large part was an attack on the College, was published in 1651, a reply came out by an associate of the College of Physicians via a translation of some of Leonard Fioravanti's works. (Fioravanti had been an Italian follower of Paracelsus.) The translation had been done by John Hester in 1596, but the new edition—in manuscript by October 17, 1651, published in 1652— was edited by William Johnson, the College's new chemist. Johnson's major addition to Hester's translation was a translator's preface and two preludes against Noah Biggs and Nicholas Culpeper.[87]

[86]James Primrose, *Popular Errours, or the Errours of the People in Physick,* trans. Robert Wittie (1651), pp. 8, 3.
[87]See Webster, pp. 312–13.

In the translator's preface, Johnson castigated empirics and ignorant practitioners in general, while praising "that honourable society of London Physicians" who "have chosen out a chemical artificer [i.e., Johnson himself], whom they have placed in their own College, and over whom they have set discreet, and learned overseers to oblige the public for their care to their medicines hereafter." In other words, no one could accuse the College physicians of ignorance or of going about their affairs at the expense of the public, even in chemical matters. Johnson attacked the elitist chemist Biggs for being only superficially learned, for he only knew his Van Helmont: "When was ever practice amongst the physicians so narrowly confined, as they kept themselves to one author?" "Yet you are so much for Helmont, as if he were the great luminary of the world."[88]

The reply of Johnson to the more leveling Culpeper was more vicious. As for the claim that "'we are prisoners, and kept in darkness, and who are our jailors but scholars'" of church and medicine, Johnson suggested that Culpeper's alternative was to "teach [unlearned men and women] a desperate unwarrantable practice!" Johnson "cannot but smile" at Culpeper's "nonsense similitudes," such as his statement that the physicians' "'covetousness outweighs their wits, as a millstone outweighs a feather.'" Going on to poke fun at Culpeper's learning, Johnson wrote that "it seemeth you rather know how to translate Latin, than transfer it into a sentence." He ended by telling the story of how a "gentleman and scholar," passing by a bookstand, picked up a book, and after perusing it, asked the bookseller if it was by Culpeper. Receiving an affirmative reply, he said that "truly Culpeper hath made cul-paper, paper fit to wipe one's breech withall."[89] That kind of reply by slander was characteristic of much of the interchange between the public critics and the defenders of the College of Physicians in the 1650s.

And yet there was an undercurrent of the new endeavors of the physicians that seemed to reflect an unease not unlike that exhibited by their critics: the new medical science would have to be more in touch with experiments, with empirical discoveries. The fact that the new researches of the physicians also promoted empirical work of a "scientific" kind made it clear that this type of debate by pamphlet over who was the most learned could not ultimately preserve the

[88]William Johnson, *Short Amimadversions* [sic] *upon the Book lately published by one who stiles himself Noah Biggs, Helmonti Psittacum* (1652), prefix to L. Fioravanti, *Three Exact Pieces* (1652), p. 2.

[89]William Johnson, *Friend Culpeper . . .* prefix to *Three Exact Pieces*, pp. 9–14.

physicians' place at the top of the medical hierarchy. The public was getting confused about what learning ought to be and about the distinctions between empiricisms. In a period in which "science" was being invented, both sides were claiming empirical evidence as support for their view on which was the superior medicine.

In 1655, therefore, another shift in the College's outward behavior manifested itself. The restoration of order in England under the Protectorate of Oliver Cromwell at the end of 1653, and the centralization of power in the hands of the major generals in 1655, gave the members of the College a new opportunity. If the College was to take advantage of the new situation to restore its power over other practitioners, it could do so by allying itself with Cromwell.

The College first debated taking action against apothecaries, who were openly practicing physic, in April of 1655, although it was finally agreed that it was impossible to take action against them just then. On October 1, the College voted Edward Alston into the president's seat, thus placing a strong Cromwellian at the head of the institution. In the months before Prujean's ouster in favor of Alston, a dispute had arisen over admitting the former Royalist and Prujean's friend, Walter Charleton, to the fellowship. In the end, the Cromwellians had their way, and Charleton was refused, while at the same time the Parliamentarian William Petty was made a fellow-in-absentia.[90] In November, Francis Glisson was made an elect. Glisson had been left in his post as Regius Professor of Physic at Cambridge during the period of the university's domination by the Parliament, and he wrote on divinity as well as medicine, including treatises on the Book of Revelation.[91] The next elect, voted in on July 9, 1657, was John Bathurst, M.P. for the Second Protectorate Parliament in 1656 and personal physician to Cromwell.

The move by the Cromwellians to take control of the College of Physicians soon paid off. In mid-March of 1656, debate began on how to control the empirics, and by the end of the month, a committee had been established to deal with the problem. The committee was composed of Drs. Ent, Bate, Staines, Paget, Goddard, Trench,

[90]Annals, 4:55b, 56a–56b, 57a, 57b, 59b, 63a–63b; William J. Birken, "The Puritan Connexions of Sir Edward Alston, President of the Royal College of Physicians, 1655–1666," *MH* 18 (1974): 370–74; idem, "Fellows of the Royal College," pp. 135–42, 167–69; and Lindsay Sharp, "The Royal College of Physicians and Interregnum Politics," *MH* 19 (1975): 112–18, 120–26.

[91]One of his brothers had been a physician to the parliamentary army of the Eastern Association, in which Cromwell had commanded the cavalry, while another brother became a member of the Cromwellian civil service.

Wilson, Coxe, Stanley, Scarburgh, and Merrett, all but three of whom can be identified as being clearly committed to the new government.[92]

The committee seems quickly to have obtained the good graces of the authorities, for by the end of April it declared that all those practitioners parading as physicians in public advertisements were to be arrested, while all other empirics were to be considered guilty by subpoena on the authority of the Exchequer, and the beadle was ordered to seek out the offenders. On June 6, the first case of illicit practice in many years was brought to the College: one Dr. Timme was warned not to practice without the permission of the College. Others were brought before the College in the next few months. To cap it all off, on November 8, a charter was obtained from the lord protector confirming the Act of 14 and 15 Henry VIII that had granted the College the power to regulate medical practice in London.[93]

Other physicians in London who were not members of the College looked on these moves with trepidation. William Rand, a physician who "identified himself with the [reforming] aims of Hartlib and Boyle,"[94] possessed an M.D. from Leiden that had not been incorporated in one of the two English universities, and he feared that the College would soon restrict his own practice and the practices of others. He wrote to Hartlib, in a letter dated August 15, 1656, proposing the creation of a group of "Graduate Physicians." These men would be M.D.s banding together to defend their interests against the physicians of the College. Rand wished Hartlib to communicate the project "only to such as you know are averse to the College . . . lest we be countermined!" He believed that the new group would attract the "more studious, modest, reserved, public, and humble spirited" physicians, while the "more ambitious, covetous, domineering, and selfish sort of physicians" would continue to try to join the College.

The "better sort" of physicians, as Rand saw it, needed to associate for two reasons. First, they had need for a common legal defense from the "suits and other molestations [of the College of Physicians] (to which all are liable)," which was to be paid for out of "a common stock, arising from a light but weekly contribution." Second, "that

---

[92]Annals, 4:60b, 61a. Stanley, Scarburgh, and Merrett are the three members who cannot be identified as Cromwellians, but all three of them were junior members of the College. For the others, see Sharp, "Royal College of Physicians," pp. 111–13; and Birken, "Fellows of the Royal College," pp. 306–7, 309, 311.

[93]Annals, 4:61a–61b; Clark, p. 282.

[94]Webster, p. 305.

in case the College shall move for a confirmation of their charter"—exactly what the College was just then doing—the graduate physicians could move as a group to have clauses inserted that would protect their rights to practice as M.D.s despite the College. It was not other M.D.s, but the "mechanics and wicked persons, as without education, [who] thrust themselves upon the practice thereof," who ought to be prohibited from practice. The "avarice and unskillfulness" of these people "can no more be charged upon graduate physicians of the universities, than upon the members of the College of London."[95]

But nothing came of Rand's scheme. It is likely that the difficulties that the College of Physicians soon encountered served notice that the other physicians would not be bothered, at least not for the present.

The reassertion of the power of the College of Physicians to regulate medical practitioners ran into a dead-end in November 1656, only a few weeks after the new charter had been obtained from Cromwell. At the end of the month, three trials took place before the court of Common Pleas sitting at Guildhall in which the College of Physicians sued Richard Barker (later Sir), William Blank, and William Trigge for illicit practice. All three were notorious empirics, and all three had caused trouble for the College since the 1630s. Blank and Trigge had been sued in higher courts, and Barker had been ordered to conform to the College in 1640,[96] but the legal and political turmoil that had surfaced later that year had caused the College to drop its suits. The restoration of stable government and the renewal of the College's charter seemed to make the time auspicious for renewing the suits against the three. The College intended to make an example of them, demonstrating its revitalized power.

The case of Trigge can serve to illustrate all three of these crucial cases. He had first been brought to the attention of the College in February 1631, at first got off, then was fined £10 and imprisoned, then fined another £25 and sent to the Fleet prison (where he bribed the warden and got out). Intermittent testimony had been taken on his practice during the next few years, but the censors were more concerned with trying to discipline the Society of Apothecaries than

---

[95]For Rand's remarks and more on the College of Graduate Physicians, see Webster, pp. 300–308, 533–34; and idem, "English Medical Reformers," pp. 35–39. The iatrochemical milieu of the Hartlib circle may have provided the setting in which Rand could write to Hartlib, but it was the particulars of the College's aggressive behavior in the spring and summer of 1656 that temporarily created the need for such an organization.

[96]Annals, 3:208a, 208a–208b, 212a–212b.

Trigge. But he was tried again in 1637, fined £20 and imprisoned in Newgate for malpractice. In trouble again in 1640 for illicit practice, he was tried by the College before the King's Bench at Guildhall, where he was defended by the radical lawyer John Cooke. He was fined £155. He tried to get a writ of error in the House of Lords, but he was turned down since the king would not sign the document. When the College tried to collect the fine in 1647, Trigge's petition against the College (signed by 3,000 people) did get him a hearing from the House of Lords, but the College won its case there.[97] With Cromwell's new charter in 1656, however, the College again hauled Trigge into court at Guildhall, confident of the outcome of the case.

Despite the new charter, Trigge's case in 1656 represented the College of Physicians as an unjust monopoly that prohibited good practitioners from treating people in London. Trigge's petition to the House of Lords in 1647 had noted that Trigge "did abundance of good to all sorts of people in and about this City when most of the College doctors deserted us" in the plagues of 1630 and 1636. "Since which time your petitioners have for above twenty years, in their several times of sickness and infirmities, taken physic from him . . . in which time, we do verily believe in our consciences, that he hath done good to above thirty thousand persons," while making his medicines himself and charging the poor nothing and others only what they wished to pay. The petition concluded that unless Trigge be allowed to continue, "many poor people must of necessity perish to death . . . for they are not able to pay great fees to doctors and apothecaries' bills which cost more than his advice and physic; nor can we have access unto them when we desire, which we familiarly have to Dr. Trigge to our great ease and comfort."[98]

Such sentiments were not only similar to the view expressed in an earlier petition to the Parliament asking that physicians (as well as divines and lawyers) be paid "out of the public treasury" so that all people would have access to medical care,[99] they also reflected the

<hr />

[97]Annals, 3:168b, 169b, 173a–173b, 188b, 189b, 208a; S.P. 16/373/4; John Cooke, *Unum Necessarium: Or, the Poore Mans Case* (1648), pp. 41–63. Cooke later conducted the prosecution of Charles I: C. V. Wedgwood, "The Trial of Charles I," in *The English Civil War and After, 1642–1658,* ed. R. H. Parry (London: MacMillan, 1970), pp. 45, 48–50.

[98]"Humble Petition of Many Thousands of Citizens . . . ," quoted in Alice Clark, *The Working Life of Women in the Seventeenth Century,* pp. 262–63; *Royal Commission on Historical Manuscripts, 6th Report* (London: HMSO, 1877), p. 176; *House of Lords Journals,* vol. 9, p. 197; vol. 10, pp. 276, 291, 332, 334.

[99]Petition of Mr. Samuel Herring, 1653, in *Original Letters and Papers of State Addressed to Oliver Cromwell,* ed. John Nickolls (London, 1743), p. 101.

judgment that the College of Physicians was an unjust monopoly, a view that had the support of a legal mind such as Sir Edward Coke's. Coke's *Fourth Institute,* published in 1648, had directed those seeking his opinion on the College of Physicians' ability to try other practitioners to his declaration in Bonham's case, in which he had declared it "null and void" for going against "right reason." A legal volume almost contemporary with Trigge's case extended Coke's declaration there to argue for free trade.[100]

In the face of the apparent injustice of the learned doctors bringing suit against such men as Trigge and the two others, Chief Justice St. John threw out the 1656 case on a technicality. He declared that the original Act of 14 and 15 Henry VIII that gave the College its corporate powers had not been registered with the king's signature and was therefore null and void.[101] Cromwell's new charter, based as it was on that act, could not overcome this declaration.

Because of this verdict the College found itself with no statutory existence. The case had a very important impact on the College's juridical powers for more than twenty years. In the face of such an overwhelming judicial decision, the College of Physicians could not hope to continue to prosecute others, no matter how much influence it had with Cromwell's government.

The physicians scrambled to try to remedy the situation. Christopher Merrett combed the archives and found the registration of the original charter with King Henry's signature, he said. On December 18, 1656, a new charter was obtained from Cromwell. At the beginning of February 1658, an empiric, Robert Combes, of Knightrider Street, was forbidden to practice, and at the beginning of March, the College heard testimony against a surgeon-apothecary, Edward Randal, who was accused of malpractice. In June, a new committee was appointed to proceed with suits against empirics—possibly to renew the suits against Trigge, Blank, and Barker.[102]

[100]Edward Coke, *The Fourth Part of the Institutes of the Laws of England: Concerning the Jurisdictions of Courts* (1648), pp. 251–52. (Also see my article "'Against Common Right and Reason': The College of Physicians versus Dr. Thomas Bonham," *American Journal of Legal History* 29(1985):301–22.); William Shepheard, *Of Corporations, Fraternities, and Guilds* (1659), pp. 12, 17, 88–89.

[101]Christopher Merrett, *A Collection of Acts of Parliament, Charters, Trials at Law, and Judges Opinions Concerning Those Grants to the Colledge of Physicians London* (1660), pp. 122–26 (who says that the judge was "Nicholas," and omits any reference to it being the court of Common Pleas); and Adrian Huyberts, *A Corner-stone laid towards the Building of a New Colledge* (1675), pp. 5–7.

[102]Merrett, *A Collection of Acts of Parliament,* pp. 122–26; Clark, p. 282; Annals, 4:70a–70b, 71a.

But as the autumn season, when the College saw to most of such business, approached, the lord protector sickened, and on September 3 he died. Political uncertainty and the threat of civil war again stalked England, and, as before, the College stopped all public prosecutions until the situation stabilized. Few of the physicians could have imagined that Charles II would be restored shortly, and that with his restoration would come the almost complete collapse of their corporation.

The professional benefits that had accrued to the physicians under Charles I included, above all, the support of the Privy Council and the Star Chamber in the College's attempts to punish and suppress other practitioners it saw as rivals or as troublemakers. The physicians, not the public, were the judges of medical practitioners under that juridical order, and could largely protect the notion that their learning in the texts yielded the best medical practices. With the meeting of the Long Parliament, however, the College began to put some distance between itself and the Crown.

When civil war broke out, the College changed its policies under new leadership. At the same time, many of its younger members were freed to take up the new science and to explore anatomical and physiological researches. Yet, with the execution of the king and mounting public attacks on physic, further reversals of College policy occurred in the early 1650s, first installing Royalist sympathizers into the leadership of the College, then putting Cromwellians there; both attempted to reassert the role of physicians in making public distinctions between good and bad practice. Throughout this period, too, the new researches continued, and they gave the College a degree of intellectual strength in its replies to its critics.

But a struggle to win public support through arguments over learning alone could never have resulted in a clear victory for the physicians. The cases thrown out by chief justice St. John in late 1656 showed that only when legal authority was added to governmental support could the physicians supervise the medical milieu and hence uphold the kind of learning they believed to be best. As events began to move toward a restoration of the Stuart monarchy, the hopes of some of the physicians for a return to their former position grew.

4

Political Weaknesses and Intellectual Threats, 1660–1672

It is a great mistake to conceive of this historical revolt [of the new science against its intellectual past] as an appeal to reason. On the contrary, it was, through and through, an anti-intellectualist movement.

Alfred North Whitehead,
Science and the Modern World

The Restoration of the Stuarts in the spring of 1660 brought renewed hope to the officers of the College of Physicians, hope that their institution would also be restored to its position of authority. Unfortunately for that hope, the 1660s brought new problems of both an institutional and an intellectual kind. The clock could not be turned back to 1640. Lord Chancellor Clarendon's influence was not strong enough to gain passage in Parliament of a bill giving statutory authority to a new College charter. Opposing the bill were the Society of Apothecaries and the Barber-Surgeons' Company. But also among the opponents of the bill seem to have been some of those infatuated with the "new philosophy." The new science had widespread support at court in the first part of the decade, as exemplified by the large number of aristocrats who signed the register of the newly created Royal Society from 1663 to 1666. Yet some physicians worried that the new science would undermine the status of learned physic by substituting for physic's academic education in the texts an interest in mere medicine's empirical cures.

The intellectual and institutional threats posed to learned physic by the supporters of the new philosophy, the virtuosi, were redoubled when a rival, the Society of Chemical Physicians, organized in the months following the defeat of the College's charter. The new society found many patrons at court, particularly the duke of Buckingham and other virtuosi. The chemists argued that intuitions and hands-on, empirical experiments in making medicines were essential to the true art of healing. So did some members of the Royal Society who practiced medicine. A coalition of factions at court, the new Society of Chemical Physicians, and the Royal Society appeared to be on the verge of overwhelming the College of Physicians. No wonder some of the physicians responded by attacking the new science or by encouraging others, especially Henry Stubbe, to do so.

The College Charter Controversy

In the first months of the Restoration, many people and groups paid homage to the new king and, claiming to have fallen from fortune's favor in the years since 1641, lobbied for a restoration of their former rights, privileges, titles, and powers. Among these importunate groups was the College of Physicians, who through the offices of Edward Hyde, soon to be Lord Chancellor Clarendon, managed to get a delegation of its members admitted into the royal presence in the middle of August. The delegation presented the king with a Latin oration on his fortunate return and the gift of a unicorn's horn, considered to be a rare but effective antidote for many ills and poisons. In a most politic manner, the members of the College stated their bitter opposition to the Commonwealth and their great pleasure at Charles's return. The president, Edward Alston, who gave the oration, was knighted on the spot.[1] The hopes of the College were high. If the Stuart king would support the College, its members might again become the shepherds of the London medical community, enforcing their privileges and preventing many of the abuses of practice that, in their view, existed around them in great numbers.

Even if the new Crown had quickly and firmly supported the College of Physicians, the new political "revolution" would not turn the clock back to 1640, to when the College's public authority had not yet begun to decline. Rather, the Restoration was legally something more like the compromise of 1641. The political result in 1660 was therefore a weakened Crown and a Parliament that tried increasingly both to gain benefits for former Royalists and to control

---

[1]Annals, 4:75b–76a; Clark, pp. 303–4.

the monarchy through governing its finances while at the same time attacking Clarendon's friendly gestures to Presbyterians and former Roundheads. The College would have to tread carefully on the confusing political groundwork of the Restoration.

While the College was testing the new government, with the intention of regaining its former powers, certain internal disputes also had to be settled. The most difficult emerged over the position of William Goddard, who had been expelled from the fellowship in 1649 for contumacy. Goddard had unsuccessfully filed suit against the College in King's Bench that same year in an attempt to regain his post. But he, too, saw the Restoration as a return to things past, and in October 1660 he requested that he be restored to the fellowship. The issue came to a vote at the regular December 24 meeting. Goddard was refused, but he tried to take his seat anyway, causing the meeting to be dissolved. On February 26, 1661, the College learned that the King's Bench ("*suprema Curia*") had ordered Goddard's restoration; the matter was referred back to the College's lawyers, who entered a return in the same court. There one of the College's lawyers argued that the fellowship "doth not concern any freehold, but a privilege occasionally made for convenience by by-law, . . . it concerns no matter of government or legal interest." The four justices agreed, finally, that Goddard's living did not depend on his fellowship, and so found in favor of the College.[2]

This case clearly established, at the beginning of the Restoration, the right of the College to govern its own internal affairs. Ironically, Goddard's case also clearly implied that the College was legally impotent to carry out its will in regulating the medical marketplace: "it concern[ed] no matter of government," because membership in the College would have no effect on Goddard's ability to practice medicine in London. The King's Bench had been convinced (by the College's own lawyer) that the College was more a learned society than a professional monopoly.

But the College had already begun to change this state of affairs. Legal and political moves were going on behind the scenes at court during 1661 and 1662, as the physicians tried to strengthen their position. As it had under previous governments, the College had friends at court, including the four royal physicians, all of whom

---

[2]Annals, 4:76a, 77a; "Doctor Goddard's Case," 1 Sid., 29, *English Reports* 82; "Doctor Goddard's Case," 1 Lev., 19, *English Reports* 83; "Doctor Goddard's Case in Assize Br. 76," 1 Keble, 75–76, *English Reports* 83; "Doctor Goddard's Case," 1 Keble, 84–85, *English Reports* 83.

were members of the College: John Baber, with influential Presbyterian connections; George Bate, who had served both Charles I and Cromwell during the revolution; Sir Edward Greaves, who had been physician to the Royalist army in Oxford and to Charles I in his captivity; and Sir Alexander Fraizer.

Sir Alexander Fraizer was the most important of them all. He was made first physician, the most senior of the appointed physicians, to Charles II on June 24, 1660.[3] He had obtained the fellowship in 1641 after first practicing illicitly, but he fled to the Continent in 1647 with the help of Colonel John Hutchinson.[4] He served the future Charles II in exile, one of the several Scots gaining influence in the intrigues of that factious court (he was in Lauderdale's group).[5] He returned to England after Cromwell's death in 1658 and was restored to his position at the College on December 22, despite some internal opposition.[6] After the Restoration Fraizer became a significant figure at court once again, along with his wife, one of the queen's dressers. He even had rooms in the middle of the Whitehall Palace maze (and began building additional rooms at Whitehall in 1677).[7]

In addition to the royal physicians, Clarendon, the lord chancellor, who had been the conduit for the College's audience with Charles in 1660, seems to have favored the College's actions. That College members felt secure in the Crown's graces seems clear from their behavior as they campaigned for a new charter between 1661 and 1664.[8]

Among the first steps that the College took after the Restoration was to publish a book outlining its legal powers. Christopher Merrett, curator of the new Harveian Museum and Library, wrote the book. In it he transcribed the sixteenth-century acts and charters that gave the physicians power over others. He also selectively included reports of cases that the College had won in court, against Buggs and Barton (empirics), and against Gardener and Bonham (physicians). The book ended with a description of the trials at Guildhall in 1656

---

[3]*Calendar of Treasury Books,* July 12, 1664.

[4]Lucy Hutchinson, *Memoires of the Life of Colonel Hutchinson* (1802–1822. Reprint. New York: Dutton, Everyman's Library, 1968), p. 240.

[5]See, for example, Edward Hyde, Earl of Clarendon, *The History of the Rebellion and Civil Wars in England* (Oxford: Clarendon Press, 1819), vol. 3, pp. 530–31, 682.

[6]*Annals,* 4:71b–72a.

[7]*Calendar of Treasury Books,* January 31, 1677.

[8]On the new charters of the Restoration, see John Leslie Miller, "The Crown and the Borough Charters in the Reign of Charles II," *English Historical Review* 100 (1985): 53–84, esp. 56–67.

that had overturned the College's statutory authority and Merrett's discovery of documents that, in his view, invalidated Justice St. John's ruling. No mention was made of Cromwell's charters of confirmation.[9]

Clearly, the College felt that its legal position had been undermined because of the 1656 ruling, and it wanted to reestablish the precedents that had been followed during the early seventeenth century and had made it strong. To do this, the College would have to return to the Crown's favor (and pass over Cromwell's support for it). A book like Merrett's, circulated among friends at court, might well help the College restore its powers.[10] A book listing the benefactors of the College, including all the kings and queens (except Edward VI) from Henry VIII to Charles II, famous physicians such as William Harvey, and gentlemen such as John Selden, was also published.[11]

A College committee established to pursue negotiations for obtaining new privileges in June of 1661 soon brought results.[12] The parliamentary act proposed in 1661 "for preventing the printing of seditious or schismatical books and papers" empowered the College to review and license all books on physic.[13] On January 23, 1663, a new charter was written, and it passed the Privy Seal in March.

The new charter of the College, styled the "King's College of Physicians in the City of London," ratified a number of its powers and clarified others. The College would be able to recover fines by action of debt in a court of record (up to ten pounds per month's practice from any illicit practitioner of physic) and sue for forfeitures of such fines. It would also be empowered to "examine, and punish practitioners in physic, and apothecaries, druggists, distillers, and sellers of waters, and preparers of chemical medicines for sale, etc. . . . by fine, amercement, imprisonment, or other lawful ways or means as the nature of the offense shall require." The College could fine a practitioner who used "unfit physic or medicine" up to ten pounds and imprison him or her for as long as fourteen days after

[9]Christopher Merrett, *A Collection of Acts of Parliament, Charters, Trials at Law, and Judges Opinions Concerning Those Grants to the Colledge of Physicians London* (1660).

[10]The College also publicly emphasized its role as a learned body by having Merrett publish *Catalogus librorum, instrumentorum chirurgicorum, rerum curiosarum, exoticarumque Coll. Med. Lond. quae habentur in Musaeo Harveano* (1660).

[11]*Collegii Medicorum Londinensium Fundatores et Benefactores* (1662).

[12]The committee was composed of the *consiliarii* (Prujean and Hamey), the censors (Ent, Goddard, Merrett, and Baber), Micklethwaite, and Fraizer.

[13]S.P. 29/39/95.

the fine was paid. The president and the censors were empowered to call before themselves any practitioners or witnesses and put them to an oath, fining them if they refused. In disputes over the College's powers, the College would be judged, not by a common law court, but by a group of "visitors": the lord chancellor, the chief justices of either bench, and the chief baron of the Exchequer (two or more sitting to make a quorum). Any fines over and above the expenses of the College for the trial of an offender were to go to the poor of the offender's parish. Other practitioners could be asked to sign a recognizance in the name of the king to the effect that they would never practice again. The king would in return for all of this receive a "rent" of six pounds annually from the College. This abridged list indicates just how extensive were the range of powers granted the College in its new charter.[14]

Before the College's new charter would pass the Great Seal, however, it needed the approval of Parliament. In the preface to the charter, the king therefore directed his attorney general to obtain in Parliament a ratification "for the preventing all controversies, that may arise." The bill was entered before Parliament in March. On April 13 a committee of the College was established to see it through.[15] Had the new charter been passed, the "King's College" of Physicians would have firmly restored to it all the powers it had possessed under Charles I, and more.

The former rival of the College, the Society of Apothecaries, opposed certain clauses in the new charter, but it sought an agreement with the physicians. The committee of the College met with representatives of the apothecaries on April 29, and the apothecaries presented a document listing their objections. The apothecaries agreed that "empirics and unskillful and ignorant men" ought not to practice physic; but, the apothecaries claimed, they themselves only prescribed for the physicians, "unless in charity and where the physician refuseth or cannot be called in." If the physicians agreed to limit their charter so as not to interfere with the apothecaries' "just privileges of vending machines at their shops," and so as not to prohibit their practice of physic in emergencies, the apothecaries would help to get the charter ratified. But in return, the apothecaries wanted no physi-

---

[14]Sloane 3914, fols. 100–103. For a very different list of the important clauses in the charter, cf. Clark, pp. 304–6.

[15]Annals, 4:81b. This committee was composed of Prujean, Ent, Micklethwaite, Fraizer, Coxe, Stanley, Whistler, Wharton, Merrett, Greaves, Croyden, and Quartermaine.

cian to keep an apothecary's shop unless he had been apprenticed to a freeman of the society for seven years; they wanted their master and wardens to accompany the physicians on their searches of apothecaries' shops; and, most importantly, they wanted to be able to administer physic in lieu of a physician and to change the prescription in light of available drugs.[16]

Another meeting between the College and the apothecaries was held on May 5 in an attempt to reach a compromise. At this meeting, the apothecaries wanted to know precisely who was to be the object of the College's attentions. If it was "such only as make it their custom[ary] profession, and undertake cures, and do ordinarily take fees for council . . . we concur with you." But they reserved certain of their own practices:

> When an apothecary either at any unseasonable time, as possibly in the nighttime when physicians may not be willing to be disturbed, or at the urgent request of the patient, or in cause of necessity at other times when a physician cannot be had presently, and the danger not admitting delay, shall in order to the preserving of the interest of the physician and the life and health of the patient, order a clister or cordial, or some other remedy . . . till a physician may be had; or [when an apothecary offers] charity to any poor people who are not able to go to a physician; in such cases, so doing it shall not be construed any offense, nor [shall] the apothecary incur any punishment.

The right of the president and the censors of the College to enter and search apothecaries' shops and to examine the persons there on oath, the lack of the power by the apothecaries to substitute substances in physicians' prescriptions, the physicians' right to keep apothecaries in their houses to sell drugs, and other objections, were also listed.[17]

The self-confident and serious tone of the Society of Apothecaries was that of a group asking to be allowed to become legitimate practitioners in instances when the physicians were not available—asking the College to acknowledge their de facto practices. The registrar of the College reported that the meeting was amicable.[18] But no agreement could be obtained; for many physicians, the apothecaries asked too much in seeking to become junior partners. If a settlement had

[16]Annals, 4:82a; Sloane 3914, fols. 92–92b.
[17]Sloane 3914, fols. 92b–93b.
[18]Annals, 4:82a.

been reached with the Society of Apothecaries, the College would have had an ally to help get its new bill passed by the Parliament. Together, the two groups could have moved against the empirics. Medical licensing might have sooner become somewhat more like it was after the passage of the Apothecaries' Act of 1815.[19] But the officers of the College balked and, relying on high-minded ideas of their former privileges, went the regulatory route alone, therefore alienating an increasingly influential group. The officers must have felt that their friends at court were powerful enough to help them get their way without the assistance of the apothecaries.

Dealing with their friends at court for a new charter, however, cost the officers dissension within the College as well as potential allies. In June of 1663 a meeting ended on an acrimonious note when Timothy Clarke and several of his fellow candidates spoke out of turn in English. The new charter named forty fellows of the College. Clarke and others saw that the new charter advanced certain new candidates to the position of fellow over more senior ones; Clarke had been a candidate, waiting to become a fellow, since 1654. The new fellows were close to people in the government of Charles II. In the shouting that followed the interruption, President Alston and Sir Francis Prujean, a *consiliarius,* rebuked the candidates and closed the meeting. The candidates complained again at the next meeting, at the end of September. This time they were more polite, and they received an answer: the officers assured the candidates that the charter could not now be altered but that no precedents had been set for the future. Clearly the officers, at least, believed that it would be necessary to make some concessions to the king, letting his favorites be advanced, in order to retain court support for the charter. At a meeting at the end of December, for example, a letter from the king was read, after which the College immediately decided that the next opening would go to the king's second physician, William Quartermaine.[20]

By early 1664 it had become clear that the College's bill would be read in the next session of Parliament (which met from March to May). On March 26 the College decided to admit all royal physicians as *sociorum supernumerariorum,* "additional fellows." On April 4 representatives of the Society of Apothecaries and the Barber-Surgeons' Company came to the College to try to work out a last-minute compromise on the new charter, discussing clauses that they believed

---

[19]See S. W. F. Holloway, "The Apothecaries Act, of 1815: A Reinterpretation," *MH* 10 (1966): 107–29, 221–36.
[20]Annals, 4:82b–83a.

infringed on their freedoms as guaranteed in their own royal charters, but the College stood firm on its intended privileges. On April 19 the College's bill was read in the House of Commons for the first time. The opposition of the apothecaries and others, however, prevented a second reading, and the bill did not proceed any further.[21]

An important indication of why the College's bill did not pass the Parliament came from a source of opposition other than the apothecaries: one of those who favored the "new philosophy," a virtuoso. The evidence for opposition from this important new group came in the form of a book by someone identified only as "T. M."[22] T. M. notes that "our House did not pass the Patent," indicating that he was closely associated with, if not a member of, the House of Commons.[23] And he remarks that he had been among the virtuosi when they discussed the "unhappy estate of the profession of physic" at one Sir Thomas's house.[24] T. M. declares that he is not surprised that the House "for the present laid aside" the College's charter, since the charter was so long, since so many "men of several sorts . . . made opposition," and since the House had so much other business and so little time to consider it.[25] He suggests that, instead of trying to get its charter passed in Parliament de novo, the College should have brought "small additional bills, praying such new powers as might enable [it] to put in execution the true intents of the first act."[26]

Yet, T. M.'s true views on the state of physic certainly are not views that were shared by the officers of the College. T. M. introduces several lines of argument that became common to the debates over physic in the 1660s. He blames the "dark ages" for destroying the unity of physic; that is, he believes that the Greeks and Romans had employed physicians who not only had prescribed but also had practiced surgery and made up drugs with their own hands, and that

---

[21]Annals, 4.83a–84a, *Commons Journals*, vol. 8, p. 546.

[22]"T. M." has commonly been identified as Christopher Merrett, apparently on the strength of Merrett's involvement in some of the ensuing pamphlet wars. That this identification is unlikely is pointed out by R. S. Roberts, "Jonathan Goddard . . . A Lost Work or a Ghost?" *MH* 8 (1964): 191. His suggestion that T. M. was Timothy Clarke seems highly unlikely to me, especially since Clarke later authored a reply to T. M.

[23]T. M., *A Letter Concerning the Present State of Physick, and the Regulation of the Practice of it in this Kingdom. Written to a Doctor here in London* (1665), p. 5.

[24]Ibid., p. 4. The only "Sir Thomas" then a member of the Royal Society was Sir Thomas Nott, also a courtier.

[25]Ibid., p. 6.

[26]That is, powers to examine apothecaries' shops, to gain the aid of magistrates in pursuing others, and to arrest and imprison offenders of the College's powers (ibid., pp. 5–6).

afterward the corruptions of a barbaric period had introduced divisions resulting in the discrete crafts of physician, surgeon, and apothecary. He respects the surgeons and apothecaries as well as the physicians, but he sees that the three corporations will not be reunited. Yet without a union of head and hand in medicine, he believes, no improvements can be made.[27]

T. M. therefore proposes a solution: the introduction of "experiments of physic" on a large scale, "in which vast design Descartes hath resolved to spend the whole remainder of his life." Reforming physic experimentally would accomplish three goals: it would make physic useful to natural philosophy, "which is so universally the design of the present age"; it would make physic better at preserving life; and it would make medicine cheaper and less hazardous than before. Since the College of Physicians was the only body with men competent to engage in such an enterprise, according to T. M., it was to undertake this venture, and in the process gain the acclaim of everyone, restoring physic to its former prestige. The College could be divided into research committees (as the Royal Society had just been, in late 1664 and early 1665). For example, one committee could be established in anatomy, and that committee could be subdivided into subcommittees to study the brain, the heart, bodily fluids, bones, etc. Comparative work between animals and human subjects could be done cooperatively, using the latest techniques of geometry, the microscope, and chemistry. All this would make medicine a science, thus increasing the public's respect for the physicians and getting them more patients at less charge.[28]

Remaking the College in the image of the Royal Society was only half of T. M.'s design, however. The other half was to have the physicians stop prescribing compound medicines made up by apothecaries. Instead, T. M. tells the physicians, they ought to buy the simples from the apothecaries and then make up the medicines with their own hands. This would make medicine cheaper, but, more importantly, it would also make the physicians experimental philosophers in medicine. They would unite head and hand, things divorced since the "dark ages." T. M. takes up most of his book giving seventeen reasons why having physicians make up remedies themselves would be good. In the course of his reasoning, he clearly valued chemical medicaments.[29]

[27]Ibid., pp. 9–10.
[28]Ibid., pp. 13–20.
[29]Ibid., pp. 21–58.

In conclusion T. M. writes, "I have so great a zeal to see something of this nature effected for the public good, that if [the College's] own particular interest, joined with it, will not prevail, I could desire it may be thought advisable to provide for it by public authority."[30] The virtuosi, then, would not support a new charter from a merely academic College of Physicians and, moreover, if the College did not reform itself, they would intervene legislatively. The implied threat of the experimentalists to try to force the physicians into the manual parts of medicine undoubtedly worried many members of the College.

T. M.'s arguments about remaking the College in the image of the Royal Society and about encouraging the experimental philosophy in order to better unite theory and practice were publicly rebutted by Timothy Clarke. He wrote a letter of reply to T. M. in 1665 (published in 1670) in which he stressed how uneducated practitioners had killed thousands of people through unsupervised practice. He admitted the importance of chemistry: "I think no man worthy the name of physician, that is not knowing in it; for it hath not only much mended the preparation of medicines, but hath produced many generous remedies, and of great use." After all, the last of the College's "dogmatical Galenists" had been Dr. Thomas Winston (a Royalist who had died in 1655) and Dr. Laurence Wright (physician to Cromwell, died in 1657). But the answer to the College's troubles did not lie in making it into a formal experimental society, for such a society would be publicly ridiculed, too. Besides, individual members of the College already carried on experiments after the example of William Harvey. No, Clarke claimed, T. M.'s plan would not work. The crux of the matter was simply to forbid unqualified practitioners from engaging in physic—to restore the full juridical powers of the College to enable it to supervise medical practitioners.[31]

In one respect, however, the College of Physicians did emulate the Royal Society: it broadened the base of its society far beyond the fellowship by adding the category of honorary fellow. During 1664 and 1665, the Royal Society was having great success in recruiting courtiers and aristocrats as members, at least in name (few paid their

---

[30]Ibid., pp. 64–65.

[31]Dr. C. T. [Timothy Clarke?], *Some Papers Writ in the Year 1664. In Answer to a Letter, Concerning the Practice of Physick in England. Published at the Request of a Friend and Several Fellows of the College of Physicians* (1670), pp. 13–39. The British Library copy identifies C. T. as Timothy Clarke on the title page in a contemporary hand (B.L. 1171.1.45[3]). The second essay is a reply to T. M., written in 1665. The introduction and first essay were rewritten to address the problems of 1670, and are taken up later in this chapter.

dues).[32] A proposal to extend the rank of honorary fellow to all sorts of people beside the royal physicians was agreed to by the fellows on September 1, 1664. Some precedent existed for this. Henry Pierrepoint, lord marquis of Dorchester, who was interested in medical research, had been made an honorary fellow in July 1658, presumably so that he could enjoy the benefits of membership in the College even though he was not a professional physician. The two gentlemen friends, Thomas Baines and John Finch, who had traveled to take their M.D.s at Padua in the 1650s, were honored by the College in February 1660 with the titles *socius extraordinarius* in memory of their close associates William and Eliab Harvey. At the time, this was stated to be an unusual situation that was to set no precedents, but half a week later, John Baber wanted Quartermaine to be made an honorary fellow. That decision was put off, but the idea had caught on.[33] Then, in March of 1664, to help muster support for the College's proposed charter, the royal physicians had been admitted *sociorum supernumerariori*.

The potentially rival Royal Society was widely extending its membership, so the officers of the College proposed to affiliate many physicians and influential people by creating a large group of honorary fellows. They did this explicitly to restore their finances and to strengthen their influence.[34] Letters were written to the professors of physic at Cambridge and Oxford reassuring them that the College was not set on a course that would undermine the privileges of the universities. At the same time, six candidates, including Clarke, who had objected to the list of members of the king's charter, were made fellows, despite the fact that this created more fellows than were allowed by statute of the College.[35]

A great many honorary fellows—seventy-three—were formally admitted at a great banquet (paid for by them) in December of 1664. The honorary fellows presented the College with silver vessels worth £100. These new fellows, with few exceptions, each paid the large sum of £20 apiece for the honorary admission. They also took a long oath in which they swore to obey the president and the elects; to uphold the honor of the College and to donate money if it was

[32]Michael Hunter, *The Royal Society and Its Fellows, 1660–1700*, pp. 182–96.

[33]Annals, 4:71a–71b, 77a–77b; cf. Clark, pp. 312–13.

[34]"Resarciendis Collegij impensis, firmandaeque Ejusdem auctoritati, consultum videbatur, viras doctos gravesque, Doctoriatus Laurea ornatos, in Collegium nostrum, Sociorum Honorariorum titulo, adsciscere." Annals, 4:84a–84b.

[35]Annals, 4:84b–85b.

needed; never to enter into a discussion or a friendship with anyone who spoke against the College; to prosecute ignorant practitioners, empirics, and impostors; to administer no poisons or abortifacients; to divulge no secrets to outsiders; to teach no anatomy by dissections, except to College members, within the seven-mile radius of London; never to bargain with apothecaries for their remedies; never to accuse a fellow physician of ignorance; to consult with other physicians, provided only that the persons called never insulted the first physician or accused him of bad practice. In a final statement, the College members were praised as always striving for the support of virtue and learning. At one blow, many physicians who might possibly be in opposition to the College had been co-opted and the College treasury had grown by the huge amount of £1,070.[36] With such a fund, and with the support of so many physicians from all around the country, the College could spend money on legal proceedings (and grease palms) to help it regain its authority.

To some extent the new tactic seemed to be productive. In mid-April of 1665, the king himself visited the College, attending the third of that year's anatomy lectures, at that time being given by George Ent. Charles II knighted Ent on the spot.[37] This seemed to indicate that the College retained the king's favor, which was essential if it was to regain its powers to prosecute others. But other events in the winter of 1664–65 were less reassuring. The king may have come to the College to show his favor only as a counterweight to other schemes being bruited about at court to create a rival organization, the Society of Chemical Physicians.

Experimentalism and the Society of Chemical Physicians

The first sign that a rival society to the College was being considered was a book that appeared in late 1664, only six months after the College's charter had been defeated in the Parliament, and about the time that the College was inducting its honorary fellows. Marchamont Nedham's *Medela Medicinae. A Plea for the free Profession, and a Renovation of the Art of Physick* was published with a dedication dated November 26, 1664. Any knowing physician would have worried

---

[36]Annals, 4:85b–87b; "Letters and Papers of Glisson," Sloane 2251, fol. 111; cf. Clark, pp. 314–15.

[37]Annals, 4:87b.

when Nedham took up his pen against the College, for Nedham had always written with a political intent and had been backed by influential men. As a young man (he took a bachelor's degree from All Soul's, Oxford, in 1637), Nedham stepped into the center of political controversy in 1643 by bringing out *Mercurius Britanicus,* a weekly newspaper presenting the Parliament's case (in response to the earlier Royalist *Mercurius Aulicus*). He soon became an associate of Milton's. He quickly lined up on the side of the Independents when the Parliamentarians began to split into factions, and he began to attack the king, to promote some radical views, and to argue for religious toleration. Sometime in the mid-1640s he also took up the practice of medicine. In September 1647 he shifted sides and became an ardent Royalist—perhaps anticipating a Royalist/Independent alliance against the Presbyterians that never materialized—and brought out the paper *Mercurius Pragmaticus* and some pamphlets for the Cavaliers. After Charles was executed, however, Nedham became one of the most important polemicists for Cromwell and the Protectorate, writing *Mercurius Politicus* as well as various pamphlets. After the Restoration he played on his earlier support for Charles I to buy a pardon and return from Holland, where he had fled. Although he had miscalculated politically in the past, his record indicated an influential pen and a nose for the latest political possibilities.[38] His book of late 1664 suggested that powerful interests were organizing against the College.

Nedham dedicated his long (516-page) book to the marquis of Dorchester, the first honorary fellow of the College and a member of Charles's Privy Council. Nedham hoped that the marquis would accept the discourse. "If you meet with any acute reflections upon the Galenic way," he wrote, "I presume they are no other than necessary for the awakening of such as silently rest in an opinion of its sufficiency." "It is for the good of mankind [that] there should be a liberty allowed in the practice of physic," he argued (as he had earlier, for a liberty in religion). Medically, he believed that many diseases were new to the world in the seventeenth century, and that this was due to the spreading of "venereous and scorbific ferments," and "vermination"; therefore, the "old way of physic" was useless against these

---

[38]On the complicated career of Marchamont Nedham, see Joseph Frank, *Cromwell's Press Agent: A Critical Biography of Marchamont Nedham, 1620–1678* (Lanham, Md.: University Press of America, 1980); and Blair Worden, "Classical Republicanism and the Puritan Revolution," in *History and Imagination,* ed. H. Lloyd-Jones, V. Pearl, and B. Worden (London: Duckworth, 1981), pp. 182–200, esp. pp. 192–99.

new diseases.[39] The solution was a new kind of medical practice, a Helmontian chemical medicine that was to be pursued without the interference of the College of Physicians.[40]

Perhaps at the urging of his seniors, Robert Sprackling, a candidate of the College, rushed to the defense of the established order with *Medela Ignorantiae: Or a Just and Plain Vindication of Hippocrates and Galen from the Groundless Imputations of M. N.*, licensed on February 24, 1665.[41] He portrayed Nedham's attack as part of a medical conspiracy against the government. His tactic was to refute Nedham's specific claims while tarring him with his past: Nedham was accused of "atheism and cruelty" and "treason and conspiracy." Sprackling suggested that Nedham objected to regular physicians because they upheld the social fabric: *they* at least had not learned "to violate the laws of the kingdom, to which their allegiance is due." Sprackling concluded with a plea for a new charter for the College. "I am not worthy," he wrote,

> to tender those many pressing and irrefrangible reasons to the public, which must at last induce (not to say more) the endeavors of Authority, to suppress and exclude by some new and effectual laws (if strict execution of the present ones be not found sufficient) that swarm of desperadoes and cannibals, which feed and live on the bodies or carcasses of their miserably deluded neighbors.[42]

This kind of rhetoric indicates that physicians like Sprackling had deep fears that the College might not retain the support of the Crown

[39]Agues, worms, new fevers, more severe women's diseases, French pox, scurvy, rickets, consumption, smallpox, and measles were among the "new diseases" he listed. Also see Lloyd G. Stevenson, "'New Diseases' in the Seventeenth Century," *BHM* 39 (1965): 1–21.

[40]Marchamont Nedham, *Medela Medicinae. A Plea for the free Profession, and a Renovation of the Art of Physick* (1665). For lengthier descriptions of Nedham's treatise, see Richard F. Jones, *Ancients and Moderns: A Study of the Rise of the Scientific Movement in Seventeenth-Century England*, pp. 206–10; and Lester S. King, *The Road to Medical Enlightenment, 1650–1695*, pp. 145–54.

[41]Sprackling's book is dedicated to Francis Glisson, "the Hippocrates of our own nation." Sprackling, whose M.D. from Anjou had been incorporated at Cambridge in 1662, went on to note that Cambridge (where Glisson was and had been Regius Professor of Physic) "can never forget, that when her theology and law lay bleeding and expiring by the swords of rebels and usurpers, physic alone preserved her perishing fame alive." One suspects that Sprackling meant to rise in the world through the favors of some of his seniors. Also see Jones, *Ancients and Moderns*, pp. 210–11.

[42]Robert Sprackling, *Medela Ignorantiae: Or a Just and Plain Vindication of Hippocrates and Galen from the Groundless Imputations of M. N.* (1665), p. 163.

at the moment when a Society of Chemical Physicians was seeking incorporation.

For, immediately after Sprackling's prickly attack on Nedham, Thomas O'Dowde published a tract in which a "copy of engagement" was printed, indicating that a powerful group of chemical physicians and courtiers were trying to incorporate a new medical institution. O'Dowde's *The Poor Man's Physician,* signed March 10, 1665, went through at least three printings in that year. As given by O'Dowde, the "engagement" read, in part:

> Whereas after sufficient experiment, it is found most true, that chemical medicines well prepared, and as well applied, are above all others, the safest, pleasantest, and most effectual means, both for conservation of health, and cure of all diseases whatsoever. And whereas some of a different practice from it [i.e., the academic physicians], as well as those many false pretenders to arcanas of this nature, do either maliciously or ignorantly hinder the clear and general understanding of the virtue and excellency of such noble preparations, and by consequence the public good. To the end, therefore, that patients may not spend themselves, their precious time, and money in vain; and also that the licentious abuses and impostors may hereafter be detected, we whose names are hereunto subscribed, do resolve and promote to our uttermost abilities, to preserve and advance the honor and credit of this profession of chemical physic. And in order thereunto, humbly to propose, and as much as in us lyeth, endeavor an obtaining of His Majesty's gracious favor by letters patents.[43]

This ringing declaration made clear the intentions of those hoping to form the proposed society to replace the academic physicians by gaining a charter for themselves.

The "engagement" was signed by thirty-four chemical practitioners. Heading the list was William Goddard, the physician who recently had been expelled from the College; two candidates of the College (John Fryer and Joseph Dey) were included, as was an honorary fellow (Edward Warner); the names of several well-known chemists, among them George Starkey and the king's chemist, Nicaise Le Febvre, appeared; and at the end was, naturally, the name of Thomas O'Dowde, not only a chemist but also a groom of the king's Privy

---

[43]Thomas O'Dowde, *The Poor Man's Physician, Or the True Art of Medicine* (1665), pp. 90–92. Also quoted in Henry Thomas, "The Society of Chymical Physitians: An Echo of the Great Plague of London, 1665," in *Science, Medicine, and History,* ed. E. Ashworth Underwood, vol. 2, pp. 62–63.

Chamber. O'Dowde apparently was an essential link between the chemists and the king.[44]

A document of support for the chemists of the proposed society was signed by thirty-eight lords and gentlemen, headed by Gilbert Sheldon, archbishop of Canterbury, and followed by George Monck (duke of Albemarle), the duke of Ormonde, the earl of Anglesey, and other peers.[45] The spectrum of support was impressive, running from the High Church archbishop, to Clarendon's friend Ormonde, to Charles II's boon companion Buckingham.[46] The document was, in effect, a list of powerful "honorary fellows" of the Society of Chemical Physicians. Yet at least two of the most powerful men at court did not sign it: The earl of Arlington and lord chancellor Clarendon (although Clarendon was later addressed in a dedication by a member of the society). Neither was a dabbler in the chemical arts, and neither was enamoured of the duke of Buckingham (who as a favorer of chemistry may well have been the main organizer of aristocratic support for the society).[47] The court was not unanimous in favoring the chemists, then, but the physicians must have worried about the clout the chemists were displaying.

The training, education, and political and religious backgrounds of the signers of the "engagement" of the Society of Chemical Physicians varied enormously. Yet on one thing virtually all the chemical physicians agreed: academic physic alone could not earn the respect of true lovers of medicine, for two reasons. First, most chemists claimed that their science had been derived from the Hermetic philosophy and was therefore more ancient and closer to God's initial revelations to

[44]George Thomson, *'Misokumias helegkos'; or, A Check Given to the insolent Garrulity of Henry Stubbe* (1671), p. 9, says that O'Dowde was the chemists' link to the king. According to his daughter, O'Dowde was dispossessed of his estates in Ireland, followed Charles I in the wars, and went into exile with Charles II, taking up chemical medicine to support himself. See his life in Mary Trye, *Medicatrix, or the Woman-Physician: Vindicating Thomas O'Dowde . . . against . . . Henry Stubbe* (1675), pp. 24–43.

[45]The list is printed in Thomas, "Society of Chymical Physitians," pp. 63–64.

[46]See the identification of the signatories given in P. M. Rattansi, "The Helmontian-Galenist Controversy in Restoration England," *Ambix* 12 (1964): 13–15. Also see idem, "Paracelsus and the Puritan Revolution," *Ambix* 11 (1963): 24–32; and Charles Webster, "English Medical Reformers of the Puritan Revolution: A Background to the 'Society of Chymical Physicians,'" *Ambix* 14 (1967): 16–41. Webster concludes that the "Society of Chemical Physicians was a defensive gesture taken after the revival of the College licensing power," while the scheme of William Rand for a College of Graduate Physicians in 1656 "was an expression of confidence by physicians who had witnessed the decline of the College of Physicians' authority" (pp. 40–41); my argument is that the cases were reversed.

[47]Rattansi, "Helmontian-Galenist Controversy," p. 15, suggests the connection between Buckingham and the Society of Chemical Physicians.

Adam than was pagan Greek medicine. T. M., too, had believed that physic had been pushed off the true path by the "dark ages" in which Galenism had ruled. But Paracelsus and, more important, Van Helmont had recovered the ancient art of chemistry as part of their reformation of knowledge, and not only had they recovered that "more ancient" way, but they had imbued it with a Christian vision of nature. The physicians who followed Galen therefore followed a corrupt, pagan way of healing; in fact, phlebotomy, a mainstay of Galenic therapy, was "Satan's device and plot to destroy mankind."[48]

Second, the chemists experimented with medicines: empiricism had been proclaimed a virtue by T. M. and was to be by other virtuosi. Using this reasoning, George Thomson of the Society of Chemical Physicians challenged Nathaniel Hodges of the College of Physicians to a trial of their rival methods of treatment: the outcome would prove which method was best.[49] Results were the fundamental criteria for judging efficacy. Again like T. M., Thomson believed that true healers should be physician, apothecary, and surgeon, as he proudly proclaimed himself to be. The final advice Thomson gave his readers was: "Be ascertained, before you meddle with a physician, that he have an intuitive knowledge of animals, vegetables, and minerals; that he is well versed in the separation of their pure crasis with his own hands."[50] A chemical philosopher such as Thomson could claim to offer the patient both the true "intuition" and the handiwork to be a curer of a better sort than any College physician.

The reasoning of Thomson and other chemical physicians betrays an anxiety on their part that was common to many beyond their ranks, a belief that the medicine of the academic physicians did not properly link experience to the world of hidden truths. These truths could be obtained only by the properly prepared believer; they were revealed, but only to one who both cared for the spirit and worked with things.[51] The search for new links between theory and experience was not new to the chemists: Sir Francis Bacon, for one, had declared that truth came through inductive experiences, through a process that involved "the true and legitimate humiliations of the

---

[48]George Thomson, *Galeno-Pale: Or, A Chymical Trial of the Galenists* (1665), pp. 93–94.
[49]George Thomson, *'Loimotomia': Or, The Pest Anatomized* (1666), p. 173.
[50]Ibid., preface.
[51]For an important argument on the connections between intuitions or inspirations and empiricism, see Walter Pagel, "Religious Motives in the Medical Biology of the Seventeenth Century," *BHM* 3 (1935): 97–128, 213–31, 265–312.

human spirit" in the face of nature, and that truth obtained this way yielded beneficial results, which should be sought out in "charity."[52]

It has been pointed out elsewhere that, intellectually, the virtuosi of the Royal Society and the Helmontians of the proposed Society of Chemical Physicians were opposed to Galenic rationalism, based as it was on anatomy, metaphors from nature as an artifice, analogical method, and reductionism. To be sure, the virtuosi and the Helmontians ultimately differed in their view of the sources of knowledge, and both Galenists and virtuosi in practice saw the world as God's artifice. Both the Galenists and the virtuosi therefore used analogies from artificial things to speak about nature, whereas the Helmontians' naturalism proposed that all a priori analogies were useless, since life was not artificial—that only the "facts" could be known, not the structure behind the facts.[53] In other words, the virtuosi were not quite the wholehearted empiricists that the Helmontians were, but on the whole the views of these two groups were closer together than the virtuosi's were to the Galenists'.

To a traditionally trained academic physician, however, the claims of the chemists and others to a closer union between the world of things and the world of mind seemed groundless. The university-trained physicians relied on discursive reasoning; they believed that the mind could rationally penetrate to the true causes of things, not through sense experiences and intuitions, but only with the aid of the powerful tools of logic and the criticism of texts. Those who relied on their experiences to guide their "intuitions" were nothing more than mere empirics, deluding the public with unfounded claims to expertise.

By the mid-seventeenth century, academic physicians tended to lump chemists and empirics together, since many chemists claimed to be finding new therapies empirically and were justifying the new therapies after the fact by their "intuitions" and various other mystical principles. In 1666, for example, Nathaniel Hodges defended

---

[52]Sir Francis Bacon, *The Great Instauration* (1620), preface. It may be that the affinities between Bacon's methods and the methods of the medical chemists were no accidents: Graham Rees has recently made a strong argument that Bacon's science derived from Paracelsian principles. See his "Francis Bacon's Semi-Paracelsian Cosmology," *Ambix* 22 (1975): 81–101; idem, "Francis Bacon's Semi-Paracelsian Cosmology and the *Great Instauration*," *Ambix* 22 (1975): 161–73; idem, "The Fate of Bacon's Cosmology in the Seventeenth Century," *Ambix* 24 (1977): 27–38.

[53]Peter H. Niebyl, "Science and Metaphor in the Medicine of Restoration England," *BHM* 47 (1973): 356–74, esp. 368–69. Also see Peter Dear, "*Totius in verba*: Rhetoric and Authority in the Early Royal Society," *Isis* 76 (1985): 145–61, and Jones, *Ancients and Moderns,* who with some reason lumps together the chemists and the virtuosi.

academic physic from chemical empirics like Thomson. "True experience is constituted of reason and sense," he argued; medical science had been founded on these principles long ago. Rational medical science, once founded, was "henceforth unquestionable by sense," since it dealt in "immutable truths" that had "the royal assent affixed to them" as "standing laws not subject to future censures." The empirical medicine advocated by the chemists was simply a wasted, misguided effort: "So then there is no cause why we should return to the first and more rude and imperfect way [of empirical trials], since the science of medicine is not only already invented and discovered, but adorned with intelligible rules and aphorisms, and thereby improved to general use."[54] Chemists, advocating therapies based on empirical experience in making medicine with their own hands, and guided only by "intuitions," were seen as empirics in another form—as being dangerous to patients and to the established academic practice of medicine.

For the moment, however, the chemists had taken the offensive, and they clearly tried to link their endeavors to the more generalized cultural support for the new science. Edward Bolnest, a chemical physician and a signer of the "engagement," quickly brought out a book to support O'Dowde's. This book, titled *Medicina Instaurata: or, A Brief Account of the True Grounds and Principles of the Art of Physick* (licensed on April 20, 1665), provides further evidence for the interests and powers of the proposed society. Bolnest dedicated his book to Buckingham. "One," he wrote, "who by your own most noble and acute genius, conceptions, observations, and constant manual operations, have not only discovered the vanity of the Galenic way, but rendered your self most perfect, as well in the practice, as theory of experimental philosophy."[55]

As Bolnest's dedication suggests, socially as well as intellectually the equation of chemical medicine with the "experimental philosophy" was not without foundation.[56] For instance, the president of the Royal Society was William, Viscount Brouncker, a man with chemical as well as mathematical interests; the man who most likely procured the Royal Society's charter, Sir Robert Moray, had been quite

---

[54]Nathaniel Hodges, *Vindiciae Medicinae et Medicorum: Or, An Apology for the Profession and Professors of Physick* (1666), p. 4.

[55]Edward Bolnest, *Medicina Instaurata: or, A Brief Account of the True Grounds and Principles of the Art of Physick* (1665), dedication.

[56]Charles Webster has argued for the connection between chemistry and the "new philosophy" in several works; see his *From Paracelsus to Newton: Magic and the Making of Modern Science*.

involved with chemistry, especially during his exile in Maestricht, and after the Restoration often worked with the king in the chemical laboratory at Whitehall. The king himself became a member of the Royal Society on January 9, 1665, as the Society of Chemical Physicians was organizing; on the same day, James, duke of York, and George Monck, the duke of Albemarle, signed the register of the Royal Society. Over the next few months, Viscount Stafford, the earl of Manchester, and the earl of Carlisle, to mention only titled aristocracy, signed on as members of the society.[57] At the moment, many members of the court were associating themselves with the Royal Society. The connection between experimental philosophy and chemistry was underlined in the pamphlets published by members of the organizing Society of Chemical Physicians.

As Marchamont Nedham said in his discourse introducing Bolnest's book, "'Tis pretty to observe" how some of the physicians of the College "at last, perceiving most of the great lords, and other noble gentlemen of learning do prefer our way before the Galenic, are not ashamed to cry out, that themselves also are chemists, and so no need of erecting a new Society upon the account of chemistry." He continued: "There is no way to redeem our profession at the hands of old women, and others, but by setting the whole frame of physic upon a new sort of operative and experimental philosophy, because the common [Galenic] methods and remedies are every where to be had in print." Chemistry being a more secret art, it would allow practitioners to carry on without their efforts being debased by common practitioners, and so would not need regulatory laws like those for which the College asked. Chemical physicians, Nedham said, welcomed new men of breeding and education, and he urged the lords and gentlemen of England to follow the example of the king by setting up private laboratories to find new medicines for the current age. They should also rid themselves of Galenic physicians, employing only chemical ones. The attempt of the College physicians to smear the chemists with charges of ignorance only because few of them had university degrees Nedham dismissed with a contempt for mere academic titles. He declared that members of the society had been well received by the king at his "council table."

Finally, Nedham returned to the physicians:

But they say, that what ever is wanting there in virtue of medicine, they can supply in the use of them by strength of wit, which is what

[57]Hunter, *Royal Society*, pp. 192–96.

they call method. Oh, here is the Diana, the great goddess Method, or the round of the mill-horse, which every one can run that hath bought Sennertius, or Riverius in English; and that is the reason why other folk spoil their trade much more than the chemists do, and for thirty or forty shillings worth of books, soon learn to become as complete methodists as themselves.[58]

Other proponents of the Society of Chemical Physicians entered the fray, also attacking the College.[59] Their books and pamphlets exhibit a contempt for mere academic learning, an enthusiasm for discovering new things and for the current fashions of court, and a belief in a union between chemistry and the new philosophy as well as in the usefulness of experimental philosophy in uncovering God's ways in nature. These ideas gave the proposed Society of Chemical Physicians great credibility and deeply threatened the College.

No senior physician of the College risked his reputation by publicly replying to the chemists, yet such challenges could not be ignored. A defense of the College was therefore directed from William Johnson, the chemist "to the King's College of Physicians in London," and the man who had defended the College from Biggs and Culpeper in the previous decade.[60] Dedicated to Lord Dorchester (who had not signed the "engagement," and who was the first honorary fellow of the college), in whom "Galen and Helmont are reconciled, and made friends," Johnson's book attacked "pseudochemists" while trying to show that the college favored both Van Helmont and Paracelsus, as well as Galen and other medical authors. "The judicious and learned do not build the praises of Galen on the disgrace of Van Helmont, but honor both according to their respective worth, and are ready to confess that the German on Galen's shoulders might possibly see more than he." Again, he tarred these chemists with the brush of sedition: "These fellows do by chemistry, just as our fanatics do in religion: both being equally ignorant, and both enemies of the truth." Johnson had least patience for O'Dowde: "It seems master O'Dowde can cure the dropsie without the removal of the symptoms."[61] In his conclusion, however, Johnson supported the proposals in T. M.'s *A Letter Concerning the Present State of Physick* ad-

---

[58]Marchamont Nedham, "Epistolary Discourse," prefix to Bolnest's *Medicina Instaurata*.
[59]See especially Thomson, *Galeno-Pale*.
[60]William Johnson, *'Agurto-Mastix,' or, Some Brief Animadversions Upon two late Treatises; . . . Galeno-Pale; . . . the Poor Man's Physitian* (1665). It was licensed May 10, 1665.
[61]Ibid., pp. 7, 3, 18.

vocating a Royal Society–like College, and supported the idea that a union of the physicians, apothecaries, and surgeons would be in everyone's interest.[62] The more old-fashioned members of the College who were not favorers of the new philosophy may very well have worried at replies to the chemists that conceded enormous virtues to experimentalism.

At this point, May of 1665, the disputes between the College and the chemists were somewhat overshadowed by the outbreak of plague. But to anticipate events: only the fiercest onslaught of the pestilence interrupted what was now a full-blown pamphlet war between the chemists and the members of the College of Physicians.

Johnson had reminded his readers that the physicians had always stayed in London to fight the plague, pointing to numerous memorial plaques in the London churches and vestries as proof.[63] George Thomson immediately responded to Johnson with *A Gag for Johnson,* and his fellow George Starkey attached *An Epistolar Discourse to . . . the Author of Galeno-pale* to Thomson's book (Starkey's discourse is dated June 21, 1665). Starkey accused the College of Physicians of abandoning the sick in the plague. "For my part, I should give my vote that none such might be admitted publicly to practice for the future, that should now desert their station."[64] Thomson wrote more directly that he resented having the College set its "dog" (its chemist Johnson) on him. But he also distanced himself from O'Dowde, writing that to speak of his friendship with him was "as arrant a truth as that you are real friends to chemistry." "If this fellow [O'Dowde] . . . deserve not to be whipped about the pig-market, and every chemist in England to have a lash at him, let any judge that is truly sensible of the loss of a good name."[65]

The physicians' tactic of exposing the "ignorance" and past histories of some of the chemists may have helped to stop the proposed charter for the Society of Chemical Physicians. But furthermore, at the same time that the society presented its case to the Crown (probably in mid-April of 1665), the possibility of another epidemic of bubonic plague loomed, and it had always been the College to which the Crown had turned for advice in such emergencies. On May 17,

---

[62]Also see Thomas's account of Johnson's book in "Society of Chymical Physitians," pp. 67–68.

[63]Johnson, '*Agurto-Mastix,*' pp. 11–12.

[64]George Thomson, '*Plano Pnigmos,*' or *A Gag for Johnson, that Published Animadversions upon Galeno-Pale. And a Scourge for that Pitiful Fellow Mr. Galen* (1665), p. 54.

[65]Ibid., pp. 29, 31.

therefore, members of the College met at the request of the Privy Council to consider what was to be done about the plague in order to advise the council and the lord mayor of London. A little book of remedies was reprinted, and delegates from the College presented one copy to the Privy Council and another to the lord mayor.[66] The College also recommended that a physician, a surgeon, and an apothecary be appointed in an official capacity by the City to help fight the epidemic.[67]

The plague grew worse daily. By June 12 the president proposed that a list of six members of the College be compiled from which the City could name men to treat plague victims. Eight were actually chosen by the College, of whom four were picked by the City to treat the ill: Nathaniel Hodges (a candidate) and Thomas Witherly, Nicholas Davis, and Edward Deantry (honorary fellows). These four stayed and treated people for the pestilence; at least two of them survived.[68] Several other physicians of the College also stayed voluntarily to help minister to the sick in this emergency—as late as June 26 a special session of the College was held that was attended by twenty members—but soon most physicians of the College (like other people who could afford it) fled to the countryside.

Not to be outdone, the members of the Society of Chemical Physicians also undertook to help plague victims. A broadsheet, licensed on June 28 and presumably tacked up all about the city, advertised the services of eight of the members, including Thomson and O'Dowde. It began by touting "medicines by them prepared, in pursuance of His Majesty's command." The text went on to speak of how the physicians "principally addicted to Galenic doctrines and medicines" had "openly acknowledged . . . in several prints" that "remedies made by chemical preparation are of greater excellence than any other." (Presumably this was an exaggeration of the remarks in Johnson's tract.) The Society of Chemical Physicians therefore wished to "congratulate our brethren, touching the unhappy controversy between us and them, touching the efficacy of medicines, is now at an

---

[66]*Certain Necessary Directions as well for the Cure of the Plague, as for preventing the Infection* (1636; another ed., 1665). Fraizer, Colladon, Greaves, and Clarke presented the copy to the Privy Council; Goddard, Whistler, and Wharton, to the City.

[67]Annals, 4:88a.

[68]Annals, 4:88a–88b. Witherly became a physician to Charles II in 1677 and soon thereafter became a fellow of the College; Hodges became a fellow in 1672 and was Harveian Orator in 1683, but he died in debtor's prison in 1688 at age 59. Davis and Deantry are unknown except for being honorary fellows and for authoring the pamphlet discussed in what follows.

end." With this sleight of hand, and the implied support of the College, the society went on to advertise that the chemical medicines they offered were the best for fighting the plague. The names of the eight members—all listed as "doctor"—and their addresses in London followed, so that "all persons concerned may repair" to those places "and be furnished with the antidotes so by us prepared, at reasonable rates, with directions how to use them in order to preservation, and in case of cure."[69]

Members of the society were advertising their remedies like any other medical empirics. But the advertised project of the society to set up a "public house or college, with public officers" underlined its intention to use the epidemic as the College had in the past—to establish its importance to the public, and hence its legitimacy.

That summer the epidemic grew fierce, and all persons of any medical skill remaining in London had plenty to do. In a pamphlet dated August 2, 1665, titled *The Resolution of those Physitians presented by the Colledge To the Right Honourable The Lord Mayor and Court of Aldermen . . . for the Prevention and Cure of the Plague,* two of the College physicians working for the City described the situation. Nicholas Davis and Edward Deantry[70] complained of overwork. Eight physicians had been nominated to the lord mayor by the College, they said, and the City had been divided into eight districts with a physician in charge of each. However, the lord mayor and aldermen had decided that four was enough to handle the situation, "whether to ease the common purse of the charge, which is incident to that service, or upon other reasons," they would not speculate. Still, Davis and Deantry were struggling to fulfill their obligations in an increasingly bad situation. They wanted to have six hours' notice from those who needed attention, presumably in order to organize their busy rounds better. "And we further desire all apothecaries, who have so near a connection to our profession, to take notice of this our resolution, and to repair to us, or any other of our profession in the town, (being not so void of physicians as generally reported) for our counsel and advice, as in former cases they were wont." The physicians were on duty from 8 A.M. until 10 P.M.

Many others, too, tried to make their reputations during the epidemic. Theophilus Garencières warned against "those that set up bills for the curing of this and other diseases," for "the wonders they

[69]The facsimile and text of the broadsheet are in Thomas, "Society of Chymical Physitians," pp. 55–57.
[70]He spelled it "D'Austry."

promise, lay an ambush to your purses"; yet he advertised his own "antidote" and cordial after attacking the remedies of chemists and academic physicians alike. Richard Kephale believed the plague to be God's wrath but advertised his "conserve" and "spirit" as "two most sovereign antidotes against the plague" nevertheless. John Gadbury took chemists and empirics to task and then put forward an astrological explanation that proposed no remedies, although it safely predicted a sharp decline in the disease in November and December. "J. V." castigated "projectors" for advertising their remedies as sure cures, spoke of the College's remedies as being "common knowledge," and protested the shutting up of the sick in their houses and the continuing of unreformed church services—the latter being the cause of the pestilence, because the cure was in godliness. Gideon Harvey blamed the disease on a "pestilential venom" in the air and recommended ways for prevention and cure that were very similar to the recommendations of the College physicians.[71]

The risks taken by practitioners in London soon became clear enough. Of the members of the Society of Chemical Physicians, at least O'Dowde, Starkey, Joseph Dey, and Robert Turner died in the epidemic. Thomson became infected but survived. William Johnson, the College's chemist, perished. Davis and Deantry are not heard of again and probably died. Untold other physicians, chemists, apothecaries, surgeons, ordinary practitioners, and traditional healers died also. The bills of mortality listed 1,050 victims of the plague in a single week ending November 7. But the numbers decreased rapidly thereafter, until by March 5, 1666, only 28 were reported deceased from plague.[72] By the spring of 1666, people were again trickling back into London.

The pamphlet war over medicine did not end with the plague, however, despite decimation in the ranks of the antagonists, although by 1666 the chemists were clearly on the defensive. John Heydon, an astrologer and Rosicrucian formerly imprisoned for plotting against Cromwell, castigated Thomson, accusing him of plagiarizing his work.[73] John Twysden, a fellow of the College, published a book

[71]Theophilus Garencières, *A Mite Cast into the Treasury of the Famous City of London* (1665); Richard Kephale, *Medela Pestilentiae* (1665); John Gadbury, *London's Deliverance Predicted* (1665); J. V., *Golgotha; or, A Looking-Glass for London* (1665); Gideon Harvey, *A Discourse of the Plague* (1665).

[72]*Oxford Gazette*, no. 1, Nov. 7, 1665; *London Gazette*, no. 33, Mar. 5, 1666.

[73]"[P]ilfering what he glories in from my several works extant, and re-baptizing my Medicines into other names, and thence adopting them his own Bratts." John Heydon, *A Quintuple Rosie-Crucian Scourge for the due Correction of that Pseudo-chymist and Scurrious Emperick, Geo. Thomson. Being in Part a Vindication of the Learned Society of Physitians* (1665).

that had obviously been delayed getting into print—it took up the debate from early 1665 in the form of a reply to Nedham's *Medela Medicinae,* and it made a reference to Bolnest's pamphlet as well. Twysden, not surprisingly, wrote that an attack on the "King's College of Physicians" amounted to an attack on the king himself; he further condemned the Society of Chemical Physicians by declaring that their attempts to gain the king's support were "by that dangerous way of innovating through subscription of hands." In other words, he wished to portray the society as a revolutionary group acting through petitions.[74]

A similar chord was struck by Nathaniel Hodges, who had served the College and the City in the plague. His dedication, to Gilbert Sheldon, archbishop of Canterbury, spoke of the "late rebellion" in which "reverend clergy" suffered at the hands of their enemies, just as the physicians had suffered "by the prevailing invasion of empirics." The physicians congratulated the clergy on restoring their profession, "and most heartily wish the Church may never fall again into the hands of empirical divines who as rudely treated peoples' souls, as the present quacks in physic do their bodies." Hodges went on to appeal to Sheldon to patronize learning, so "that the profession of physic and legitimate physicians will after a long confusion be separated and distinguished from the dregs of illiterate practitioners." Concluding the dedication, Hodges appealed to the archbishop for help in restoring the College's regulatory powers: "As there are diseases in the state, so wholesome edicts may in time happily be provided to deal with their most obstinate complications."[75]

The book attacked a number of problems. It tore at empirics, the Society of Apothecaries, the licensing of empirics by bishops, and the Society of Chemical Physicians. It ended with a thirty-page account of the recent plague and how Hodges and other College physicians had stayed to fight it; as a reward, Hodges argued, the magistrates ought to protect the College against its enemies.

In what turned out to be the last piece in this stage of the debate, the chemist George Thomson replied to Hodges at the end of another book. His defense, like that of other chemists, was that experience, not theory, improved medical practice. Avoiding the term *empiric,* he nevertheless proudly wrote of things "I visibly and experimentally have found to be true, what I have handled with these hands, and seen

[74]John Twysden, *Medicina Veterum Vindicata: Or an Answer to a Book, entituled Medela Medicinae* (1666); On Twysden, also see King, *Road to Medical Enlightenment,* pp. 154–60; and Jones, *Ancients and Moderns,* pp. 212–13.
[75]Hodges, *Vindiciae Medicinae.*

with these eyes." He deeply resented being called a "fanatic, one of an anarchical principle, who have always (as my friends can testify) been loyal to my sovereign." At the same time, he spoke of the College physicians as *dogmatists*—like *empiric,* a term derived from ancient Greek quarrels over medical knowledge. Moreover, he challenged Hodges to put their two methods of practice to a trial by treating two different groups in one of the hospitals by the two methods. Thomson thought that this would prove Hodges and the College to be the worse healers. On the basis of whose cures were best, he emphasized, the world would see that the learned physicians were the truly illegitimate practitioners.[76]

In late 1666 the College might well have mounted a strong counterattack in the councils of the Crown and restored their juridical powers had not several things occurred. First, Christopher Merrett, the College's caretaker of the Harveian Museum and Library, had left his lodgings at the College during the plague. While the building was vacant, someone had broken in and forced the iron chest that held the College's valuables. All the silver plate and coin, valued at about £1,000, most of it recently collected from the honorary fellows, had been stolen. At one stroke, the hoard that the College could have used to help accomplish its goal of getting a secure statutory right to prosecute all others had disappeared. From the College's point of view, this represented an unmitigated disaster. A new strategy would have to be developed for enriching the institution before it could proceed to attack interlopers.

A second disaster struck a few months later. The College held its first meeting after the plague at the end of June 1666. A couple of weeks later, Sir Francis Prujean, who had seen the College through difficult times, died, and Sir Alexander Fraizer, the king's first physician, took his place as elect. Before any regrouping of the College could occur, however, the fire of London raged through the city. It burned down the College building, including the museum, the laboratory, and the library. Only a few of the College's records and books were hurried out in time to be saved. The institution was further impoverished and was without a place to meet or to carry on the work of academic medicine.[77]

Finally, one of the College's most influential patrons at court, Lord Chancellor Clarendon, fell from grace. The program that Clarendon

---

[76]Thomson, '*Loimotomia.*'
[77]Annals, 4:89b–90a.

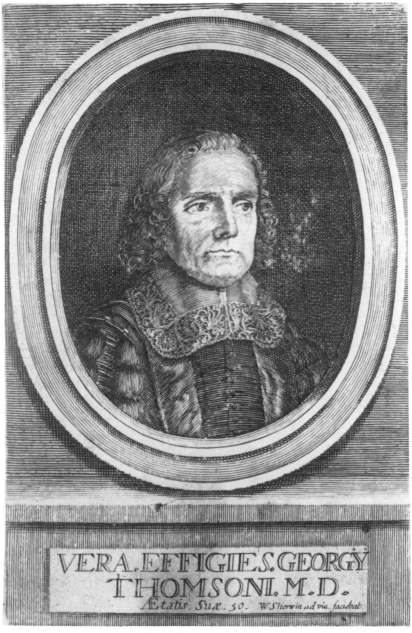

VERA. EFFIGIES. GEORGY
THOMSONI. M. D.
Ætatis. Suæ. 50. W. Sherwin ad viu. faciebat

Plate 6. Portrait of George Thomson. Engraving, by W. Sherwin, 1670. Courtesy of the Wellcome Institute Library, London.

had undertaken for restoring a limited monarchy collapsed under the dual strains of Cavaliers, who wanted the court to bring them the benefits they believed Royalists deserved, and M.P.s, who disliked any central government. The mismanagement of the Second Dutch War and the machinations of the duke of Buckingham finally brought Clarendon down in the summer of 1667. With Buckingham's influence on the rise, the College was threatened by the rivals he supported.

Deepening Divisions and the Widening Threat of the New Philosophy

As it had before in periods of political change, the College of Physicians elected a new group of officers immediately following Clarendon's downfall, trying to regain whatever influence it could. At the College's September 1667 meeting, a new slate of officers was elected. Sir Edward Alston, who had guided the College as president since it had tried to reassert itself in 1655, was demoted to *consiliarius;* Baldwin Hamey, Jr., was voted out of his position of *consiliarius* and replaced by Sir George Ent; and Francis Glisson became president. Hamey also lost his position as treasurer to John Micklethwaite. The College was increasingly divided on what policies to pursue for the good of physic; the new officers began to move the College toward what it had been in the late 1640s, a learned society not unsympathetic to the new science.

That the College was deeply divided in the later 1660s is indicated by the way in which the decision of where to rebuild the College after the fire was made. A committee had been established at the September 1667 meeting to negotiate a new lease so the foundations for a new building could be laid.[78] But former President Alston went ahead on his own, or with the support of his faction within the College, and in the spring of 1668 he purchased a location in Canon Street on behalf of the College. A private meeting of the other, and official, College faction was called on September 11, 1668; gathering at Glisson's, this faction cancelled the plan to build on Canon Street.

At the College's next meeting (September 30), a dispute loudly broke out between the two groups. As ceremony required, the outgoing president, Glisson, placed the insignia of office in the hands of

[78]Annals, 4:90b. The committee members were Staines, Micklethwaite, Whistler, and Merrett.

his predecessor while a vote was taken on the new president. Alston seized his opportunity. Temporarily president by possession of the insignia, he moved for an adjournment before the vote could be taken in an attempt to remain president by a kind of technical coup. The elects refused to leave, however, and, except for Alston, unanimously voted to restore Glisson to office. After acrimonious shouting on Alston's part, and some soothing words on the parts of others, Alston was finally persuaded to give up his attempt to take over the College. A large committee was then formed to look into Alston's land and other lands, to find the most suitable place for building.[79]

The internal troubles centering around Alston indicate the passions that surrounded the two factions. The ousted group, which had ruled the College since 1655, had been vociferous in its opposition to empirics and cautious in its endorsement of the new science. When the Royal Society first began to think about a meetingplace in late 1660 and turned to the College of Physicians, the officers had refused to let it meet on the College's premises.[80] A man like Baldwin Hamey, Jr., loved letters deeply: the Annals of the College are sprinkled with Greek tags during his tenure as registrar—his Latin is of a difficult neo-Ciceronian style. After the Harveian Museum and Library was built, he had gone to it regularly to read instead of to engage in the experimental research being done there by some of the younger physicians. Hamey was best known for his arguments over interpreting Greek passages in Hippocrates and Aristophanes. He and his friend Edward Alston never published anything on the new physiology, although that certainly did not prevent Hamey from also becoming friends with George Ent, Christopher Merrett, and Thomas Wharton—all men who valued both letters and the new researches. Hamey was willing to tolerate the new science in the College as long as it did not threaten the preeminence of academic learning, for the College was "his mistress and favorite," as his grandnephew put it.[81] In the

---

[79]The committee members were: the elects (Staines, Alston, Glisson, Ent, Micklethwaite, Hamey, Bate, and Prujean), the censors (Ent, Goddard, Croyden, and Wharton), and Coxe, Stanley, Merrett, Waldron, and Collins, Jr. The dispute with Alston was not easily resolved. A committee was authorized to get out of the lease he had signed (Annals, 4:92b–93). In November 1668 the College resolved that since Alston had negotiated and signed the lease, he was to sign the release; but Alston refused (Annals, 4:93b–94a). As it turned out, Alston's actions cost the College £150, paid in February 1669 to the owners of the land in order to break the lease (Annals, 4:94a–94b). Alston died on December 24, 1669.

[80]Margery Purver, *The Royal Society: Concept and Creation*, pp. 132–33.

[81]Ralph Palmer, "The Life of the Most Eminent Dr. Baldwin Hamey" (1733), R.C.P. 337.

wake of the conflict over the Society of Chemical Physicians, however, tolerance for the new philosophy began to look almost suicidal.

The new officers, on the other hand, reflected the same attitudes that had surfaced during the period of weakness in the College twenty years before: they represented the interests of the new science. All had been active members in the Royal Society before 1665 and carried out research in medicine along experimental lines. Physicians like Glisson, Ent, and Micklethwaite also had acquired large practices among the upper gentry and the aristocracy, who favored the "new philosophy."[82] These new experimental physicians, less interested in acting as a regulatory body, took over the direction of the College at a time when the social prestige of empirical science seemed assured.

Intellectually, the new officers welcomed views like that of George Castle, an M.D. and recent graduate of All Souls College, Oxford. Castle published *The Chymical Galenist* and dedicated it to Thomas Millington, a candidate of the College and a fellow of the Royal Society. He argued that the new anatomical and chemical discoveries had transformed physiology and pathology but not the therapy practiced by the academics. "Much of the therapeutic part of physic is like dials and almanacs," Castle wrote, "which agree as well with that of Copernicus', as Ptolemy's hypothesis." He remarked that physic could be in danger from either too much subservience to the ancients or too great an addiction to new fashions, but that the learned physicians "need not (I think) in our age, apprehend any danger to physic from an over-fondness of antiquity. The growing evil, is the other extreme, a fancy of rejecting the wisdom of the ancients, for the follies and whimsies of some phantastical pseudo-chemists." The extended metaphor Castle used was that, just as the ancient geographers did not know about America and so were unsatisfactory, so Galen did not know of recent discoveries and so was not completely correct; yet to finance voyages of anyone on the mere chance that he might discover something would be as silly as to support fully any chemists on the chance that they might do some good. He went on to defend the researches of the academic physicians as the most valuable, to refute the views of Nedham and other chemists, and to defend such Galenic principles as temperaments, humors, critical days, and pulse

---

[82]See, for example, the consultation over the earl of Shaftesbury's illness in 1668 by Glisson, Ent, and Micklethwaite, in Kenneth Dewhurst, *Dr. Thomas Sydenham (1624–1689): His Life and Original Writings* (Berkeley and Los Angeles: University of California Press, 1966), p. 38. Dewhurst follows others in calling the three "royal physicians"; they may have been consulted by the king, and certainly his courtiers consulted them, but none of them was a regular physician: see appendix 3.

lore.[83] Not all of Galenic medicine was defended, and research was praised highly in Castle's book, but the mere chemical empirics were strongly condemned. Just so the new leaders of the College had argued since their experimental work on rickets in the late 1640s.

Yet to physicians who did not welcome the new philosophy, the Royal Society seemed to be ever more a potential rival to the College of Physicians, both intellectually and institutionally. After the fire, Christopher Merrett (a member of both groups) had proposed that the Royal Society and the College of Physicians join together to build a common meeting hall, although the proposal was rejected, first by the College and, after having been accepted, also by the Royal Society.[84] Not long afterward, in 1667 and 1668, the officers of the Royal Society floated a proposal to build a "College" of their own, although this never gained the support of the full society, either.[85] By the early 1670s it was even rumored at Oxford that the Royal Society was endeavoring to grant degrees.[86]

The Royal Society was also certainly taking seriously research that physicians had formerly considered part of their own domain.[87] According to one analysis, medical experiments were the second largest category of experiments (next to "physics") undertaken at the Royal Society; added to experiments in natural history and chemistry, which were also undertaken largely by medical men, medical interests accounted for 43 percent of all experiments; 44 percent of all papers read at the Royal Society were on medicine and natural history. Another evaluation of the activities of the Royal Society confirms that the Royal Society's interest in anatomy and physiology was second only to its interest in "physics," although investigations of medicines per se took up little of the society's attention.[88]

[83]George Castle, *The Chymical Galenist: A Treatise Wherein the Practise of the Ancients is reconcil'd to the new Discoveries in the Theory of Physick* (1667), sigs. A4v, A5, pp. 1–2, 134–70, 181 ff.

[84]Christopher Merrett, *A Short Reply to the Postscript, etc., of H[enry] S[tubbe]* (1670), p. 2.

[85]On the proposal to build a College adjunct to the Royal Society, see Michael Hunter, "A 'College' for the Royal Society: The Abortive Plan of 1667–1668," *Notes and Records of the Royal Society* 38 (1984): 159–86.

[86]Purver, *Royal Society*, p. 72.

[87]See A. Rupert Hall, "Medicine and the Royal Society," in *Medicine in Seventeenth Century England,* ed. Allen G. Debus, pp. 421–52; idem, "English Medicine in the Royal Society's Correspondence: 1660–1677," *MH* 15 (1971): 111–25.

[88]R. P. Stearns, "The Relations between Science and Society in the Later Seventeenth Century," in *The Restoration of the Stuarts: Blessing or Disaster?* pp. 72–73; Robert G. Frank, Jr., "Institutional Structure and Scientific Activity in the Early Royal Society," *Proceedings of the Fourteenth International Congress of the History of Science*, vol. 4 (Tokyo, 1975), pp. 92–93.

Additionally, many virtuosi, like John Aubrey, collected empirical recipes from the "folk" or anyone else who seemed to have ideas about curing.[89] By the early 1670s, the interests of the virtuosi in curing empirically were enough a part of their public image to allow one popular playwright to mock them for it.[90] As Robert Boyle put it in 1663:

> Nor should we only expect some improvements to the therapeutic part of physic from the writings of so ingenious [a] people as the Chinese; but probably the knowledge of physicians might be not inconsiderably increased, if men were a little more curious to take notice of the observations and experiments, suggested partly by the practice of midwives, barbers, old women, empirics, and the rest of that illiterate crew, that presume to meddle with physic among ourselves.[91]

He suggested that medicine's task was to improve the efficacy of cures, and that cures were to be found out by empirical trials rather than by learned discourse—he was moving physic in the direction of mere medicine. As a matter of fact, the tone of the second part of Boyle's book, with its emphasis on chemistry as a proper method to improve medicine, was bound to generate ill feelings on the part of many academic physicians.

Other members of the Royal Society attacked learned physic even more explicitly. William Petty, for instance, held that a physician should be trained in a practical knowledge of surgery, botany, and chemistry and should have an "understanding" of French and Latin; he did not need to be expert in books and languages. He held some members of the College of Physicians in contempt and wondered "whether of 1000 patients to the best physicians, aged of any decade, there do not die as many as out [of] the inhabitants of places where there dwell no physicians," going on to suggest trials of therapies by experiment. Physicians should learn anatomy, he wrote, but their art also consisted in making "friends of patients and families[?], and of women, midwives and nurses."[92]

Several other "experimentators" not only held such opinions but

---

[89]Michael Hunter, *John Aubrey and the Realm of Learning*, pp. 43, 96, 107, 109, 139, 196.
[90]Thomas Shadwell, "The Virtuoso," act 4, sc. 6.
[91]Robert Boyle, *Some Considerations Touching the Usefulnesse of Experimental Naturall Philosophy, Propos'd in Familiar Discourses to a friend, by way of Invitation to the Study of it* (Oxford, 1663), pt. 2, pp. 220–21.
[92]*The Petty Papers*, ed. Marquis of Lansdowne (London: Constable, 1927), pp. 168–86, 191–92.

openly attacked learned medicine in public. Everard Maynwaring published *Medicus Absolutus . . . The Compleat Physitian, Qualified and Dignified* (1668), a book arguing for the importance of chemical physicians and of the new philosophy. An anonymous treatise, apparently the same as that issued two years later by Jonathan Goddard under a modified title, argued for physicians taking up chemical medicines and making up medicines with their own hands so as to rectify the "abuses" of the apothecaries.[93] Daniel Coxe, a chemical physician and member of the Royal Society, quickly followed suit with an anonymous treatise arguing that physicians should make their own medicines, not have them made up by apothecaries.[94]

Ostensibly attacks on the apothecaries for intruding into the practice of physic, all three books in fact echoed T. M.'s book. For example, Coxe accused the apothecaries of "designing" against the physicians, of making mistakes in their prescriptions, of being ignorant of Latin, of being unacquainted with materia medica, of relying on wholesalers for many compound drugs, of substituting drugs on hand for ones listed in the physicians' prescriptions, and of being ignorant of chemistry.[95] Not only the complaints about medical abuses by the apothecaries but also the historical assumptions about the problems in physic being due to the divisions in medicine growing from the "dark ages" had their parallels in T. M.'s work.[96] The main remedy for the situation, putting the apothecaries out of business by having physicians all make their own drugs with their own

---

[93]This *Discourse Concerning Physick, and the many Abuses thereof by Apothecaries* (1668) does not seem to be extant. Since the work was reviewed in the *Philosophical Transactions* (no. 41 [Nov. 16, 1668], pp. 835–36), and since Anthony Wood ascribes that tract to Goddard (*Athenae Oxoniensis,* ed. P. Bliss [London, 1817], vol. 3, col. 1029), I take this book to be a lost one of Goddard's rather than a "ghost" (see Frank H. Ellis and Leonard M. Payne, "Jonathan Goddard: *Discourse Concerning Physick . . . A* Lost Work or a Ghost?" *MH* 7 [1963]. 188–90; and R. S. Roberts, "Jonathan Goddard," pp. 190–91). One may infer from the review in the *Philosophical Transactions* that the contents are almost identical to Goddard's later *A Discourse setting forth the Unhappy Condition of the Practice of Physick in London* (1670), in which Goddard says he had the manuscript ready five years earlier. This tract is the only one of the medical pamphlets noted in this chapter to be reviewed in the *Philosophical Transactions,* for reasons that may be suggested by the argument that follows.

[94][Daniel Coxe], *A Discourse wherein The Interest of the Patient in Reference to Physick and Physicians is Soberly Debated* (1669). Coxe had been granted a dispensation to take the M.D. at Cambridge in 1667 (S.P. 44/27/146) and was awarded his M.D. by royal mandate in 1669.

[95]Ibid., pp. 13–29.

[96]These pamphlets have generally been treated as a controversy separate from the debate over the Royal Society, a mistake in my opinion. See, for example, Charles F. Mullett, "Physician vs. Apothecary, 1669–1671: An Episode in an Age-Long Controversy," *Scientific Monthly* 49 (1939): 558–65.

hands, was a solution first proposed by T. M., too, and seemed far more drastic than the "problem" presented by errors made by apothecaries (which might be better remedied by closer regulation).

Others perceived that these mostly anonymous attacks on the apothecaries had a hidden agenda. The letter of "A. N." to "T. O." (an M.D. of Cauis College, Cambridge) indicates the minor furor one book (probably Goddard's) was causing. The book had only been out for a fortnight when T. O. asked A. N. to send him a copy—it obviously was being widely discussed, possibly because it had been reviewed in the *Philosophical Transactions*. A. N. wrote that not only "scholars and citizens" but also "persons noble, illustrious, and of the best and highest quality" were reading it and talking about it. The talk was apparently so deep that A. N. refused to put it on paper: "Considering the circumstances now are such and so different as writing is from speaking, I have reason enough to beg your excuse if I decline from [telling you how the book had been received]." But he went on to point out its odd qualities in a sophisticated way. The general rumor had it that the author was trying to introduce new methods of making up medicines, when the old methods were fine. Additionally, "I charge it generally with injustice, or an under attempt of not invading but subverting the rights" of the duly incorporated Society of Apothecaries. A. N. also thought the book guilty of "indiscretion," since it was in the interests of both apothecaries and physicians to unite against mountebanks and quacks, not to fight each other. The final general charge against it was that it was not "enough authorized: I find not the suffrages of the honorable and learned College of Physicians in London added thereunto."

Two more particular matters of the argument puzzled A. N. First, why was the author "partial in his design" by singling out the apothecaries, when surgeons, chemists, mountebanks, and "quacks of all sorts" could also be blamed in a similar fashion for setting up as rivals to the physicians? Second, the physicians themselves could be accused of bad practice: "Why did he so carelessly (not to say unskillfully) calculate an accusation against the apothecaries which will (in the almanac phrase) serve as well for the medicine of the physicians as of the apothecaries?"[97] Why indeed, unless the apothecaries were not the real issue of the pamphlet? To some contemporaries, at least, the author seemed rather to mean to try to prod the physicians into being

[97]"A. N. to T. O.," Sloane 631, fols. 168–77.

more like the virtuosi than to solve the problem of practicing apothecaries. Again, the echoes of T. M.'s book are strong.

Within a year, Christopher Merrett, one of the new officers of the College and a longtime supporter of experimental research and the Royal Society, reiterated the arguments of the previous books. He, too, picked up the cudgel against the apothecaries, and he proposed the same solution as the others, explaining that Goddard's book "was too large for every one's reading, and in some things too short."[98] Merrett expanded the list of medical abuses by the apothecaries. He wrote that his public attack on so well-organized and vocal a group of men as the apothecaries would do harm to his practice, but that he preferred the "public good, and the honor of my profession before my own private profit." He had been forced to write because the apothecaries were acting wrongly on three counts. First, they were making bad medicines and generally committing "more frauds . . . than in any other trade."[99] Second, they harmed patients by prescribing too much medicine, and medicines priced too high, thus causing poorer people to run to the mountebanks for help.[100] Third, "as to the physicians in general, [the apothecaries] endeavor to extirpate them, and some have been so bold to say, they hope in [a] few years to see never a physician in London and to profess they will scramble with them for practice."[101] The answer Merrett proposed for these troubles, seeing as how the College could not then hope to delimit the apothecaries' actions legally, was to boycott the apothecaries by having all physicians make their own remedies. Half his book is devoted to pointing out the advantages to physic of the physicians becoming more knowledgeable in this way.[102]

Jonathan Goddard reissued his book under his name with a license dated January 19, 1670, but it had been written five years earlier, during the disputes over the College's charter. He may have felt that it gave too much aid and comfort to the organizing Society of Chemical Physicians and so had refrained from printing it at that time, for like Coxe and Merrett he argued that physicians ought to make their

[98]Christopher Merrett, *A Short View of the Frauds, and Abuses Committed by Apothecaries; As Well in Relation to Patients, as Physicians: And of the only Remedy thereof by Physicians making their own Medicines* (1669; the imprimatur is November 13, 1669, although the later *Lex Talionis* says it was issued on January 16, 1668/9), pp. 6–7.

[99]Ibid., pp. 5–13.

[100]Ibid., pp. 13–18.

[101]Ibid., pp. 19–25.

[102]Ibid., pp. 25–53.

own medicines, as the chemists were arguing in late 1664 and 1665. But in the meantime Goddard had been circulating his book among friends. Coxe called him "the judicious author" of the "late excellent discourse concerning the state of physic and the regulation of its practice." What his argument added to that of Merrett and Coxe was more detailed precedent: like T. M., he wrote that the ancient physicians had not used apothecaries but had made up their own medicines.[103]

These three physician members of the Royal Society seemed to be intentionally trying to deflect criticism of the experimental philosophy onto the apothecaries, the physicians' more traditional rivals. The physicians who supported the new science saw the worry of their more academic colleagues and tried to separate the issue of the control of medical practice from the intellectual threat of the new philosophy. It was not the empiricism of the new science but the practices of their medical rivals that posed the threat to physic, these physicians were claiming. The only way to counter that threat was to have the academic physicians become more empirical—exactly what the chemists and virtuosi were arguing. Needless to say, those who feared that the experimental philosophy would undermine academic medicine were not taken in by this sleight of hand.

Compounding the suspicions of the more traditional physicians were the statements of the official spokesman for the Royal Society. Thomas Sprat's cautiously written *History of the Royal Society of London,* brought out in 1667, tried, not entirely successfully, to deflect criticism from that body.[104] Sprat, chaplain to the duke of Buckingham, seemed to extend to chemical empirics the endorsement of the Royal Society. He praised chemists who "look after the knowledge of nature in general" as well as chemists who "seek out, and prepare medicines." From the labors of these men, "the true philosophy is like to receive the noblest improvement."[105] Sprat tried to set the minds of outsiders at rest about the intentions of the Royal Society, but in a curious way, a way that would not in the least have eased the minds of anxious physicians. "For what suspicion can divinity,

[103]Goddard, *Discourse Concerning Physick.*

[104]For a recent account of the relationship of Sprat's work to the Royal Society's goals, see P. B. Wood, "Methodology and Apologetics: Thomas Sprat's *History of the Royal Society,*" *British Journal for the History of Science* 13 (1980): 1–26.

[105]Thomas Sprat, *The History of the Royal Society of London* (1667), p. 37. Sprat had less patience with "such [chemists], as search after riches, by transmutations, and the great Elixir." On the generally defensive tone of Sprat's book, see Jones, *Ancients and Moderns,* pp. 221–35.

law, or physic, or any other course of life have, that they shall be impaired by these men's labors, when they themselves are as capable of sitting amongst them as any others?" In other words, the Royal Society could not be accused of undermining academic physic as long as physicians were free to join the society! Such a defense must have looked preposterous. Sprat also noted, "Of our physicians, many of the most judicious have contributed their purses, their hands, their judgments, their writings."[106] Statements like these must have made Christopher Merrett, Jonathan Goddard, and other members of the College of Physicians who did participate in the Royal Society and who urged more empiricism in physic seem like traitors to their profession in the eyes of their more conservative colleagues: they gave aid to an institution that encouraged a new empiricism inimical to the purposes of the College.

Joseph Glanvill's heated defense of himself and the Royal Society even more clearly indicates the kinds of problems that purveyors of the experimental philosophy were creating for academically trained physicians. Glanvill, a young clergyman, had apparently been made a member of the Royal Society in return for his flowery dedication to that body in his *Scepsis Scientifica* (1665; the imprimatur is dated October 18, 1664), a somewhat revised version of *The Vanity of Dogmatizing* (1661).[107] According to Glanvill, his views had led a much older and established vicar in his diocese, Robert Crosse, to attack him behind his back. When they confronted each other, Crosse wanted to get Glanvill's views on Calvinism versus Remonstrantism (that is, his views on predestination)—but this Glanvill thought incapable of resolution, so he "declined the bait" and tried to shift the subject to the new philosophy. When the young clergyman refused to discuss such a basic theological tenet, Crosse burst out with the accusation of "atheism."[108] Glanvill decided to defend his reputation by publishing *Plus Ultra: Or, the Progress and Advancement of Knowledge Since the Days of Aristotle* (1668), a book rousing men to advance the new philosophy over "notional" and "disputing" Aristotelianism. The Royal Society was introduced into the argument as a prestigious body that cultivated the new philosophy without undermining religion (the "proof" being that many ecclesiastics were members of

---

[106]Sprat, *History of the Royal Society*, pp. 66, 130.

[107]On Glanvill's works, see his *The Vanity of Dogmatizing: The Three Versions*, with critical intro. by Stephen Medcalf, and a reply to Medcalf by S. Talmor in *History of European Ideas* 1 (1981): 175–83.

[108]See Nicholas H. Steneck, " 'The Ballad of Robert Crosse and Joseph Glanvill' and the Background to *Plus Ultra*," *British Journal for the History of Science* 14 (1981): 59–74.

it). Henry Oldenburg and John Beale, members of the Royal Society, both initially encouraged Glanvill in his project, but Glanvill's intemperate defense of his own honor led him to make some heated remarks in the book, from which Beale soon disassociated himself.[109]

One of the most ill-considered remarks came in Glanvill's first chapter. The Royal Society, he wrote, acknowledges that some ancients had "wit" and useful knowledge, but it denies them "absolute empire" over human knowledge. He then proceeded beyond this straw man of modern subservience to the ancients to attack the ancients in toto:

> But besides this, the modern experimentators think, that the philosophers of elder times, though their wits were excellent, yet the way they took was not like to bring much advantage to knowledge, or any of the uses of human life; being for the most part that of notion and dispute, which still runs round in a labyrinth of talk, but advanceth nothing. And the unfruitfulness of those methods of science, which so many centuries never brought the world so much practical, beneficial knowledge, as would help towards the cure of a cut finger, is a palpable argument, that they were fundamental mistakes, and that the way was not right.[110]

When a local physician by the name of Henry Stubbe heard at the dinner table someone quote the "proof" that ancient learning was of no value because it did not teach anyone how to "cure a cut finger," Stubbe burst out angrily that "whatever defects there were in those received principles, no physician . . . could deny them to be exceeding useful." Afterward Stubbe read Glanvill's and Sprat's books and decided to reply to them in print, although his own books were at first blocked from reaching the public—by the Royal Society, he said.[111] At least that is Stubbe's own account of his involvement in a pamphlet war over the Royal Society.[112] A great many pages of his

---

[109]Henry Oldenburg, *The Correspondence of Henry Oldenburg*, ed. A. Rupert and Marie Boas Hall, letter nos. 672, 833, 893, 905, 915.

[110]Joseph Glanvill, *Plus Ultra; Or the Progress and Advancement of Knowledge Since the Days of Aristotle* (1668), pp. 7–8.

[111]Henry Stubbe, *The Plus Ultra Reduced to a Non Plus* (1670), preface; idem, *Legends no Histories: or, A Specimen of Some Animadversions Upon the History of the Royal Society* (1670).

[112]According to James R. Jacob, Stubbe was drawn into the attack on Glanvill by Crosse (*Henry Stubbe, Radical Protestantism and the Early Enlightenment*, pp. 78–79), a plausible argument although built on slender evidence and only a part of the story, in my view. It seems to me that the local quarrels only reached print when influential figures in London encouraged Stubbe to go public: see the discussion that follows.

two initial books, finally published in May and June 1670, were devoted to showing how absurd were the claims of the virtuosi and their followers to have overthrown medical diagnostics and therapeutics derived from ancient sources.

Although recently Stubbe's motives for attacking the Royal Society have been ascribed to a hidden radicalism,[113] he has usually been portrayed as a somewhat intemperate upholder of orthodoxy in religion and physic.[114] That he may have been set to the work by Baldwin Hamey, one of the ousted officers of the College, has also been noted.[115] Hamey undoubtedly believed that the Royal Society was infringing on the prerogatives of the College of Physicians and that the "power appeared on oneside infinitely superior to that on the other." He may, then, have "found out" and "retained"[116] Stubbe as others were retained to defend the College on other occasions. (The College's chemist, William Johnson, and Nathaniel Hodges and Robert Sprackling, two candidates, had earlier defended the institution, and Hamey's protégé, Charles Goodall, later set a young Oxford graduate to work attacking an opponent of the College's on the promise that Goodall would set him up in medical practice in London.)[117]

Stubbe may very well have hoped to practice in London instead of near rural Bath, where he then was. He may have wished to impress the physicians who were worried about the Royal Society, Hamey being one of the most important of them. His earlier patron, Sir Alexander Fraizer, first physician to the king, also seems to have had a hand in Stubbe's work, promising him "a letter of thanks" for what he did against the Royal Society.[118] One of Stubbe's books contains a very flattering dedication to Fraizer and declares that the book was written at the urging of "some persons of great learning, and of no common repute," while one of Stubbe's adversaries wrote "of my

---

113Jacob, *Henry Stubbe.*

114Jones, *Ancients and Moderns,* pp. 244–55; R. H. Syfret, "Some Early Reactions to the Royal Society," *Notes and Records of the Royal Society* 8 (1950): 207–58; and in the same volume, idem, "Some Early Critics of the Royal Society," pp. 20–64.

115Harcourt Brown, *Scientific Organizations in Seventeenth-Century France (1620–1680),* pp. 256–57; Syfret, "Some Early Reactions," pp. 255–56; idem, "Some Early Critics," pp. 25–27.

116Palmer, "Life of the Most Eminent Dr. Baldwin Hamey," page inserted between pp. 90 and 91. The inserts in Palmer's manuscript are common (for example, between pp. 84 and 85 and between pp. 54 and 55), and all but the last lines of the insertion between pp. 90 and 91 (not part of the quotation) are in his hand and in the same ink as the rest.

117Richard Boulton, *A Letter to Dr. Charles Goodall* (1699).

118Henry Stubbe, letter to Robert Boyle, in Boyle's *Works,* vol. 1, p. 59.

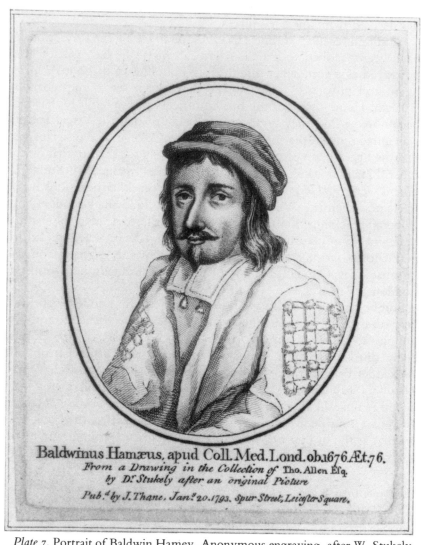

Plate 7. Portrait of Baldwin Hamey. Anonymous engraving, after W. Stukely, 1793. Courtesy of the Wellcome Institute Library, London.

grand enemy your patron."[119] Still, Stubbe insisted that "I was no way hired or mercenarily engaged to do what I did," and that "Sir Alexander Fraizer neither incited me against you, nor knew of the undertaking."[120]

Be that as it may, there is evidence that Stubbe either shared or accepted others' opinions about the virtuosi's attacks on physic. An unattributed manuscript in the British Library contains jottings of replies to the pamphlets of Goddard, Maynwaring, and Merrett as well as phrases later used by Stubbe.[121] The bulk of the manuscript copies out evidence from various texts to show that the ancients did indeed have separate professions of apothecaries and physicians. But it also contains direct rebuttals of the experimentalists' pamphlets and remarks on the machinations of the Royal Society. "To Boyle," it says, "you proclaim more compendious ways of compounding [?] [medicines] may be found [chemically]. . . . Why do you condemn the cautiousness of Galenical physicians[?]" "To Goddard: Did his brethren the experimentators first disparage the ancient practice of physic as inutile [and] censure the comp[any] as useless, and advance O'Dowde's College. [The] R[oyal] S[ociety], they are [a] common enemy as to all literature." It then mocks the attempts of the virtuosi to give medical advice. "I suppose Mr. Boyle, Maynwaring and Merrett set out books like bills on posts to tell where you may have arcanas." "All, all affaires are in danger of their encroachments. They desire all the secrets of professions shall fall into their knowledge."[122] Just so, Stubbe wrote that the Royal Society "promoted the Anti-College of pseudo-chemists, encouraging O'Dowde and his ignorant adherents in opposition to the physicians," and he wrote of "our common enemies the Royal Society."[123] Whether these notes were

---

[119]Henry Stubbe, *The Lord Bacons relation of the sweating-sickness examined* (1671), dedication and preface; George Thomson, *A Letter sent to Mr. Henry Stubbe* (1672), p. 4.

[120]Letter of Stubbe to Thomson, printed in Thomson, *Letter sent to Mr. Henry Stubbe*, p. 11.

[121]Sloane 1786, vols. 116–28. The manuscript is unattributed in the British Library's catalogue to the Sloane Collection, although the printed *Index* of 1971 lists it under Stubbe's name. It clearly is not in Stubbe's hand (or Hamey's), and the contents suggest that it was written in late 1669 or early 1670, after Goddard but before Stubbe's *Campanella Revived* (with a preface dated May 16, 1670). Possibly Stubbe had an amanuensis; more probably the jottings are of a physician as yet unidentified.

[122]Sloane 1786, fols. 116b, 118b, 119, 116.

[123]Henry Stubbe, *Campanella Revived*, "To the Reader" (dated May 16, 1670) and "Postscript" (dated June 14, 1670). Other remarks are similar to some in Stubbe's *A Censure upon certain passages contained in the History of the Royal Society* (Oxford, 1671), and Michael Hunter has noted yet others in Stubbe's *Plus Ultra Reduced to a Non Plus* (1670), as quoted in his *Science and Society in Restoration England*, p. 125.

given to Stubbe to help him compose his works or not, they indicate that Stubbe's views of the Royal Society were held by others, as well.

While the bulk of Stubbe's argument against the Royal Society was in large part a defense of the College, matters became more complicated when members of the Society of Apothecaries entered the fray to defend themselves from what they also saw as abuse by the experimentators Merrett, Goddard, and Coxe. Merrett and the others had started a debate that nearly united the physicians and the apothecaries against a common enemy, the Royal Society, as Stubbe had hoped. The apothecaries read Merrett's book at a meeting of their court in February 1670.[124] On March 28 a committee of apothecaries came to the College to ask if the recent books had been published with the College's encouragement or consent: they wished harmony to exist between the two corporations, but they would take offense if the College was behind the books.[125] The learned physicians were able to reassure the society about their own desire for harmony, and they and the apothecaries set up joint committees to try to reach an amicable settlement on the issues that divided them. In the meetings that followed, apothecaries tried to have Merrett and Goddard removed from their College fellowships.

A pamphlet by apothecaries entitled *Lex Talionis* soon came out attacking Coxe, Goddard, and Merrett.[126] The tract accused Merrett of proceeding in his book "contrary to religion, the laws of the land, and common charity"; it then tried to show point by point how the pamphlets by the three were full of lies, how it was the physicians who abused medicine, how the apothecaries were fully able to practice, and finally, by referring to the new medicine of Harvey and Willis, how the old ideas were wrong, as was any institutional structure that defended the old medical hierarchy.

By the time a final meeting was held between the committees of the College and the society, on June 21, the apothecaries were willing to propose that if no physicians would make compound medicines or pretend to any "private arcanum," they would join the College in procuring an Act of Parliament "for the regulating of physic, where-

---

[124]Underwood, p. 356.

[125]Annals, 4:96b–97a; and Underwood, pp. 116–18, 356–58.

[126]*Lex Talionis; Sive Vindiciae Pharmacoporum: Or a Short Reply to Dr. Merrett's Book; and Others, written against the Apothecaries* (1670). The authorship of *Lex Talionis* was (and is) disputed, being variously attributed to Stubbe and Marchamont Nedham, among others. Neither seems to me to be a plausible candidate, however. Probably Gideon Harvey was right in saying that it was coauthored by a "cabal" of four or five apothecaries (Gideon Harvey, *The Accomplisht Physician* [1670], p. 91).

by to suppress all empirics and illegal practitioners and makers of physic, as common enemies to both." *Lex Talionis* had poisoned the atmosphere, however, and a compromise was not struck. As in 1664, the College replied that it wanted all its own rights and privileges upheld, as well as the rights and privileges of the apothecaries as the College interpreted them.[127] The virtuosi had succeeded in keeping the physicians and the apothecaries divided enough to prevent the two groups from counterattacking, but they failed to convince the physicians or the apothecaries that the experimental medicine of the virtuosi was best for the professions.

The pamphlets continued. Gideon Harvey the elder published a book soon after *Lex Talionis* that included a hastily appended "lash for *Lex Talionis*." Gideon Harvey was not a member of the College of Physicians or the Royal Society. But he claimed that the good doctors of the College "and their art have of late years been rendered subject to the same fate [as] religion and the law not long before, of being subverted by the ignorance and ambition of such whose brain is as subject to vapors, as the climate wherein they live." Empirics, practicing apothecaries, and practicing surgeons troubled Gideon Harvey. Referring to *Lex Talionis,* he angrily wrote that though a "scurrilous cabal" had tried to defame Drs. Merrett, Goddard, and Coxe, it had succeeded only in "the bespattering of themselves" with "all the filth and dirt the sink of their imagination stunk of," and "defiling their own nest."[128] Christopher Merrett, too, soon replied, comparing his earlier book and *Lex Talionis* point by point, and showing how *Lex Talionis* made misleading statements. Merrett believed that one or more members of the Society of Apothecaries had written the book: "If they are the authors of it, they have done most impudently, in publishing a paper at such a time, when they make overtures to the College." But he noted that the apothecaries had put out a rumor that Henry Stubbe had written *Lex Talionis*.[129]

Stubbe quickly replied to Merrett in a postscript to his *Campanella Revived* (1670), and Merrett shot back with *A Short Reply*.[130] Merrett defended the Royal Society. He wrote that, contrary to Stubbe's opinion, the Royal Society had never tried to take over the College—

[127]Annals, 4:97a–97b; Underwood, p. 358.

[128]Harvey, *The Accomplisht Physician*, preface, p. 91.

[129]Christopher Merrett, *Self-Conviction; or an Enumeration of the Absurdities, Railings against the College, and Physicians in general . . . and also an Answer to the Rest of Lex Talionis* (1670), pp. 1–2.

[130]Merrett, *A Short Reply to the Postscript, etc., of H[enry] S[tubbe]*; pp. 27 to 42 point out likenesses between Stubbe's published views and those of *Lex Talionis*.

although he himself had proposed after the fire that the College and the Royal Society build a common hall. He also denied that the Royal Society ever encouraged the Society of Chemical Physicians. He continued by denying that the physicians were withdrawing their support from the Royal Society.[131] After other denunciations and distortions of Stubbe's position, Merrett ended by accusing him of being "a brother apothecary," which was an absurd statement, although Stubbe was vigorously trying to reconcile the physicians and apothecaries.[132]

Stubbe wrote in a letter to Merrett dated August 16, 1670, "If you will desert the Royal Society, and endeavor to adjust the differences, rather than widen them betwixt physicians and apothecaries, [I will help bring my friends to be friends of yours]." "Let us not, out of passion against the Apothecaries, destroy our selves, and give advantage to that multitude of quacks, under the protection of the Royal Society, and the pretence of making their own medicaments."[133] Other works, too, urged the alliance of apothecaries and physicians.[134] The medical controversies had become inextricably linked to the controversies over the new philosophy.

Some physicians saw the changes as giving rise to an anti–intellectual climate, and so did members of church and university.[135] Henry More's *Divine Dialogues* (1667) expressed the view that the experimental philosophy only encouraged atheism. The archbishop of Canterbury, Gilbert Sheldon, may finally have taken to heart Nathaniel Hodges's earlier dedication urging him to see the relationship between the chemical empirics and the religious empirics of the interregnum: the dedication speech of the Sheldonian Theatre at Oxford in 1669 by Robert South, probably intended to please the archbishop who had built it, lumped together Cromwell, religious fanatics, the Royal Society, and the new philosophy.[136] Also in 1669, Meric Casaubon published his *Letter . . . to Peter DuMoulin Concerning natural experimental philosophy,* which criticized the new science.[137] When

[131]Ibid., pp. 1–3.

[132]Ibid., p. 42.

[133]Letter of Stubbe to Merrett published in Joseph Glanvill, *A praefatory answer to Mr. Henry Stubbe* (1671), pp. 204–6.

[134]*Medice Cura Teipsum! or the Apothecaries Plea . . . from a Real Well-wisher to both Societies* (1671).

[135]See Hunter, *Science and Society,* pp. 136–61.

[136]Purver, *Royal Society,* pp. 70–71.

[137]Michael R. G. Spiller, *'Concerning Natural Experimental Philosophie': Meric Casaubon and the Royal Society* (The Hague: Martinus Nijhoff, 1980); also see the essay review of Spiller by Michael Hunter in *Annals of Science* 39 (1982): 187–92.

still other critics of the Royal Society linked the new philosophy to Catholics like Campanella, Van Helmont, Gassendi, Descartes, and Mersenne,[138] they were drawing on a campaign of religious slander associating Puritan radicalism and Jesuitism common to the period.[139] And yet in December of 1667 the duke of Buckingham, the favorer of the chemists and a virtuoso himself, launched a scheme for religious comprehension in which his instrument was the intellectual eminence of the Royal Society, John Wilkins (who was soon to gain the bishopric of Chester by the duke's will).[140]

The perception among many learned men that the experimental philosophy constituted a threat to the knowledge on which a stable political, medical, and religious order was based may help to explain why the Royal Society entered a period of decline in the late 1660s and early 1670s. One student of the early Royal Society has noted that few physicians remained active in the institution in this period— contrasting sharply with the activity of its first years.[141] Another's look at physiological work done at the Royal Society finds that almost no demonstrations of that sort were performed for a decade after 1667.[142] The "crisis of the Royal Society" of the later 1660s and the 1670s was caused by the withdrawal of physicians, among others, from the society.[143] The decline of physicians' participation in the new science seems not to rest entirely on the deaths of a few men or on the dispersal of a research community.[144] The decline was also caused by the burdens of private practice[145] and, perhaps most im-

[138]Purver, *Royal Society*, p. 157.

[139]The view that Puritanism was a Jesuitical plot to divide and destroy true Protestantism went back to Elizabeth's reign but was advanced more energetically than ever after the outbreak of civil war. See Ian Thackray, "Zion Undermined: The Protestant Belief in a Popish Plot During the English Interregnum," *History Workshop*, no. 17 (1984): 28–52; and John Leslie Miller, *Popery and Politics in England, 1660–1688* (Cambridge: Cambridge University Press, 1973), esp. pp. 86–90.

[140]On Buckingham's comprehension scheme, see Maurice Lee, *The Cabal* (Urbana: University of Illinois Press, 1965), pp. 175–86.

[141]Hunter, *Royal Society*, pp. 36–37.

[142]Theodore M. Brown, *The Mechanical Philosophy and the 'Animal Oeconomy': A Study in the Development of English Physiology in the Seventeenth and Early Eighteenth Centuries*, pp. 80–82, 104.

[143]For other explanations of this phenomenon, see Hunter, *Royal Society*; Lotte and Glenn Mulligan, "Reconstructing Restoration Science: Styles of Leadership and Social Composition of the Early Royal Society," *Social Studies of Science* 11 (1981): 327–64.

[144]This is the argument of Robert G. Frank, Jr., *Harvey and the Oxford Physiologists: A Study of Scientific Ideas and Social Interaction*, pp. 275–94.

[145]Michael Hunter, "Early Problems in Professionalizing Scientific Research: Nehemiah Grew (1641–1712) and the Royal Society, with an Unpublished Letter to Henry Oldenburg," *Notes and Records of the Royal Society* 36 (1982): 189–209.

portantly, by the fact that the new science was being seen as a growing threat to the prestige of the academic physicians, hence preventing for a time the recruitment of new talent among the young physicians to the Royal Society.

Nevertheless, the declining fortunes of the Royal Society helped
not a jot in restoring the fortunes of the College of Physicians or
medical regulation. The late 1660s and early 1670s were a low point
for the College institutionally and intellectually. The situation "indeed wholly deterred me from breeding one of my sons a physician,"
wrote Timothy Clarke, a fellow of the College. "Alas sir, we live in
an age where to prescribe any bounds is to violate magna charta" he
sighed; it "is humor now to affect, to be wisest out of the sphere that
God, nature, and education have placed us in." "Young blades,"
truant and debauched at the universities, spoke of experiments only
to "disturb the gravest societies with their impertinencies" and to
"silence the most learned."[146]

Thomas Wharton, a member of the College who had stayed in
London during the plague of 1665, echoed his colleague's statements
by advising a young man in 1673 not to enter the profession of physic:
there were "swarms of quacks, mountebanks, chemists, [and] apothecaries" trying "to overthrow all our settled and approved practice of
physic, especially in London."[147] The same was true outside of London, however: the physician Robert Wittie wrote a letter from York
dated March 21, 1671/2, that said: "We have of late become extraordinarily startled through an invasion upon our profession by abundance of quacks both within these walls and without."[148]

The heart of the problem remained: the College's officers neither
could nor would do anything to prosecute others. The pamphlet war
between Merrett and the apothecaries eventually petered out.[149]
Henry Stubbe and the chemist George Thomson carried on an argument over phlebotomy, with Stubbe defending this Galenic (and
Willisian) therapy and Thomson attacking the practice in part by
resorting to that ultimate authority on the new science, Francis

---

[146][Timothy Clarke?], *Some Papers Writ in the Year 1664*, preface, pp. 1–3.

[147]Quoted in John J. Keevil, "The Seventeenth-Century English Medical Background,"
BHM 31 (1957): 412.

[148]R. Wittie, "Letter to 'brother' [physician], Mar. 21, 1671/2," Sloane 1393, fol. 12.

[149]The last pamphlets were *Medice Cura Teipsum! Or the Apothecaries Plea* (1671), and the
reply of C. W., *Reflections on a Libel, Intituled, A Plea for the Apothecaries* (1671).

Bacon.[150] But as long as the Crown seemed unwilling or unable to support the College in enforcing its regulatory powers, such public debates only damaged the preeminence of the physicians.

The decade or so after the Restoration of the Stuart monarchy in 1660 was full of ironies for the College of Physicians. The restoration of royal authority and the College officers' apparent alliance with Clarendon seemed to augur well not only for a restoration of the College's regulatory authority, but for an extension of it. The authority of the Crown was not enough, however, given the new political conditions in England: the clock could not be turned back to 1640, and so, without an alliance with the apothecaries, the College's new charter went down to defeat in the Parliament of 1664. This led to a rash of pamphlets criticizing the College and an attempt to establish a rival Society of Chemical Physicians in early 1665. The plague and the fire further weakened the College. Then, in 1667, a new group of officers tried to win public respect by allowing empirical science. Other physicians, however, soon discerned the new science to be the enemy in their midst.

The problem was clear by 1668. The challenge of the empirical science promoted by members of the Royal Society and others could not be entirely co-opted by the learned physicians if they wished to stress a knowledge of the academic medical traditions as being important to physic. They could not control a scientific medicine; such a medical program allowed empirics to claim that experimentalism was better than the education of the learned physicians. The professional claims of the learned physicians rested on the belief that their rather old-fashioned medical learning, inculcating a broad knowledge of man and his environment, led to a better practice than the practice of the empirics, who promoted specific cures. Some physicians had been led to take up scientific research during the interregnum in the belief that this could be used to advance medical learning. But by the later 1660s, it had become clear to some that the new science might undermine the status of learned men as often as it might better it. By 1670 the lack of any medical regulation in London and the deep factional splits within the College of Physicians over whether to

[150]George Thomson, *'Aimatiasis'; or, The True Way of Preserving the Bloud* (1670); Henry Stubbe, *An Epistolary Discourse Concerning Phlebotomy* (1671); Thomson, *'Misokumias helegkos'; or, A Check Given to the insolent Garrulity of Henry Stubbe* (1671); Stubbe, *The Lord Bacons relation of the sweating-sickness examined* (1671); Thomson, *A Letter Sent to Mr. Henry Stubbe* (1672).

support the new science or the attacks on it had created a medical milieu in which any healer could practice openly and claim the support of the new science for that practice. The profession of physic had sunk to its lowest point since the formation of the College of Physicians 150 years earlier.

The Restoration had begun with high hopes on the part of the physicians for regaining their former authority and prestige. By the early 1670s, every hope had been dashed. By 1670, after years of wrangling, the virtually bankrupt and publicly ridiculed College of Physicians had only managed to draw up plans for a new building— plans but no hope of them being realized unless money could somehow be had. Its authority to regulate medicine was shot and decaying. It was apparent to almost all physicians by 1670 that the power of the College could not be restored until its legal authority was regained, and that could not happen until the Crown grew stronger and decided to support the College. But by the end of 1672, new political winds were blowing that might let the College exercise again some of its former strength.

5

The Restoration of the
Old Order, 1672–1688

We have thought good for the prevention of great damages and inconveniences, which our loving subjects may be exposed to in their healths . . . to will and require you the President and Censors of our said College . . . to do your utmost to prosecute and suppress all such unlearned and unlawful practicers of physic, as shall presume to act contrary to our said letters patents, and the laws of the realm in that case provided.

James II, June 1687

The nadir reached by the College of Physicians in the early 1670s threatened to extinguish the institution itself as well as to end all possibilities of medical regulation. But the College managed to limp forward over the next few years and, as the Crown began to intervene more directly in local affairs for the "public good" in the later 1670s, the College's authority increased. The pattern is similar to the pattern that developed under the early Stuarts: as the Crown sought to solidify its strength, it favored dependent individuals and institutions that in turn benefited from direct lines of patronage and authority radiating from the king. During the reign of James II, the College's ability to regulate medical practice was not only fully restored, but also extended and enhanced. The growth of medical regulation in the 1670s and 1680s depended, again, to a great degree on the changing political climate.

The College and the Common Law

The most important internal business facing the College in the early 1670s was to start the rebuilding program. But money was scarce and the officers had to find a way to raise funds. A committee went to see the marquis of Dorchester, who at that time was in Charles's Privy Council, to request a large donation from him. Back dues from all members were to be collected, also. This proved difficult, however, and in July 1672 the College had to approve a set of rules pertaining to those who had not paid.[1] Money problems persisted for several years.

In the meantime, the Society of Apothecaries built a laboratory in 1671 and a physic garden in 1673.[2] The apothecaries graciously presented their chemical medicines prepared in their new facility to the College for viewing and approval, but the potential for open hostility between the two institutions remained. In September of 1674, members of the College were complaining that the Apothecaries' and Barber-Surgeons' companies had already rebuilt their halls, while the College was still trying to find the money to get started.[3]

Moreover, the physicians of the College continued to be troubled by those who posed an intellectual threat to academic medicine. By the middle of the seventh decade of the century, almost no academic physicians remained in practice who had been educated before the acceptance of Harvey's discovery of the circulation of the blood or the impact of Helmontian chemistry. All of the academic physicians recognized that the new physiological and therapeutic discoveries were having an impact on medicine, especially by promoting the notion that something in the blood, perhaps "ferments," caused diseases.[4] The College of Physicians preserved the interest in chemistry and anatomy it had evinced in the 1650s by employing a chemist and by continuing to hold anatomical lectures.[5] Yet the chemistry and the physiology of the College physicians were meant to support the physicians' academic therapies.

The views of Thomas Willis were especially important to the new generation of academic physicians. He linked the recent anatomical discoveries to physiological views that stressed chemical processes,

---

[1]Annals, 4:99b–100a, 103b–104a.

[2]"Sundry Account and Memoranda Book, Apothecaries Company," Guildhall MS no. 8204, 1671. The laboratory was set up by selling shares to members, and there was talk of selling shares to the public.

[3]Annals, 4:105a–105b, 108b–110a.

[4]See Audrey B. Davis, *Circulation Physiology and Medical Chemistry in England, 1650–1680.*

[5]After William Johnson's death in the great plague, Nicaise Le Febvre, the king's chemist-in-ordinary, was allowed to serve the College (Annals, 4:90a); in 1673 the College hired one Hewke (Annals, 4:107a–107b), who served as its chemist until 1679.

and he linked these in turn to medical therapies that conserved many of the traditional Galenic practices, such as phlebotomy. Writing in Latin, Willis adapted the academics' therapeutics and, most importantly, their stress on learned reasoning, to the new medical environment.[6]

However, those who argued that the best therapies were rooted in nonacademic medicine continued to pose a threat to the physicians' medical prestige, for it was difficult for outsiders to distinguish between academic physic and learned medicine. In the later part of the seventeenth century, the name of Hippocrates rather than Galen conjured up intellectual excitement and an aura of the frontiers of knowledge. The change is significant, for Galen's reputation had come to rest on his medical rationalism, while that of Hippocrates stemmed from his empiricism. At least that is how Paracelsus, Francis Bacon, Van Helmont, and others portrayed Hippocrates, and by the middle of the seventeenth century that is how most people thought of him: the collector of case studies, the compiler of medical details, the inductivist—the early founder of true methods of natural history whose achievement had been devalued by the rationalist practitioners following him.[7]

Moreover, the man who was gaining a reputation as the true English Hippocrates was Thomas Sydenham. Sydenham did have an M.B. from Oxford, and he was a licentiate of the College, but he did not have an academic M.D., nor was he a fellow. Rather, he had strong antiacademic sentiments, believing that medicine ought to be taught by apprenticeship, not by books. When he was asked what someone should read before embarking on a practice, he is said to have replied *Don Quixote,* a book that would protect anyone from seeking illusions of the mind. Sydenham had first begun to practice while serving with the parliamentary cavalry during the civil wars, years before he earned his M.B. As for the anatomical physiology that had been developed by the learned physicians, he believed that it had increased their reputations for learning but had not helped advance the course of medical therapy. As he and his friend John Locke wrote in 1668,

[6]Thomas Willis, *Diatribae duae medicophilosophicae quarum prior agit de fermentatione . . . Altera de febribus* (1659); idem, *Pharmaceutice rationalis* (1674). See the thoughtful essay by Don G. Bates, "Thomas Willis and the Fevers Literature of the Seventeenth Century," *MH,* suppl. no. 1 (1981), pp. 45–70.

[7]See the chapter "The Modern Hippocratic Tradition," in Wesley D. Smith, *The Hippocratic Tradition* (Ithaca: Cornell University Press, 1979), pp. 13–60.

Anatomy no question is absolutely necessary to a surgeon and to a physician who would direct a surgeon to incision, trepanning, and several other operations. . . . But that anatomy is like to afford any great improvement to the practice of physic, or assist a man in finding out and establishing a true method, I have reason to doubt.[8]

Biggs, Thomson, and other rivals of the College's academic physic could not have put the case against anatomy better.

Like other empirical practitioners, then, Sydenham argued that the art of medicine consisted of finding cures for diseases, which could only be done through long experience and trial, not through understanding the workings of the body in health. Sydenham became an early founder of medical nosology, which attempted to classify diseases by describing their symptoms in detail. In other words, he believed that diseases were ontological entities, not imbalances in a body's humors.[9] In terms of the stress he placed on the role of experience in discovering medical therapies and his view that diseases were ontological entities, Sydenham closely resembled the chemical opponents of academic physic.[10] When Henry Stubbe wrote against the empirical threat to academic medicine, he lumped "the Merretts and the Sydenhams" together.[11] The more empiricist classificatory medicine pursued by the English Hippocrates and his friends and followers, as well as Helmontian chemical medicine, pointed up the dangers to learned physic that were implicit in the proliferation of nonacademic medical practitioners who were able to offer coherent views of why they undertook the therapies they did.

Nor was it easy to revive powers of coercion that had been dormant for some time. But in December of 1672, the College registrar recorded that a committee had been appointed "viz., all the censors, [and] Dr. Croydon, Dr. Hodges, Dr. Collins, Junior, and Dr. Allen, to advise with Sir William James [the attorney general], and who else they please about the prosecution of an empiric." Additionally, "liberty to go to the treasurer for moneys to maintain the suit" was

---

[8]Quoted in Kenneth Dewhurst, *Dr. Thomas Sydenham (1624–1689): His Life and Original Writings* (Berkeley and Los Angeles: University of California Press, 1966), p. 85. Also see idem, "Locke and Sydenham on the Teaching of Anatomy," *MH* 2 (1958): 1–12.

[9]On the centrality of therapy to Sydenham's thinking and Sydenham's stress on "experience," see Lester S. King, *The Road to Medical Enlightenment, 1650–1695,* pp. 113–38.

[10]See Peter H. Niebyl, "Science and Metaphor in the Medicine of Restoration England," *BHM* 47 (1933): 369–72.

[11]Henry Stubbe, *Campanella Revived* (1670), p. 22.

authorized.[12] Clearly establishing their statutory power to sue others in a common law court was essential if the verdicts of 1656 were to be overcome.

Within the next year and a half, the College had found someone to test its regulatory power on, for in September of 1674, "Captain" John Bourne petitioned the king "desiring a nolle prosequi." He complained that he was "being prosecuted by the College of Physicians in London under 14 H. VIII for practicing without their license, he having a license from the bishop of London, since he did so in ignorance of the said statute."[13] Bourne persuaded the Crown to stop the College's prosecution.

Later in 1674, however, the Crown had a new minister in Thomas Osborne, earl of Danby. His policies helped the College restore its authority, as can be seen in a letter to the College from Charles II in February 1675: the king insisted that no one be admitted to the College as an honorary fellow except an M.D. from Oxford or Cambridge, unless he had "first taken the Oaths of Allegiance and Supremacy and having been by you afterwards examined and approved according to your statutes."[14] Medical qualification and proper obedience to the laws were urged as necessary to medical practice—just what the College had been arguing for years. In January 1675, the mayor of London ordered all "constables, headboroughs and all other His Majesty's officers and ministers" within London, Westminster, Middlesex, Surrey, Kent, and Essex to prevent the setting up of shops by apothecaries until they had been made freemen of the London society.[15] Whether pressured by the Crown, the College, or the Society of Apothecaries, the Lord Mayor also indicated a renewed interest in controlling at least some medical practitioners.

In June of 1675, therefore, the College reiterated its decision to try to prosecute empirics in court, and at the same time it debated treating the poor at no charge in order to undercut criticism that the empirics were needed by people who could not afford a physician's

[12]Annals, 4:105a–105b.
[13]S.P. 29/361/245. Until the Bill of Rights in 1689, the nolle prosequi was part of the king's dispensing powers: since breaking the king's law wronged the king, he could choose not to consider himself wronged and hence grant a "no prosecution." Bourne, who continued to be troubled by the College in the 1680s, did have a license from the bishop of London that had been granted in 1662 (J. Harvey Bloom and R. Rutson James, *Medical Practitioners in the Diocese of London, Licensed under the Act of 3 Henry VIII, c. 11: An Annotated List, 1529–1725*, p. 40).
[14]Annals, 4:111a–111b.
[15]"Mayoral Precepts and Orders to the Apothecaries Company, 1661–1747," Guildhall MS no. 8296.

fee.[16] All members agreed that both of them were good ideas, although no one was sure how to effect the free treatment of the poor.

The discussion caused "C. D.", an apothecary, to publish an open letter dated October 25, 1675, that criticized the physicians of the College on the issue of high fees. If they were not lowered, he claimed, "Dunce Jones of Moor-Fields, Fletcher of Gutter-lane, Gray the quacker, and the rest of that impudent crew of illiterate quack-salvers, that stain almost every pissing-place, and hansome-post, with their detestable lies, and cheating papers, may in time erect a College, and defend their impudence *cum privilegio*."[17] The apothecary C. D. was threatening that if the College members insisted on resuming the prosecution of others without at the same time reducing their fees (a highly doubtful proposition), they might end up with a new rival corporation, as the Society of Chemical Physicians had been in 1665. The number of broadsides, pamphlets, and other advertisements from competitors in the mid-1670s makes it clear that they made their way in the medical marketplace in large numbers.

Since the prosecution of Bourne had failed because of the king's nolle prosequi, in late 1675 the officers of the College picked another practitioner on whom to try its powers: Adrian Huyberts, a man who threatened to organize just such another "College" as C. D. had threatened. He was arrested and sued in King's Bench by the College under the Act of 1523 for twenty months' illicit practice. At £5 per month, the total amount sued for was very large: £100. If the College could make its charges stick in this case, it would deliver an example to many others.

According to Huyberts, after he had prepared his defense in King's Bench, the College shifted the case to the court of Marshalsey, a move that cost Huyberts money and made him spend more time attending to legal business than to his medical practice. But after a time, on advice from his counsel (Weston), Huyberts got the case moved back to King's Bench on a plea of habeas corpus: "It being the great artifice of the Collegemen, by tumbling me from court to

---

[16]Annals, 4:112a–112b, 113b.

[17]C. D., *Some Reasons, of the Present Decay of the Practise of Physick in Learned and Approved Doctors, in an Answer to a letter lately Received from A. B. Doctor of Physick . . . with some Remedies Proposed to Amend it* (1675). Two years earlier, an anonymous tract titled *An Essay for the Regulation of the Practice of Physick, Upon which Regulation Are grounded the Composure of All Differences Between Physicians and Apothecaries* (1673), possibly also written by an apothecary, had repeated hopes for cooperation between the two companies. The more strident tone of C. D. probably reflects increasing tension as the College was becoming more assertive.

court, to tire out and ruin me, and terrify all others, if they can."[18] The case finally came to trial on Friday, January 28, 1676.

Before the trial, however, Huyberts published a pamphlet to vindicate himself before the public and to vilify the College. In *A Cornerstone laid towards the Building of a New Colledge,* he argued, as Trigge and others had twenty years before, and as Coke had fifty years earlier still, that the acts supporting the College were null and void: no English Parliament would have passed a law of the sort that empowered the College to try other practitioners. "It cannot enter into any English heart to imagine, that our ancestors would entail upon us by law so great a slavery, so manifestly contrary to Magna Charta and to all the fundamental laws and liberties of the subject." He believed that some of the junior fellows of the College wanted to harass him because one of them was jealous of his practice: Huyberts had cured some people whom the physicians could not. A second reason for the College's suit against him, Huyberts believed, was that he was a chemist. Third, he was not a member of the College, "nor will I ever be." A final reason for the suit, he believed, was that he styled himself a "doctor." The title itself meant little, but he had such contempt for academic titles that he felt that he could use the term as well as any member of the College, even though he had refused to take a medical doctorate when he had the opportunity.[19]

Huyberts's contempt for the academic physicians of the College is clear. Regarding the physicians' intellectual grounds for claiming superiority, he noted that "such collegiate establishments or corporations of physic, have been great hinderers of the progress of this art [of medicine] throughout all Europe, and still are."[20] He quoted Francis Bacon and Marchamont Nedham to prove that medicine was not advanced by reading the Greeks and Arabs.[21] "I can here challenge them, and do, in view of the world, to nominate any one particular improvement, that their society hath made in the art of curing, since their first incorporation, and I will prove the contrary." Improvements in anatomy, the pride of the College, did not count as improvements in medicine proper, for they did not contribute to

---

[18]Adrian Huyberts, *A Corner-stone laid towards the Building of a New Colledge . . . in London. Upon the Occasion of the vexatious and oppressive proceedings acted in the name of the Society called the Colledge of Physicians: for the Better information of all men . . . It being an Apology for the better education of Physicians* (1675), pp. 32–33.

[19]Ibid., pp. 4–5, 2–3, 16–17, 24–31.

[20]Ibid., p. 24.

[21]Sir Francis Bacon's *The Advancement of Learning* and Marchamont Nedham's *Medela Medicina. A Plea for the free Profession, and a Renovation of the Art of Physick* (1665).

better cures. Anatomy was only a showy trick of the physicians to make others think that they were learned, like a mountebank's tricks "to entertain spectators, and amuse the world, [in order] to uphold some repute among such as are ignorant, and draw on customers." He quoted Boyle's *Experimental Philosophy* as saying that in " 'those new discoveries [in anatomy, not] any thing has been done, to better the cure of diseases.' " Chemistry was the best way to find new cures—even the physicians of the College were admitting it these days.

Huyberts's recommendation was therefore to "rely upon the common law" to let anyone practice who claimed he or she could do good, and to leave the law to punish only those who harmed patients.[22] Setting up a College to judge others was contrary to the spirit of Englishmen; it was also ridiculous, since there were no certain rules of practice and any rules there might be were constantly changing due to improvements in medicine.[23] Huyberts's stance captured and refined most of the arguments against medical regulation that had been in circulation since the civil wars. His would make an excellent test case of the College's authority.

Judicial sentiment had changed in the twenty years since 1656. When his case came to trial, Huyberts pleaded that the Act of 14 and 15 Henry VIII ratified by the Act of 1523 lacked the royal assent—the same plea that had gotten Trigge and others off in 1656. The justices of King's Bench, however, decided that "though the statute roll be but a transcript of the bill, it hath always been accepted as the law," and the College won the case for the full judgment of £100.[24] Huyberts then petitioned the Crown for a writ of error, to have his case reviewed in the House of Lords.[25] When this failed, he was locked up as a prisoner of King's Bench until he discharged the debt. He petitioned the king to release him at the end of 1676, almost a year after the trial. But Walter Charleton tipped off the College, and the officers counterpetitioned Charles II to keep Huyberts imprisoned.[26] Huyberts was finally set free—whether because the king wished it or because he paid the fine is unknown—and was sued again in 1681. The College also won a suit against one "Needham" in 1677, proba-

---

[22]Huyberts, *A Corner-stone*, pp. 25, 15, 26–27.

[23]Again he quoted Bacon's *Advancement of Learning*, which classifies medicine as an "Art Conjectural."

[24]"Colledge of Phisitians and Cooper or Hubert," 3 Keble, 587–88, *English Reports*, vol. 84.

[25]S.P. 29/281A/74 (incorrectly listed as "1670?").

[26]The petitions are given in full in *Annals*, 4:131b–133b.

bly Marchamont Nedham, who had helped stir up the Society of Chemical Physicians over a decade previously.[27] The College's test cases had been successful, and were probably worth the legal expenses. The College could begin to move against others in the courts, the first step toward restoring corporate medical regulation.

Yet all attempts by the College to restore its legal powers of coercion would ultimately be in vain as long as the king and his courtiers felt that they could intervene in the prosecutions whenever they wished. This they did frequently in the late 1670s. For example, Lord Arlington, the lord chamberlain, wrote to the College in 1678 that

> His Majesty hath commanded me to acquaint you that he would have you stop further prosecution of Mr. Russell concerning his practice of physic: In regard of His Majesty hath admitted him into his service, he having been a practitioner about this city for the space of thirty years; and remained here in time of the great plague, and did great good to the public at that time; of which I desire an account from you, that I may inform His Majesty of your compliance herein.[28]

With orders like this from the Crown, the College could only use its powers of suit against unprotected practitioners, a not wholly satisfactory situation.

Undoubtedly some tension and misunderstanding remained between the Crown and the College in the 1670s. Dr. Edmund King presented a letter in 1676 from Charles II requesting that the College make him an honorary fellow. (He was a surgeon who practiced chemical medicine and who had come to the attention of the king, obtaining a Lambeth degree in 1671; he would be knighted in 1686.) The College refused the king's petition after some debate.[29] In 1677 Charles II paid a royal visit, not to the College, but to the new laboratory of the Society of Apothecaries.[30] Other troubles surfaced, as well: in 1676, three physicians demanded the right to practice in London by virtue of their Cambridge degrees alone; in February of 1678, two physicians demanded the right to practice lithotomy and to cure dropsy victims, respectively, in accordance with Charles's decree of June 12, 1672, that immigrants from the United Provinces

---

[27]"The Colledge of Physitians and Needham," 3 Keble, 672, *English Reports* 84.

[28]Annals, 4:143a. Russell had been licensed by the king in August 1667 (*Calendar of State Papers Domestic, Domestic Correspondence,* July 1667, vol. 211, 123).

[29]Annals, 4:120a–121b; S.P. 44/27/199.

[30]"Sundry Account and Memoranda Book, Apothecaries Company," Guildhall MS no. 8204, 1677.

would be given the same privileges as Englishmen.[31] A fundamental change of policy by the Crown was required before it and the College could see eye to eye on medical regulation. That change occurred after the Exclusion Crisis of 1679.

A Reassertion of Regulation

As the English Crown grew stronger and less penurious in the later 1670s, suspicions regarding its political and religious goals also grew. The turmoil that resulted from the Popish Plot in the autumn of 1678 threatened to bring down the government. The crisis did bring down Danby, but Charles II managed to weather both it and the Exclusion Crisis of 1679 in good order, dismissing opposition leaders from the government in 1680 and soon thereafter embarking on a period of rule without a Parliament.

The decline in parliamentary power and the rise in royal authority in the end helped the College to restore medical regulation, for it had always been more successful in gaining friends at court than in warding off opposition from rivals in the Parliament. Moreover, like the Crown, the College was suspected by the Parliament of harboring members of the papist conspiracy. On March 29, 1679, the College received the following message from the House of Lords:

> It is ordered by the Lords Spiritual and Temporal in Parliament now assembled that the governors or principal members now in town of the several societies of Doctors Commons, the College of Physicians, and the Heralds' Office, do forthwith, bring into this House the names of such members of their respective societies as are papists or reputed papists and that they do [as] soon as regularly they can expel out of their several societies all such persons as shall not give testimony of their being Protestants by going to church, receiving the sacrament, and by making such oaths, and making and subscribing such texts and declarations as are appointed by any law for distinguishing Protestants from papists; and that none be hereafter admitted into any of the said societies that shall not do the same.

Charles II followed this order by issuing letters patent to the College to administer the Oath of Supremacy and the Oath of Obedience. The College instructed its Catholic members John Betts and Thomas

---

[31] Annals, 4:116a–116b, 127a–127b.

Short to take the oaths at the next meeting. But too few members were present—perhaps purposefully—at that meeting to make up a quorum, and so Betts and Short never had to take them.[32]

The political situation also caused some differences between members of the College that showed up outside the meetings of the group. For instance, the Catholic Thomas Short greatly increased his practice by taking on many of the aristocrats who left Richard Lower after Lower sided with the Whigs.[33] The factional splits in the College could be papered over during a period of relative weakness, but within a few years, as political tensions heightened and royal authority grew, they were bound to surface again on questions of College policy.

Contributing to future disputes was the intellectual diversification of the College of Physicians in the late 1670s and early 1680s. For nearly a decade, few collegiate physicians had participated in the activities of the Royal Society. But the Royal Society was becoming more active again in the later 1670s and was attracting renewed public interest.[34] A number of physicians began to be active in the society once again,[35] and some of them were soon made members of the College. The College seems to have been reaching out to those who would bring it into touch with the latest intellectual fashions.

Several among the physicians active in the Royal Society were either recruited to the College or were given a weightier role in the College around 1680. Nehemiah Grew, an important naturalist and one of the most active members of the Royal Society in the later 1670s and early 1680s (as well as secretary to the society from 1677 to 1679 and a member of its council in 1675 and 1677 to 1683), was made an honorary fellow of the College of Physicians in 1680, an honorary

---

[32]Annals, 4:134b–136a.

[33]W. R. Munk, *The Roll of the Royal College of Physicians*, vol. 1, 1518–1700, pp. 354–56. Lower had in turn taken over the practice of Thomas Willis (Kenneth Dewhurst, *Thomas Willis as a Physician* [Los Angeles: William Andrews Clark Memorial Library, 1964], p. 16), and Short's practice came to John Radcliffe on Short's death in 1685. (Short was said to have died by poisoning after spreading the rumor that Charles II had been poisoned to death.)

[34]See Lotte and Glenn Mulligan, "Reconstructing Restoration Science: Styles of Leadership and Social Composition of the Early Royal Society," *Social Studies of Science* 11 (1981): 327–64; and Michael Hunter, "Reconstructing Restoration Science: Problems and Pitfalls in Institutional History," *Social Studies of Science* 12 (1982): 451–66.

[35]Mulligan and Mulligan, "Reconstructing Restoration Science," p. 337, table 2; and Michael Hunter, *The Royal Society and Its Fellows, 1660–1700*. The manuscript index to the "Classified Papers" in the archives of the Royal Society bears out the point about M.D.s participating actively in the society until 1668 or 1669 and then again after about 1675.

fellow only, since he possessed a Leiden M.D. that had not been incorporated at Oxford or Cambridge because of his nonconformity.[36] Martin Lister was another important naturalist member of the Royal Society. He practiced medicine in York from 1670 to 1683 and corresponded frequently with the society, to which he was elected a member in 1671. Then, in 1683, he obtained an Oxford M.D. on the recommendation of the chancellor and moved to London, where he became an active participant in the society's meetings (and a member of its council from 1683 to 1685). Lister was made a candidate of the College in 1684. Edward Tyson, an important naturalist and comparative anatomist, joined the Royal Society in 1679 and became very active (he was a member of the council in 1681, 1683, and 1685). He obtained his M.D. at Cambridge in 1680 and became a candidate of the College the same year.

Somewhat less renowned men followed a similar pattern. Frederick Slare took his M.D. at Utrecht in 1679 and returned to England and incorporated it at Oxford in 1680. He joined the Royal Society the same year, becoming a very active member (and a councilman in 1682 and 1684). The College admitted him as a candidate in 1681. Thomas Allen, who had been made a fellow of the College in 1671, had been active in the Royal Society in the late 1660s but then had ceased to attend its meetings. In the late 1670s, however, he again became active in the Royal Society and also took the position of censor in the College in 1674, 1679, and 1682. Less active members of the Royal Society who were also members of the College of Physicians were Andrew Clench (fellow Royal Society, 1680, fellow College of Physicians, 1680), Walter Mills (F.R.S. 1682, F.C.P. 1683), and Thomas Novell (F.R.S. 1681, F.C.P. 1680).[37] Other active and inactive physician members of the Royal Society joined the College of Physicians under special circumstances in 1687. Many of these physicians made their way through the channels of the Royal Society first, joining the College afterward.

Although the College of Physicians did not have a "unified intellectual strategy"[38] in the later 1670s and early 1680s, some fellows

---

[36]Michael Hunter, "Early Problems in Professionalizing Scientific Research: Nehemiah Grew (1641–1712) and the Royal Society, with an Unpublished Letter to Henry Oldenburg," *Notes and Records of the Royal Society* 36 (1982): 189–209.

[37]Information on the activity of physician members of the Royal Society is taken from Hunter, *Royal Society*.

[38]The phrase is Theodore M. Brown's, in his *The Mechanical Philosophy and the "Animal Oeconomy": A Study in the Development of English Physiology in the Seventeenth and Early Eighteenth Centuries*, pp. 167, 177–78. Brown believes that an intellectual "unification" took place in the College and was the necessary prerequisite for the regulatory activities of the later 1670s and early 1680s.

had been following developments on the Continent and in England with interest. The works of Steno, Malpighi, and Borelli on the Continent made approaches to medical theory based on the mechanical philosophy viable. Walter Charleton's anatomy lectures of 1679 at the College were in an "iatromechanical" vein.[39] Other members of the College remained old-fashioned vitalists or simply noncommitted practitioners who lacked a strong philosophical orientation. Martin Lister, for example, encouraged Edward Tyson's work on insects "though some of late of our people have bespatted this kind of study, as despicable and unbecoming a physician."[40] The 1680s may not have been a period of intellectual consensus in the College, yet supporters of new medical philosophies derived from the new science were allowed to enter the College and participate in it. It seems likely that an attempt to play to the latest intellectual fashions in which the court participated (although to a lesser degree than in the 1660s) led the College to become more intellectually diverse around 1680.

Then, as the immediate political crisis passed around 1680 and the government grew stronger, the College of Physicians acted to make itself legally stronger, too. Many of its senior members, including its president, Sir John Micklethwaite, were physicians to the king and his courtiers and so could use their influence to increase the political support of the College. The College also sought the opinion of counsel (Sir Francis Pemberton) on the ability of the College "to constitute different orders of men in their own faculty," among other things.[41] Receiving a positive reply, the College reinstituted the process of admitting honorary fellows, thus increasing its support among physicians who had not become members by the normal channels.[42] Also, in October of 1680, Sir John Holt (later chief justice

---

[39]Brown (*Mechanical Philosophy*, p. 175) believes that these lectures were "the College's formal announcement of total support for the iatromechanical approach to medicine"; I believe that intellectual diversity, even among "iatromechanists," was the rule of the day. For a discussion of various approaches to medical theory in the period, see Lester S. King, *The Philosophy of Medicine: The Early Eighteenth Century* (Cambridge: Harvard University Press, 1978).

[40]Quoted in Mulligan and Mulligan, "Reconstructing Restoration Science," p. 333.

[41]"Opinion of Counsel on the power of the College to constitute different orders of men . . . ," R.C.P., box 9, env. 172.

[42]In September 1680, the following persons became honorary fellows: Robert Wittie, John Windebank, William Stokeham, William Burnett, Nehemiah Grew, Henry Sampson, Daniel Coxe the elder, Christopher Love Morley, John Master, Francis Bernard, Thomas Gibson, John Garrett, and Jones. Their political and religious views ranged from Whiggery to staunch Royalism, from Catholicism to nonconformity; their medical and scientific views from old-fashioned notions to contemporary mechanical ones.

of King's Bench) was consulted by the College about its proceedings in the court of Chancery against a fellow, Christopher Merrett.[43]

In November of 1681 the censors took more testimony against illicit practitioners and decided to prosecute in other courts Adrian Huyberts, Frederick Harder, and Charles Blagrave. Interference came from the royal court, but this time to no avail. The earl of Arlington wrote a letter on Frederick Harder's behalf. When a few months later, in June 1682, a letter in the name of the king was addressed to the College in order to stop its prosecutions of Gerard Van Mullen, however, the College replied firmly:

> We humbly beg leave to inform Your Majesty, that we are bound by solemn oath, by law, and by the duty we owe both to Your Majesty and to the safety of your subjects, by due course of law to prosecute all empirics, and other illegal practitioners of physic whatsoever in London, and within seven miles thereof. . . .
> We therefore humbly beseech Your Majesty to leave this matter wholly to the due course and determination of Your Majesty's laws.[44]

By the elections of 1682, a clear turning point had been passed in the College's attempts to regain its regulatory authority. A further shake-up among the officers occurred, and in December the College ordered the names of all duly elected members to be published.[45] Legal advice was sought, and opinions were rendered on a number of questions. The College's lawyers (Bollenson and Saunders) agreed that practitioners could not legally practice by virtue of medical degrees from Oxford or Cambridge or of a bishop's license alone. Moreover, they found that "if any person goes to an empiric or an unlicensed physician and acquaints him with his sickness, or carries his urine, and receives a medicine from him for it with advice [on] how to use it, and pays money to such [an] empiric thereupon," the College could prosecute that practitioner.[46] On the basis of these opinions, the officers of the College believed they could sit as a court

---

[43]Annals, 4:159a, 161b. Merrett carried on a longstanding dispute with the College, trying to regain his position as Harveian Librarian. He was expelled in September of 1681 on the grounds that he did not come to a meeting to which he had been summoned.

[44]Annals, 5:1a–2a.

[45]Annals, 5:6b; the new officers were Thomas Coxe (president), Daniel Whistler (elect), and Samuel Collins, Sr. (registrar).

[46]"Legal Opinion on several cases relating to the College of Physicians . . . ," R.C.P., 2012/54–55; "Legal Opinion re propriety of the College of Physicians issuing licenses to practice outside of London," R.C.P., 2014/1.

once again. The president and the censors soon began to do so for the first time in more than twenty years.

The political climate also favored the College, for 1682 saw the beginnings of a renewed attack by the Crown on the chartered corporations.[47] First striking at the City of London, the Crown moved to gain clear-cut control of all corporations, both to exert more control over their personnel (and thereby also to influence elections to the Parliament) and to control the administration of justice better.[48] The City had again become the catalyst for parliamentary agitation against the Crown from 1679 to 1682, many in Parliament believing that the City's financial struggle to avoid bankruptcy would never succeed as long as it was governed by a pro-court set of aldermen. The attack on the corporations may not have been done with an "ideology" of "absolutism" in mind.[49] But many corporations that did not elect M.P.s, including the London livery companies, were remodeled. And in the remodeling, the Crown clearly favored loyal subjects, through quo warranto proceedings coming to control more closely the affairs of the kingdom.[50] The City companies were purged of Whigs. In this atmosphere, bodies that acted as agents of the Crown would obviously be favored, and the College officers sought to take advantage of the situation.

Moreover, at least one important element of public opinion favored the College's resurgence. Edward Chamberlayne, a doctor of laws, published the fourteenth edition of a book titled *Angliae Notitia, Or the Present State of England*, in 1682. It included a section on the College of Physicians that specified that "no man, though a graduate in physic of Oxford or Cambridge, may, without license under the said College seal, practice physic in London or within seven miles of the City. . . . Whereby also they can administer an oath, [and] fine and imprison any offenders." Chamberlayne then listed the members of the College by name. He ended with an expression of his opinion that probably reflected the views of at least a few others:

---

[47]On the background to the incorporations, see Shelagh Bond and Norman Evans, "The Process of Granting Charters to English Boroughs, 1547–1649," *English Historical Review* 91 (1976): 102–20; and Robert Tittler, "The Incorporation of Boroughs, 1540–1558," *History* 62 (1977): 24–42.

[48]See Jennifer Levin, *The Charter Controversy in the City of London, 1660–1688, and Its Consequences,* pp. 2–21.

[49]John Leslie Miller, "The Potential for 'Absolutism' in Later Stuart England," *History* 69 (1984): 187–207; idem, "The Crown and the Borough Charters in the Reign of Charles II," *English Historical Review* 100 (1985): 53–84.

[50]Miller, "Crown and the Borough Charters," p. 56; Levin, *Charter Controversy,* p. 87.

Besides the worthy persons mentioned in the list above, there are diverse physicians that have good practice in London, although they never had any license, which is connived at by the College, and so is the too much practice of empirics, mountebanks, pretended chemists, apothecaries, surgeons, wise-women, etc. In which piece of folly, the English surpass all the nations of Christendom.[51]

Here was a clear public mandate for the College to act aggressively to clean up the medical marketplace.

By 1683, therefore, the College bore down harder. It voted for the first time to fine any member who consulted with an empiric £10.[52] Most of its meetings were taken up with hearing complaints and with taking actions against various illegal practitioners. Most remarkably, at the autumn elections John Knight became a third *consiliarius*—only two were allowed by College statute. But Knight was Charles II's favorite surgeon and had been granted an M.D. by the king's mandate before he became a licentiate of the College in 1675. The close alliance between College and Crown that had been lacking since 1640 apparently was becoming reestablished. Furthermore, the College obtained another legal opinion from Justice Holt specifying that the College could prosecute anyone in King's Bench who practiced within seven miles of London without the "express license under the common seal" of the College.[53]

Of course, ordinary practitioners did not much like the situation. Nathaniel Merry published a book full of the familiar grievances: scholastic medicine was inferior to chemical medicine; the College was not suing Merry and others for malpractice (since they practiced well) but for illicit practice, which was a perversion of English law; the anatomical discoveries of the physicians did not help the cure of diseases any more than painted glass helps light get into a room; since chemical medicine was not developed when the College was first chartered, the College ought not to govern chemists any more that fletchers, bowyers, and bow-string makers ought to regulate gunsmiths; and, finally, the physicians' methods of treatment were harmful to the patient.[54] Someone else who disliked the College's actions tried to undo them by putting about the rumor at court that

[51]Edward Chamberlayne, *Angliae Notitia, Or the Present State of England* (14th ed., 1682), pp. 275, 277–81.
[52]This became a College statute in 1684.
[53]"Legal Opinion re Power of College over Extra-Licentiates," R.C.P., 2014/2.
[54][Nathaniel Merry], *A Plea of the Chymists or Non-Colegiates: Or, Considerations Natural, Rational, and Legal, in Relation to Medicine* (1683).

the College's last Harveian Oration had been seditious in some manner. The bishop of London was asked to look into it, but he found the address "quite different from what was represented and the address full and proper without any alteration."[55]

By 1684 the College of Physicians had begun to get its affairs in order. It was undertaking measures to get out of the last of the debts incurred from the rebuilding of the College. Sir John Cutler came to its assistance.[56] That summer, Charles Goodall published *The Royal College of Physicians of London Founded and Established by Law* in two volumes.

Dedicated to Francis, Lord Guildford, the lord keeper of the Great Seal, Goodall's book was clearly intended to make public all the pieces of law granting the College regulatory power. Goodall took up a theme promoted for several decades by many physicians of the College: "We have to deal with a sort of men not of academical, but mechanical education," he wrote, "who being either actually engaged in the late rebellion, or bred upon some mean and contemptible trades, were never taught the duty they owe God or their sovereign, to their native country or the laws thereof." Goodall therefore hoped that Lord Guildford would help to defend the College, which had been established by royal grants and acts of Parliament, "thus rudely assaulted by barbarous and illiterate mechanics."[57]

Since Goodall's volumes are almost always considered an objective account of the legal powers of the College, even being used in contemporary legal declarations,[58] an investigation of how Goodall composed his book is in order. In volume one, Goodall published in full the acts and charters of the sixteenth century governing medical practice and the charters granted to the College by James I (October 1618) and Charles II (March 26, 1664). He also gave the full text of the Society of Apothecaries' charter. He did not indicate that neither James I's nor Charles II's charters had been ratified by Parliament, nor did he hint at charters issued by Cromwell. What he published seemed to be clear (and royal) authority given to the College over the apothecaries and other practitioners of physic.[59] Goodall then reported a number of

---

[55]S.P. 29/429/180.

[56]Annals, 5:28b–29b. Cutler's "gift" later turned out to be a loan, much to the College's dismay.

[57]Charles Goodall, *The Royal College of Physicians of London Founded and Established by Law*, 2 vols. (1684), sig. A4.

[58]"The College of Physicians against Salmon," 5 Mod., 327, *English Reports* 87.

[59]Goodall, *Royal College*, pp. 1–146.

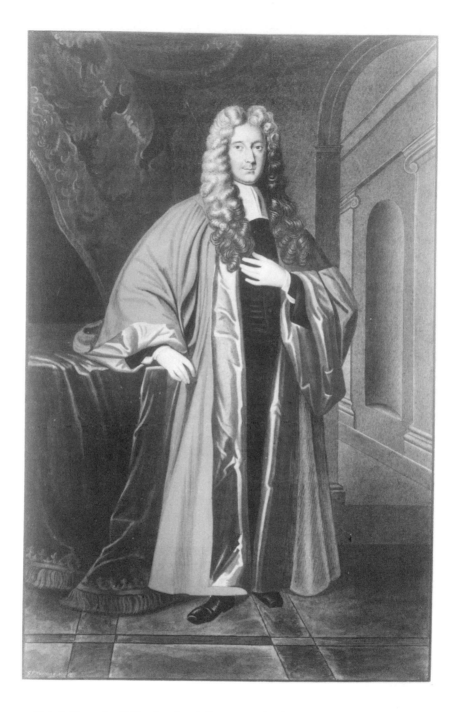

Plate 8. Portrait of Charles Goodall. Watercolor by G. P. Harding, 1810, after
T. Murray. Courtesy of the Wellcome Institute Library, London.

legal cases.[60] He gave no indication of the 1656 trials that so seriously damaged the College's ability to act against others, or of the case of Goddard in 1661 and 1662 that did not restore Goddard to the fellowship because the case concerned "no matter of government." Assorted statutes concerning the College's power over university graduates in physic, and exemptions for College physicians from watch and ward, the militia, and so on were also printed.[61] The impression that these testimonies leave on the reader is of a strong and fully empowered body of physicians granted complete regulatory powers. Only the omitted things could explain why the College had not acted on this seemingly clear authority for over twenty-five years. But the sins of omission no doubt meant that the book made a good impression on jurists, courtiers, public officials, and Goodall's colleagues.

In his second volume, Goodall tried to reinforce this good opinion by recounting how the College had in the past driven certain empirics from London and by supplying information on the lives of eminent College fellows. And he repeated, addressing the College, that the "primary cause of [its] incorporation [was] the restraining and suppressing illiterate, inexperienced, and unlicensed practitioners," while the secondary cause was to encourage learned practitioners.[62] Goodall tried to show how these goals had been achieved, thus creating the impression of a group of strong and successful physicians acting in the public interest to expel unlearned practitioners from London. The men given short biographies by Goodall had been or were researchers—again, the court's respect for advances in learning influenced the College's public image.[63] Goodall's account is accurate insofar as it goes, but by selecting evidence and accounts it creates an impression of the College of Physicians that is misleading—although successful.

This book, plus the actions of the Crown, moved the College ever more closely toward the position it had occupied in the 1630s.[64] As it

[60]Ibid., pp. 147–224. The cases were: the *College* v. *Gardiner, Bonham, Butler, Buggs, Huyberts,* and *Nedham.*

[61]Ibid., pp. 275–88.

[62]Ibid., vol. 2, p. v.

[63]Goodall writes of Linacre, Bartlot, Freeman, Owen, Caius, James, Goulston, Harvey, Glisson, Micklethwaite, Wharton, and Willis; and of those still living at the time, Whistler, Ent, Scarburgh, Charleton, Croune, Lower, Needham, and Sydenham (the only licentiate among the group).

[64]The same process was occurring in other corporations with regulatory authority: see particularly Cyprian Blagden, *The Stationers' Company: A History, 1403–1959* (London: George Allen and Unwin, 1960), pp. 152–72.

had in the past, the College rearranged its officers in the autumn of 1684 to take advantage of the situation. Sir Thomas Witherly, a physician to the king, became president; Sir Charles Scarburgh, also a royal physician and a firm supporter of strong royal government, became a *consiliarius;* and Peter Barwick and John Betts the Catholic became elects. The embarrassing fact of former President Whistler's embezzlement of College funds in 1684 was quietly investigated and passed over in silence.[65] The rival London corporations of apothecaries and barber-surgeons were on the political defensive, having been forced to spend about £200 apiece getting their charters renewed by the Crown.[66] More importantly, Charles II died in February of 1685, making his brother, James, king; and James II wished even more than Charles to bolster the authority of the monarchy.

The College and James II

James II had been one of the most important of his brother's advisers since 1679; given the opportunity to rule, he pushed even harder for an authoritative central government. From his father's execution, James came to believe that kings should always be firm and that only ill-willed rebels would oppose a steady king.[67] As king, he began to build up the standing army that William III and Marlborough would later use so effectively against France. A Catholic, James sought to have Catholics granted full liberties. He also continued the attack on the corporations in order to ensure the loyalty of these significant units of administrative authority. If the College of Physicians needed a firm hand at the tiller of government in order to restore its full capabilities to prosecute its rivals, then the College could look forward to a bright future with James II in charge.

The alliance between the king and the College was forged formally, not simply through the influence of the royal physicians. On October 19, 1685, the College learned that its charter would be called in by quo warranto during the following term. The members of the College decided not to wait, but to hand the charter over immediate-

---

[65]Annals, 5:26b; Daniel Whistler, "Inventory of his goods, chattles, and debts, 1684," R.C.P., box 9, env. 109.

[66]"Collection of Copy Acts and Ordinances, together with other papers relating to the regulation of the Apothecary Society, 1618–1743," Guildhall MS no. 8293; "Miscelleaneous Papers of the Barber-Surgeons' Company, 1612–1763," Guildhall MS no. 9833.

[67]John Leslie Miller, *James II: A Study in Kingship,* p. 11.

ly and voluntarily, asking for changes in their favor. During 1686, as the charter was being redrawn, only two meetings were held: one to admit more fellows (the College had decided to go from forty to sixty or even eighty, and to admit no one except faithful subjects— "*fidelis subditus*"), the other to reply to a letter from Robert Spencer, earl of Sunderland, one of James's closest advisors.[68]

As he had during the reign of Charles II, Sunderland had written to try to stop the College's prosecution of an unlicensed practitioner, Nathaniel Merry (who had written a treatise against the College in 1683): "He being particularly recommended to me for an honest and ingenious man, I thought it not amiss to desire your favor towards him, in your discharging him from his present confinement." But negotiations were going well for the issuance of a new charter, and the College respectfully refused Sunderland's request, explaining that it had been "informed that [Merry] is a person of no learning, of a mean and mechanical education, having done much hurt to the King's subjects by his ignorant and evil practice." Therefore, instead of releasing Merry (he had been imprisoned for refusing to pay a fine of forty pounds to the College), the College hoped to gain His Lordship's help against Merry and other "unlawful and unskillful practitioners: especially considering that our prosecutions of this nature are undertaken only for the public service, with great trouble and charge and no advantage to ourselves." President Witherly and Sir Thomas Millington formally (and no doubt respectfully) presented the College's reply to Sunderland, who then left Merry's fate up to the College.[69]

The College also published a short pamphlet condensed by Goodall from his *The Royal College of Physicians,* probably for distribution at court. The pamphlet countered charges of monopoly by stating that an unlimited number of Englishmen could be licentiates, so that "no person can be excluded out of the College, or debarred from practice, but such as are so wholly illiterate and unskillful, that they dare not adventure to submit themselves to the examination and judgement of . . . the College . . . though the President and Censors be men strictly sworn to do justice to all persons." The pamphlet continued:

From hence it manifestly follows, that the College of Physicians is very far from be[ing] a monopoly, since it cannot reject any of the King's subjects who are duly qualified for the exercise of all, or any part of

[68] Annals, 5:51a–53b; *Entry Book,* 71/194.
[69] Annals, 5:54a–55a.

physic; and therefore, all pretenders to secret medicines, or to the practice of physic, without license first had from the College, are justly prosecuted and punished as public cheats and impostors.

An outline of the legal powers of the College followed, and the conclusion clearly aligned the College with privilege and the "public good":

> We are also fully resolved, for the public good, to encourage and protect those two necessary instruments of physic, the surgeons and the apothecaries . . . so long as they shall contain themselves within the limits of their own professions; and in short, to do all other things necessary for the vindication and perpetuating of the faculty of physic, that so the young students in our universities, may not be discouraged from applying themselves to the study of a science, so useful to the commonwealth; nor that the profession be invaded by the vulgar, which hath been the usual support of the younger sons of the gentry of this kingdom.[70]

By February 1687 all the College's points had been accepted by the crown, and the College gained the right to "license the printing and publishing of books, etc. relating to physic and surgery," while the law officers drew up a new and much stronger charter.[71] That new charter was presented to the College during a feast on April 12, 1687. Under the new order, the Crown did not bother to present it to a Parliament for ratification as it had in 1664.

In the words of James II, the new charter gave the College all its former rights "together with other privileges and more ample authority for suppressing all illiterate and illegal practitioners of the art of physic in our City of London and seven miles distance." In June, James II issued letters expanding on this "more ample authority"; these letters were kept secret until after they were officially signed, in July.[72] In part, the letters said that James

> will[ed] and require[d] you the President and Censors of our said College and your successors, in pursuance of our said letters patent, as also of the laws and statutes of our realm, forthwith to do your utmost

---

[70][Charles Goodall], *A Short Account of the Institution and Nature of the College of Physicians, London. Publish'd by Themselves* (1686), pp. 2–3, 7.
[71]S.P. 44/56/362; 44/337/201.
[72]Annals, 5:58a–60b.

diligence to prosecute and suppress all such unlearned and unlawful practitioners of physic, as shall presume to act contrary to our said letters patent, and to the laws of the realm in that case provided.

Not only did the College regain all its old privileges and more, but it also received a mandate from the Crown to act on them.[73] Also, the number of fellows was doubled from forty to eighty, and the fees were increased, resulting in an immediate income for the College of £1,695.[74] For what more could the officers of the College have wished?

Yet, the College did receive an even better authorization. In order to make sure that everyone understood that medical regulation by the College of Physicians was now a matter of concern to the Crown, James's letters went on:

And for your encouragement we do require all our judges, Justices of the Peace and others whom it may concern to countenance and assist you the President and Censors in your prosecution of such offenders according to law; and for the more effectual doing thereof, you are as occasion shall offer to demand the aid and assistance of the Lord Mayor and Aldermen of our City of London, whom by our letter we have required to give you all countenace and assistance in the execution of our royal will and command, not doubting but that you will be careful to suppress such offenders and answer the trust in this case committed to you.

Copies of the letters prepared by James went to the lord mayor of London and "to all Justices, Mayors, sheriffs, bailiffs, constables, head-boroughs, and all other His Majesty's officers and ministers to whom this shall appertain, within the City of London, [the] suburbs and liberties thereof, and the limits within mentioned, and to every and either [each] of them."[75]

Not surprisingly, the College wasted little time in seizing the initiative, first by enacting new statutes governing the behavior of members and then by undertaking prosecutions for the violation of those statutes or of the new authority given its members over other practitioners by the charter and letters of James II.

[73]The charter of James II is reprinted in Clark, pp. 418–25.
[74]"Rationes Accepti et Expensi in Collegio Medico. Londinensium," R.C.P. 2073, fols. 35–36.
[75]Annals, 5:58b–60b.

The statutes were stricter than ever before, and they became a bone of contention in future years. They declared that no member of the College could write Latin directions for the use of medicine on a prescription (to prevent the apothecaries from learning physic); that no member could send his prescriptions to an apothecary who had been in trouble with the College; that no surgeon or apothecary could join the College without first having renounced his respective guild; that any member who did not pay his subscriptions, fees, dues, or fines could be expelled from the College; that those expelled could gain readmission only by acknowledging their faults and paying their fines; that no College member could print anything without the permission of the College (to avoid having members advertise their practices); that a ten-man committee of delegates would see to the College's profit and dignity; and that steps be taken to prevent anyone from being able to defraud the College. Other statutes restricted the consultations between members of the College (including licentiates) and nonmembers.[76]

The College faced other institutions with renewed confidence. At the end of August, the lord mayor agreed to cooperate with the College by proclaiming James II's order at Guildhall.[77] By October, the newly elected *comitia censorum* was hearing cases in extraordinary numbers, numbers that were unprecedented in the College's history (see appendix 2, table 1).[78] As before, most of this activity struck at illicit practitioners (see appendix 2, table 3). In addition, in November of 1687, the College sent a letter to the bishops of England informing them that the College would now be censoring all books pertaining to physic, and in January of 1688, the College received permission from the Crown to publish the letters of James authorizing such extraordinary support for the College.[79] Moreover, in 1688 the College's lawyers advised that everything the College was doing was entirely legal and was supported by the new charter.[80]

All in all, the College that appeared during 1688 was a body that was more inclusive, both in terms of the numbers of men listed as

---

[76]Annals, 5:60b–65a.

[77]Annals, 5:61a–63a.

[78]The president was Sir Thomas Witherly, a royal physician; the body of censors consisted of John Betts and John Elliott, both Catholics, and Robert Pitt and John Bateman (Pitt having been made a member by James's charter, Bateman being known as one of the authoritarians in the College).

[79]Annals, 5:68b–69b; S.P. 31/4/4; 44/337/382.

[80]"Opinions on Legal Powers of the Censors," R.C.P., 2003/22–26; "Legal Opinions [of Serj. Creswell Levinz] re confirmation of College statutes, etc.," R.C.P., 2012/6–8.

fellows by James's charter and in terms of the somewhat lower standards of preparation in academic physic exhibited by some of the new fellows. The College's intellectual vitality (if not its academic composition) did rise perceptibly with the infusion of a number of physicians who were active in the Royal Society. Among the new fellows in this category who were named in James's charter were Walter Needham, Henry Paman, Robert Pitt, Hans Sloane, Tancred Robinson, and Richard Robinson. But few of them had endured the long study in the texts at university necessary to gain an academic M.D.

At the same time, the College was a more disciplinarian institution, both in the way in which its members were regulated and in the way it prosecuted outsiders. When the institution no longer stood for the highest standards of academic learning in physic and yet imposed its will as never before, there were bound to be strong objections. But as long as James II ruled, they were not voiced.

The College found itself obligated, however, to do something to benefit the realm other than simply expelling other practitioners if it was to live up to royal expectations for the public good. An active College of Physicians was supposed to benefit the public. Therefore, in July of 1687, it was decided to have all members give free medical treatment at their residences to paupers of London parishes and all other parishes within the College's seven-mile jurisdiction. This practice would undercut the business of empirics, apothecaries, and surgeons, as well as make the College an instrument of charity. But in August of 1688, it was reported that this system was not working, because the physicians did not want to pay for the medicines they gave out, and if patients merely got a prescription for expensive medicines, they would not bother to come to the physicians. It was therefore decided that many of the medicines would be made in the College's own laboratory, that the room next-door would be set aside as a repository, and that these steps would be funded by subscriptions and run by a committee.[81] This plan of action soon became central to the designs of the College.

As might have been anticipated, the new activity against other practitioners and the inclusion of many new fellows by virtue of their being named in James II's charter caused some friction among College members. Andrew Clench, for example, was an independent soul who did not believe that the College ought to regulate practitioners. Although a fellow, he had accused other fellows of ignorant and unsound practice for the second time in 1682, for which he had

[81] Annals, 5:60a–60b, 86a–86b.

been fined eight pounds. In 1683 he had promised not to be so friendly with the empiric Samuel Haworth. Then, in early 1687, soon after
the College had received its new charter, Clench was still refusing to
pay his fines, and he angrily accused the censors of bad behavior—
after which he was expelled. He continued to make abusive refer-
ences to the "new College." By December of 1687, however, the
College and the Crown forced him to present a letter of apology or
face being driven from London. His first letter was not accepted
because it was not submissive enough. Clench appealed to the lord
chancellor but was forced to swallow his pride and submit a more
abject apology to the College in February, which regained him his
seat.[82] Such tactics alienated some of the more libertarian members of
the College, especially those having empiric or apothecary friends
and associates.

Internal divisions in the "new College" were brought about by
other matters, too. In August 1687 the censors renewed visitations to
apothecaries' shops, something College members had not done for
many years. Another decision was made regarding the apothecaries
in August, but no information is recorded in the Annals, since it was
to be kept secret. In December it was proposed that the inspections of
shops include an inspection of the apothecaries' records in order to
ascertain whether anyone (including fellows) had dealings with empirics. But this proposed method of controlling the medical marketplace caused "some heats" to arise "between some of the members of the College, fitter to be forgotten than registered."[83]

On March 28, 1688, the lord chancellor was forced to intervene in
the College's affairs, since he had been given petitions from the
Apothecaries' and Barber-Surgeons' companies against the censors'
aggressive actions. He privately told the College that "the occasion of
his visiting was the great outcry in the town of the physicians injuring
both the surgeons and apothecaries." He clearly sympathized with
the physicians, but he "could not refuse" to look into the complaints.
In April 1688 the College sent a delegation to the chancellor to explain its position at greater length. The "heats" between members
continued: Richard Lower and Charles Scarburgh engaged in a bitter
quarrel in May 1688. It is likely that Lower, a Whig (and a man

[82]Annals, 5:8b, 18b, 57a–57b, 66a, 71a–71b, 72a–74b. Clench was murdered in 1692 by
a lawyer who was angry about the price of rents Clench charged tenants in one of the many
properties he owned in London.

[83]Annals, 5:63a, 61a, 71a–71b. The apothecaries' shops had not been formally visited by
officers of the College since the early 1660s.

whose father had suffered for his Quaker beliefs), disliked the College's activities against other practitioners, while Scarburgh, a Royalist and a physician to James II, encouraged them.[84] But whether these internal divisions might have led to difficulties for the College soon became moot. The long shadow of impending political turmoil again touched the physicians.

Unluckily for the authoritarians in the College of Physicians, James II's moves toward tightening the reigns of government were making his position difficult after the religious blunders and "absolutist" activities of 1687.[85] By the spring of 1688 it was becoming clear to James and his advisers that he could not continue to press for the kind of government he envisaged. The birth of a male heir and the acquittal of the Seven Bishops in June made his position almost untenable. As members of his government defected during the summer, James tried frantically to reverse some of his policies. Whether the College would have continued to receive the wholehearted support of James's government in the years after 1687 and 1688 soon became immaterial. In November, William of Orange landed an army and conquered England with hardly a shot fired. James's officers and soldiers slipped over to the other side. Once again, the College would have to find its way in a new political environment.

The strong governments that existed during the last years of the reign of Charles II and during the reign of James II supported the College of Physicians' attempts to restore its coercive powers of medical regulation in London. These governments hoped to control the realm better by extending the influence of corporations and individuals tied closely to the Crown. As the academic medicine of the physicians became less Galenic and more open to currents of empiricism, chemical medicine, and physiological research, it became ever harder to make the public aware of the distinctions between learned medicine and the medicine of the physicians' rivals. Institutional distinctions therefore became especially important to the more conservative members of the College. They took advantage of the Crown's willingness to exercise and extend its authority in order to exercise and extend their own. But with the revolution of 1688, the College entered a new period of confusion and factionalism before the political and intellectual climate turned squarely against the authoritarian academics at the end of the reign of William III.

[84]Annals, 5:76a–79a, 80a–81a; Clark, p. 449.
[85]I here follow the account of James R. Jones, *The Revolution of 1688 in England.*

6

The Decline of the Old Medical Order, 1689–1704

> "College of Physicians! What of them? by your leave, Doctor, I think the Company of Apothecaries very substantial men, and are able to buy twice your College. They are moneyed-men; and have an Interest almost everywhere. College of Physicians! they are learned men, they say, but what's that to money? Hah! Hah! Hah!"
>
> "Tom Gallypot" (modeled after John Badger),
> in Thomas Brown, *Physick lies a Bleeding,
> or the Apothecary turned Doctor*

The Glorious Revolution slowly brought a new political order into being, one in which Parliament had substantial influence in the councils of the Crown. For one hundred and fifty years, medical regulation had flourished under strong monarchs and had been forced into quiescence during times of political turmoil. The Crown remained outwardly strong under William III, especially under the period of the Whig Junto, but the ever louder voices in Parliament of the spokesmen for the City medical corporations, combined with both the continually growing respectability of nonacademic medicine and the loss of Collegiate influence in the rapidly expanding military services, boded ill for the College of Physicians' authority. The apothecaries were even found to be a "profession" by the House of Commons.

Even worse, the corporate solidarity of the institution was riven by factions to a greater degree than ever before. Both to benefit the public and to undermine the Society of Apothecaries, the officers of the College created the dispensary in the midst of their attempts to retain their corporation's authority. But not all fellows agreed with this and other steps taken to regain the power of the College. Moreover, after the Glorious Revolution many fellows opposed the older traditions of academic physic, while others of them objected to the new statutes of their institution and their enforcement. The notion that the College was a bastion of academic excellence in physic had been undermined by the large number of quickly educated physicians who had been admitted under the charter of James II. The institution seemed intent on enforcing discipline to rules but seemed to lack the moral authority to make it clear that this was for the good of physic. As a result, several physicians went so far as to make common cause with the College's opponents.

The House of Lords spoke against an important part of the College's regulatory power in the Rose case of 1703–04. Despite the law, the Lords allowed apothecaries the right to practice medicine. The decision signaled the nearing end of real medical regulation in London. The decadence of the old medical order was plain to all not much more than a decade after the revolution of 1688.

In the Aftermath of the Glorious Revolution

After William's November invasion and the flight of James to France, members of the College of Physicians faced deep uncertainty about their legal rights and privileges in the new constitutional order. The members of the College became increasingly divided on the direction the institution should take. In the immediate aftermath of the Glorious Revolution, the foremost question that divided the physicians was whether the "new College" of James II had any legal existence at all: a proclamation of October 17, 1688, had declared that all the corporation charters remodeled by James through quo warranto would be nullified, returning the corporations to the status quo ante. The charter the College operated under—the legally weak old charter that had been ratified by the Parliament during the reign of Henry VIII or the unratified charter of Charles II or the new charter of James II that had given the College both firmer police powers and twice the number of fellows—would make a significant difference to the institution and to other practitioners.

The answer to the problem of under which charter the College would act was in part a legal problem, but it was also a problem of policy. Fundamental choices concerning the very nature of the institution, therefore, divided the members, particularly since half the members would be forced out if the new charter was declared invalid. One of the first items of business for the College officers was to procure legal advice on whether the new charter was still valid. If it was, the members also needed to know whether they could retain eighty fellows and whether they could enforce the new statutes that they had enacted against disobedient members.

The College's attorney in the winter of 1688–89 was one of the best: Creswell Levinz, a Tory justice who had been dismissed from the bench under James II but who also had been one of the six justices who had defended the Seven Bishops. The considered opinion of this conservative but constitutionally concerned attorney was that the proclamation about James's remodeled charters did not apply to the College; although he did not put his reasons in writing, Levinz may have believed that the proclamation only applied to corporations that involuntarily submitted to quo warranto proceedings. Levinz also declared that the College could keep the number of fellows at eighty and require the obedience of its members to the statutes it had passed in 1688.[1] Opinions regarding the powers of the College to act against members and other practitioners were also solicited, and not only Levinz, but also Sir John Holt, soon to be chief justice of the King's Bench, declared in the affirmative for the College.[2]

After obtaining this expert legal counsel, the College took up the issue of the authority under which it would continue in a general meeting on March 19, 1689. A majority of the fellows (many of whom had been created fellows by the charter of James II) voted to continue to act under James's incorporation. A committee was therefore appointed "to take care" that it was not "accidentally included among [the] other charters that are likely to be vacated" by the new Parliament.[3]

The physicians then took their case to the public by publishing a broadside arguing that their institution could act under the authority that the last king had granted it. The new charter had merely restored the privileges of the charter of Charles II, it claimed. "And we humbly conceive that our late augmentation of fellows would not have met with any dislike, had it not happened at a time when the general surrender of charters gave a national offense; nor hath the College any

[1] "Legal Opinions [of Serj. Creswell Levinz] re confirmation of College statutes, etc." R.C.P., 2012/6–8.

[2] "Opinions on legal powers of the Censors, 1688," R.C.P., 2003/22–26 (Serjeants Pemberton, Levinz, and Holt, and Mr.s Bollenson and Finch).

[3] Annals, 5:96a–97a. The committee was composed of Millington, Gordon, Lower, Goodall, Elliott, Bateman, and Gill.

privileges granted contrary to law, or the common interest of the nation." A College with more members and greater strength, the physicians declared, "more encouraged the public good."[4]

But the "new College" took the course of maintaining the policies of the last years without internal unanimity and against the opposition of outsiders, as well. In January of 1689, Parliament had entered a petition of the Society of Apothecaries that opposed the searching of their shops by the officers of the College. Such searches, the apothecaries argued, were "to the prejudice of the Corporation and also of many patents."[5] The College in turn petitioned the parliamentary Committee on Grievances.[6] As in the past, however, petitioning Parliament brought out divisions within the College.

The first leader of the opposition to the institution created by James II was, surprisingly, the current president of the College, George Rogers. Rogers was trained in the old manner. His father had been a physician before him; the younger Rogers had studied physic at Padua, his father's alma mater, and had obtained his M.D. in 1646 at the age of twenty-eight; since the early 1680s he had held significant positions as an officer of the College. And yet Rogers objected to the charter of James II, not because he did not favor a College that acted against empirics (he did),[7] but apparently because the charter arbitrarily admitted so many new fellows, many of whom were not educated in the old manner.

The kind of medical training and practices a person took up was an issue that had always concerned the College, but it was a particularly significant issue at the end of the seventeenth century. More "doctors" than ever had degrees from foreign universities or mandated degrees from one of the two English universities, neither of which paths represented a training in traditional learned physic. Instead, notions of new "experimental" medicine were popular, even more than they had been during the 1660s. Many of the fellows admitted under the charter of James II were "moderns" in medicine.[8]

---

[4] *The Case of the College of Physicians*, London (1689).

[5] Quoted in C. R. B. Barrett, *The History of the Society of Apothecaries of London* (London: Elliot Stock, 1905), p. 110.

[6] Annals, 5:97a–97b.

[7] Rogers's *Oratio anniversaria . . . in commemorationem beneficiorum a Doctore Harveio* (1682) vigorously condemns illicit practitioners who, it states, were undermining academic physic.

[8] See Joseph M. Levine, "Ancients and Moderns Reconsidered," *Eighteenth-Century Studies* 15 (1981): 72–89; and G. S. Rousseau, "'Sowing the Wind and Reaping the Whirlwind': Aspects of Change in Eighteenth-Century Medicine," in *Studies in Change and Revolution: Aspects of English Intellectual History, 1640–1800*, ed. Paul J. Korshin, pp. 129–59.

One example of the kinds of problems some of the new "experimental" physicians were causing is provided by the case of John Colbatch, who was knighted by George I in 1716. A native of Worcester, he began as a practicing apothecary who experimented with chemical remedies. He opposed the then-popular notion that all diseases were caused by acids in the blood and that therefore the best remedies were alkalies. He had found that when he administered alkalies, they did little good, except for preparations of steel and antimony, which were, he discovered, in fact acidic.[9] Experimenting further, he found acidic remedies to be good in many cases, and so he developed a universal external remedy and a universal internal remedy of acidic kinds to be given to those suffering from wounds. He managed to get an appointment to the army of William III in Flanders and tried out his cures on wounded soldiers, basically applying a mild acid to the wounds and then bandaging them rather than trying to suppurate them. He claimed that all but one soldier were cured by this treatment, although this success led to jealousy on the part of surgeons, who tried to poison him and his friends (one of whom died).[10] He also advocated eating acidic food (oranges and lemons) to cure scurvy. All these remedies he ascribed to the "experimental philosophy" begun by Boyle.[11]

But not only surgeons called Colbatch's cures into doubt; so did well-educated physicians who thought that dividing the world into acidic and alkaline diseases and cures was far too simple. A long and bitter controversy over Colbatch's ideas ensued.[12] Both sides made public appeals through pamphlets. The appeal to the public of the new and "experimental" treatments of the nonacademic physicians, couched in simple schemes and backed by seemingly apparent evidence, continued to undermine the traditions of academic physic.

Worse, some of these nonacademic physicians had been introduced

[9]John Colbatch, *A Physico Medical Essay, Concerning Alkaly and Acid* (1696), preface.
[10]John Colbatch, *Novum Lumen Chirurgicum: Or, A New Light of Chirurgery* (1695), pp. 7–11.
[11]Colbatch, *A Physico Medical Essay,* chap. on scurvy and conclusion.
[12]"Letter from C. Bernard to Colbatch," Sloane 1783, fols. 80–81; John Colbatch, *Some Farther Considerations Touching Alkaly and Acid* (1696); idem, *A Treatise of the Gout* (1697); S. W., *An Examination of the Late Treatise of the Gout* (1698); Colbatch, *The Doctrine of Acids in the Cure of Diseases Farther Asserted* (1698); Francis Tuthill, *A Vindication of some Objections Lately Raised against Dr. John Colbatch his Hipothesis* (1698); Colbatch, *A Relation of a very Sudden and Extraordinary Cure* (1698); William Coward, *Alcali Vindicatum: Or, The Acid Opiniator not guilty of Truth* (1698); Thomas Emes, *A Dialogue Between Alkali and Acid* (1698); Charles Leigh, *A Reply to John Colbatch, Upon his late Piece, Concerning the curing the Biting of a Viper by Acids* (1698); Richard Boulton, *An Answer to Dr. Leigh's Remarks* (1698); idem, *An Examination of Mr. John Colbatch his Treatise of the Gout* (1699).

into the College by the charter of James II and had a majority of the votes. A number of physicians of the College were gaining reputations not by emphasizing their academic learning but by underscoring their special views of disease or their witty and worldly conversation. John Radcliffe, for example, who had been made a fellow by virtue of the charter of James II and was enjoying a large and lucrative aristocratic practice, bragged that he completely lacked medical books in his private library (which was something of an exaggeration, by the way).[13] Samuel Garth and Richard Blackmore acquired reputations as wits and poets and consulted with patients in coffeehouses, not unlike some empirics. On the other hand, Richard Mead and John Freind took the high road, attaching themselves to the new science by becoming medical "Newtonians." The continuing reinvigoration of the Royal Society in the 1690s also created some worry, since, as before, "science" and "empiricism" seemed linked in the public mind. In 1696 Hans Sloane placed the imprimatur of the Royal Society on his new book ahead of that of the College of Physicians (he was a fellow of both institutions), which caused consternation among the officers of the College.[14]

Matters had not yet reached the point they would in the early eighteenth century, when Richard Mead and John Woodward fought a well-publicized sword duel in the streets of London over their different views of medical therapy.[15] But by the 1690s the threats of the 1660s had become real: academic medicine counted for much less in the eyes of the public than the latest "scientific" or literary fashions. Almost any literate practitioner could seize on these fashions to build a practice—unless, in the virtual absence of intellectual boundaries, the College could make disciplined membership the crucial distinction between good and bad practice.

On March 11, Rogers called a meeting of the elects (who had all been elevated to the rank before 1687) to discuss what should be done about the new charter and the new members. Naturally enough, the other fellows, many of them new, objected to this select meeting, and Rogers was forced to admit his error in trying to get policy approved by the elects only.[16] The divisions between the two groups deepened quickly.

[13]Campbell R. Hone, *The Life of Dr. John Radcliffe, 1652–1714; Benefactor of the University of Oxford* (London: Faber and Faber, 1950).

[14]Annals, 7:28.

[15]Joseph M. Levine, *Doctor Woodward's Shield: History, Science, and Satire in Augustan England.*

[16]Annals, 5:95b–96a.

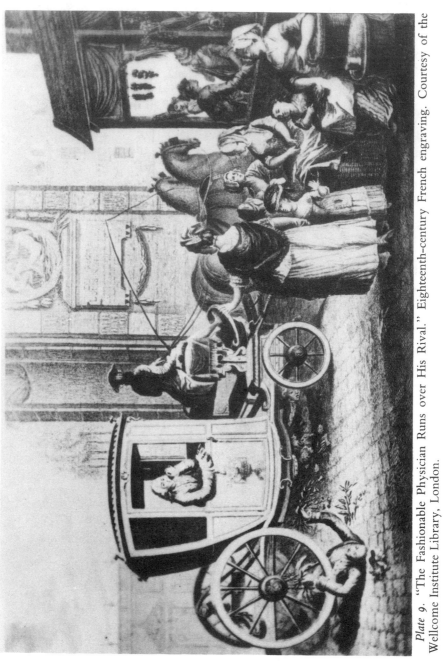

Plate 9. "The Fashionable Physician Runs over His Rival." Eighteenth-century French engraving. Courtesy of the Wellcome Institute Library, London.

Perhaps to protect themselves from an internal remodeling of the College, the majority of fellows, over Rogers's objections, entered a bill in the Parliament asking for an explicit confirmation of James II's charter. The bill declared that "Their Majesties are graciously inclined not only to give all due encouragement to the judicious and learned professors and practitioners of the necessary and useful faculty of physic, [but] also to take the most effectual care of the safety and health of their subjects." Therefore, "by reason of the increase of the number of inhabitants in and about the City of London" it was "expedient" to increase the number of fellows of the College to eighty and to double the number of elects. The bill listed each college member by name and confirmed the government of the College as stipulated in the current statutes, including the power of the censors to call forth persons to testify about medical practice. The committee of the House of Commons did not much like the "new College's" bill, but the House of Lords consented to consider it, giving it a first reading on June 7.[17]

But the "new College" faced embarrassment and parliamentary suspicion when in June two of the fellows who had been admitted under the new charter were caught circulating a declaration of James Stuart from Ireland: they were arrested and treason proceedings were begun against them.[18] Within a month, the House of Lords ordered the College to report to them the names of papists, reputed papists, or "criminals" in their ranks. The names of seven fellows were turned in as "criminals or reputed criminals" (apparently Jacobites), but no "papists" were reported. Probably if they had been, the list would have been much longer, for at the next meeting, the College was disconcerted when it learned that "a proviso was added to the said bill by the Committee of the House of Lords, that all members of our College should take the Sacrament according to the Church of England." As the registrar noted, "this being a surprise unlooked for," the committee appointed to follow the progress of the bill through the House of Lords "are desired to take all care they can about that affair." At the same time, however, seventy members took the new oaths and subscribed to the declaration on an "Act for Abrogating of the Oaths of Supremacy and Allegiance and Appointing other Oaths."[19]

---

[17]"Proposed Act of 1689," in *Historical Manuscripts Commission, 12th Report* (London, 1890), app. 6, pp. 121–29; *House of Lords Journals*, vol. 14, p. 235.

[18]Robert Gray and John Elliott; see Clark, pp. 371–72.

[19]*Annals*, 5:99b–101a; the names of the reported "criminals" were Betts, Sr. and Jr., Waldegrave, Conquest, Mendez, Gray, and Elliott.

But Rogers and his colleagues tried to obstruct the College's actions. Early in June, a rumor began circulating that the president had ordered the College's suit against Edward Tyson stopped—Tyson was a fellow who refused to obey the statutes passed in 1688. Rogers had also neglected to summon a meeting of the College to transact important business relating to the impending bill. Moreover, at the end of July, Sir Thomas Millington, the treasurer, reported that the president had sent him a letter forbidding him to pay to the College's solicitor or to anyone else money for getting the bill passed in the House of Lords. Rogers tried to prevent a vote being taken on the issue, but Goodall got up and proposed that the treasurer pay "the solicitor's bill of charges for the College bill now depending in Parliament," and his proposal passed, twenty-seven to five.[20]

Rogers and his colleagues did more than obstruct the internal business of the "new College," however; they went so far as to petition Parliament against their colleagues' bill. On June 12, five days after the College's bill had been entered in the House of Lords, the Lords heard a petition from the "president and ancient fellows" of the College praying that "they may be heard, before the passing of [the] Bill." Their petition argued that the College had been acting under the charter of Henry VIII until the reign of James II, "when Sir Thomas Witherley and others by threats procured a surrender of the charter to the King, and though the surrender was not enrolled, a new charter was obtained which destroyed their rights and privileges." After the revolution that expelled James, the petitioners had been advised that the new charter was void. Therefore, "about three months since," they, with others,

> caused a College [meeting] to be summoned to settle themselves upon the old foundations; but the new members, some of whom are known to be papists, together with some of the old ones, who contrived the surrender, opposed [the] petitioners, and kept possession of the College by force under the color of the new charter, and endeavored by petition to the Commons to get their new charter confirmed. . . . Since then, the same persons who procured the new charter, joined with the new fellows, have procured a Bill to be brought into their Lordships' House, under pretence of better settling the College, in opposition to the petitioners' rights, as well as the universities'.[21]

---

[20] Annals, 5:99a–99b.
[21] "Proposed Act of 1689"; *House of Lords Journals,* vol. 14, p. 241.

The "ancient fellows" who signed this petition undoubtedly had different motivations for opposing the "new College," but the two fundamental issues of the enactment of overweening internal statutes and the admission of poorly educated fellows brought them together: "The petitioners' rights, as well as the universities'," were at stake. Rogers, John Lawson, and John Downes had all been educated at Padua at mid-century (although Downes finally took his M.D. from Leiden) and then had incorporated their degrees at Oxford or Cambridge; Humphrey Brooke (an elect), Richard Torlesse, Josiah Clerk, Edward Browne, and Thomas Alvey all had traditional M.D.s from one of the two English universities; and Richard Morton, Jr. (who had a mandated Oxford degree of 1670 on the recommendation of the Prince of Orange), Edward Tyson, and John Atfield (an M.D. of Caen who had incorporated his degree at Oxford in 1661) were having individual disputes with the College.[22] As an inclusive body that admitted those who lacked long academic educations, yet an active one that imposed internal discipline by strict statutes as well as by prosecuting outsiders, the "new College" seemed to devalue an academic education in physic while subordinating the behavior of all practitioners to merely institutional rules.

Despite these objections, however, the "new College's" bill obtained a positive hearing in the House of Lords, and was passed on July 10.[23] The Commons took up debate on the bill sent to them from the upper house on July 24, and the College majority published several short pamphlets in support of their legislation, putting their requests forcefully.[24] The House of Commons was still considering the matter on September 30.[25]

But by early October the "ancient fellows" and the City companies of barber-surgeons and apothecaries had gotten the ratification of James's charter voted down. The attempts of the majority of fel-

---

[22]Morton had been one of the four left off the College list by James's charter, Tyson was being prosecuted for disobedience to the statutes of 1688, and Atfield was being threatened with expulsion.

[23]The House of Lords heard counsel for and against the College's bill on June 22; had it read in the House for a second time on June 25; accepted a petition of the Barber-Surgeons' Company against it on that day; heard arguments by all sides in committee on June 26 and 29 and July 3 and 4, the opposition now being joined by the Society of Apothecaries; reported the bill out of committee to the floor on July 4, and passed it on the third reading, July 10 (*House of Lords Journals*, vol. 14, pp. 252, 253, 254, 268, 272).

[24]*Commons Journals*, vol. 10, p. 234; *Reasons for Passing the Physicians Bill* (1689); *Answers to the Objections Against the College-Bill* (1689); *The Physicians Reply to the Surgeons Answer* (1689).

[25]*Annals*, 5:102b.

lows to secure their corporation had had a quite unintended result: greater confusion than ever reigned on the questions of who was a fellow and how the College could police itself and others. The alliances between some members who opposed the "new College" and outsiders, particularly in the Society of Apothecaries, would continue to plague the authoritarians.

Under the brief leadership of a new president, Walter Charleton, the College of Physicians set about reordering its affairs and trying to regain some unanimity, although matters only quieted for a while; there was no true reconciliation between groups. A committee composed of four old and four new fellows was set up to settle the differences between the two factions.[26] The committee reached a compromise on the figuring of the seniority of the members that was adopted by the College at the end of November 1689. But many members continued to push for forthright actions under the statutes of 1688 against members and outsiders both, in order to reassert College authority.

An account of one conversation at a meeting on November 12 suggests the kind of issues being debated by the two groups. Dr. John Bateman suggested to another fellow that any member expelled from the College ought to forfeit his degree and everything else making it possible for him to practice in London. The anonymous fellow to whom Bateman suggested this line replied that it seemed "very hard, that men who had made their acquaintance in and about London should upon the pique of some men against them, be reduced to seek their bread amongst strangers." Bateman repeated his views, the other tried to rally supporters to his side, and President Charleton finally calmed them all down only by saying that "we cannot hinder them practicing" because of the precedent set by the cases of Christopher Merrett [and William Goddard] in previous decades.[27]

Because the new fellows and their friends retained a majority, members of the College did vote to pay the expenses for the defeated bill (about £82) out of institutional funds. They also agreed to suspend the requirement of an English M.D. for those fellows admitted under the charter of James II. In early December, they further decided to set the number of fellows at eighty (although not to double the number of elects), and to admit all M.D.s, even those not of the two English universities, until that number was reached. This stance was

---

[26]Annals, 5:104b; the four old members were Millington, Morton, Brooks, and Torlesse; the four new, Needham, Bernard, Blackburne, and Blackmore.

[27]"At the Committee of the College November 12 1689," Sloane 1789, fol. 160.

fundamentally to undermine the idea that the College represented the highest academic standards in physic—a problem that was to haunt the "new College" for years.

The majority of fellows also decided to continue to take testimony against illicit practitioners, but that "prosecution [would] be suspended till time convenient." Such a time would be reached when the College received some legal or political confirmation of its authority to take action against its rivals. The "new College" therefore set up a committee to prepare still another bill for submission to the Parliament guaranteeing it its old rights in that regard.[28]

The proposed new bill would have ensured that the new government would support the College when it acted against illicit practitioners. It was in the public interest, these physicians argued, to make sure that all practitioners were properly qualified. But London had been invaded by "intruders . . . merely illiterate empirics and unlearned men and women," as well as by those who were "learned, but irregular and adverse to government." The College had tried to stop their practices, but it could not

> discover their practice upon particulars, for they avoid proof [by] writ[ing] no bills [i.e., prescriptions], neither are any bills found written by the apothecaries, whom they use, neither will those upon whom they practice and such as entertain them testify against them. May it please you therefore that it may be enacted, that either they shall write bills and sign them as Collegiate physicians do or that some apothecary may write what they dictate, for some of them . . . cannot write; that so their practice may appear whether good or bad. Or that it may be lawful for the College to sue them upon common fraud or testimony of other sufficient men.[29]

But the political conditions were not ripe for getting this petition granted in the Parliament. In 1690 the Parliament seemed incapable of resolving the medical disputes of the capital by siding with any single

[28]Annals, 5:105b–107a, 103a, 104a; the committee was composed of Stokeham, Millington, Griffith, Needham, Hulse, Bernard, Bateman, Blackburne, and Blackmore.

[29]"Petition of the College to Parliament for Suppression of Ignorant Practitioners," R.C.P., box 4, env. 48. The College also sought to make it clear that not writing prescriptions would be the equivalent of "evil practice"; that the physicians had the right to inspect the apothecaries' wares and to destroy the bad ones; that they could outlaw books they disliked; that they could have dead bodies for public dissections; that they could increase the number of elects; that they could prohibit the practice of graduates in medicine from Oxford and Cambridge if they were not members of the College; and that they would be free from bearing and providing arms.

group. The fellows of the "new College" found that the Barber-Surgeons' Company—which had been instrumental in defeating the College's bill of 1689—was promoting a bill of its own that would grant surgeons the right to administer internal medicines in certain cases without consulting physicians. By appealing to the public and lobbying the Commons, the College managed to get the bill stopped, even though it did not manage to get its own bill passed.[30] Other proposals to change medical regulation in London of a more radical nature were also stopped.[31] Although not all of the differences among the members of the College were resolved, then,[32] for the most part the College entered a period of inward hesitancy and little outward activity under Charleton's presidency.

As the College watched and waited for legal and political direction, it recruited few new members and prosecuted very few others (see appendixes 1 and 2). It did advise the rapidly growing army and navy on medicines for use by the surgeons assisting the troops in the first years of what would be the Nine Years War, and it suggested various physicians for the officers.[33] But generally Charleton and other cool heads restrained the members who yearned to attack their rivals aggressively before the College's powers were clarified by the Parliament or by the Crown.

Apothecaries and Their Physician Friends against the "New College"

Attempts to reinvigorate medical regulation began yet again in 1692, when the Whigs became dominant in William and Mary's councils. As they had been so often before, changes in policy were signaled by changes in the leadership of the College. Thomas Burwell became president, and Samuel Collins and Sir Thomas Witherly (who had been president during the autocratic years under James II)

[30]Annals, 5:107a, 118a–119a; *A Short State of the Case Between the Physicians and Surgeons* (1690); *Commons Journals,* vol. 10, pp. 336, 342, 344, 445, 446, 451, 453, 458, 478, 482; "Papers Relating to Disputes and Suits Between the Society of Apothecaries and the Barber-Surgeons' Company," Guildhall MS no. 8290.

[31]Hugh Chamberlen, *A Proposal for the Better Securing of Health. Humbly Offered to the Consideration of the Honourable Houses of Parliament* (1689). Chamberlen argued for a yearly tax on households which would pay for free medical services to all Londoners and be administered by seven local Colleges of medicine that would each include physicians, surgeons, and apothecaries.

[32]In October 1690, Blackburne complained that the statutes of the College were contrary to the laws of the land: Annals, 5:118a.

[33]Annals, 5:153b–152b[*sic*]; 6:4–5, 6–7, 8, 11–12.

became the two *consiliarii*. The previous president, George Rogers, had resigned his position as elect in 1691, as had Sir Charles Scarburgh and Peter Barwick (who was well known for his cures of fevers and smallpox and apparently less concerned about upholding College policies than some of his colleagues). Voted into the vacant spots were John Lawson, who had opposed the College's bill in 1689 but had become reconciled to the "new College," and Sir Thomas Millington, a royal physician. The reshuffling of men at the top brought new policies to the College—or, rather, a return to its former aggressive policies. Yet the officers and fellows who promoted and carried out this regulatory activity found themselves frustrated at almost every turn.

The campaign against illicit practitioners got off to a fast start. Soon after the College's election in 1692, the new officers ordered "that the names of empirics and those that practice illegally be taken by the beadle and brought to this Board [of censors at] the next censors' meeting in order to [begin] their prosecution."[34] In 1693— perhaps not coincidentally after the formation of the junto that was willing to advocate unpopular policies so as to keep public order during the war—the number of hearings of cases of illicit practitioners reached great heights (see appendix 2, table 1). The College also placed the following advertisement in the *London Gazette:*

> Whereas many and great complaints have lately been made at the Censors' Board, in the College of Physicians Warwick Lane, of injury done to Their Majesties' subjects within the City of London and seven miles compass, by illegal and ignorant practitioners in physic; this is to give notice that all persons, or their friends so aggrieved, may apply to the Censors, who meet the first Friday of every month, at the College, and are authorized by acts of Parliament to punish such offenders.[35]

The new group's policies also continued to link prosecuting illicit practitioners with enforcing internal discipline. The new leaders wished to break the social and, particularly, the medical links between members of the College and outsiders. Such a policy meant emphasizing the College's controversial 1688 statutes on several issues. The College's lawyer had found that under the College's 1687 charter, a number of the 1688 statutes could be enforced, among them the College prohibition against members publishing short ad-

[34]Annals, 6:33.
[35]Annals, 6:134–37.

vertisements (although not books); the College requirements that members date and sign their prescriptions (so that they could not be used again by the practicing apothecaries) and pay their dues and fines (or face expulsion); and the College prerogatives of refusing membership to those who had not repudiated membership in another company and refusing to provide consultation to those who were expelled from the College.[36] Between 1692 and 1700 the new officers named or fined as troublemakers under these statutes forty members of the College, most of them fellows (the rest were licentiates), and took several to outside courts.

The College officers' actions against John Pechey were meant to be an example to others but soon led to vehement internal quarrels. Pechey, a licentiate since 1684, is first mentioned as being harassed by the College in 1689, when he was sued for back dues. He had already become a member of the "repository" practice, in which he and three other licentiates prescribed to walk-in patients free of charge and then sold them the medicines they stocked,[37] and he associated with several illicit practitioners, as well. He was obviously seen as a potential troublemaker: he is mentioned in a note that includes notices of suits against several empirics.[38] A follower of Sydenham's empiricist medicine and a translator and editor of his works in English, Pechey expressed his medical views succinctly in one of his many books:

> I believe nothing has so much obstructed the improvement of the art of physic, as the late unaccountable humor of romancing on the nature and the causes of diseases: for in our modern authors, the greatest part of the paper is wasted about flourishing a whimsee, to make it pass for a probable supposition. . . . Whereas reason and argument are not the true tests of physic, nor indeed of any thing else, when experience, the great baffler of speculation, can determine the matter.

Therefore, Pechey concluded, his book (and his practice) "must ex-

---

[36]"Legal opinions [of Serj. Creswell Levinz]."

[37]Their practice was advertised in *The Oracle for the Sick* (1687), a short book in which the patient could underline the answers to questions and draw a line to the seat of his pain on a woodcut of the human body and send the completed questionnaire in by mail; the diagnosis would be made at the "repository" and mailed back to the patient. The copy of this book at the Wellcome Institute Library has a different title page than does the copy in the British Library, so there seems to have been more than one printing of the pamphlet.

[38]Annals, 5:110a.

pect but cold entertainment with the speculative physician," either "ancient" or "modern."[39]

But the College's suit against Pechey at Guildhall under the statutes of 1688 to recover his back dues was thrown out in late 1692 when the lord chief justice discovered that the College statutes had not been dated, and hence it could not be clearly shown that they were in force before Pechey was sued. In 1693 the beadle of the college was ordered to demand Pechey's "quarteridge" dues, but Pechey again refused to pay. When in February of 1694 Pechey was summoned to a *comitia censorum,* "he answered very peremptorily, that he had the better of the College in a suit before, and bid them begin when they pleased. Whereupon this Board ordered him to be arrested *de novo,* and prosecuted according to law." The suit was scheduled to be brought to court in November 1694, although no record of it ever coming to trial is extant.[40] Just as had happened when the "new College" tried to get the charter of James II ratified in Parliament and failed, the legal decision that the new statutes could not be enforced led to internal confusion.

By the spring of 1693, in the wake of Pechey's case being thrown out of court, a virtual rebellion was underway within the College. A meeting of the full College was called for April 1693 during which all the College's statutes were to be read aloud so as to establish a verifiable date for their public promulgation—but most of the candidates and licentiates boycotted the meeting. One of the things the College officers wanted to obtain from the candidates and licentiates was information against "unfaithful and illiterate practitioners." This many were reluctant to give, since so many had friends and associates among these practitioners. They therefore engaged in a kind of passive disobedience against their authoritarian superiors by refusing to testify against their colleagues who were not of the College. At the end of June, the candidates and licentiates were called in so that the statute *"de conversatione morali"* could be read to them, but again, few appeared.[41]

Anger against the "new College" was manifest in the rumors and slanders some members were spreading about the leaders. Edward

[39]John Pechey, *The Store House of Physical Practice* (1695), preface. Also see G. C. Peachey, "The Two John Peacheys, Seventeenth-Century Physicians: Their Lives and Times," *Janus* 23 (1918): 121–58.

[40]Annals, 6:13–14, 70–71, 86–88, 105, 171–74.

[41]Annals, 6:60, 62–64, 71–73.

Baynard, for example, was furious at an "oversight" that left him off the list of members. Baynard, who had studied medicine at Leiden but had taken his M.D. in 1671–72 from King's College Aberdeen, had established himself first in Preston, then in Bath and London, becoming an honorary fellow in 1684 and a fellow in 1687 by virtue of the new charter. He was, however, left off the College's "catalogue" that was printed in the spring of 1693. He seems to have begun to denounce the College publicly, for in early April he was summoned to a *comitia censorum,* but he refused to wait to be called in. He left the following note to the president, a note of high enough tone to cause the registrar to copy it into the Annals:

> I am a gentleman, and no footman, so do not understand waiting beyond the time of your summons. If you or the censors have any further business with me, you must send a further summons, and be more punctual to your time, than to this, otherwise I shall not obey it. I am as you please yours or not your servant.

When he finally appeared before the censors, he loudly complained about being left off such a potentially important medical list. After some discussion, the censors decided that the catalogue was not official, but Baynard threatened "to bring a visitation [from the government] upon the College" for not including him. Not mollified in the least, he was brought before the censors again on May 9 on the charge that he had called the president "the son of a whore."[42]

Other members of the College who did not like its new policies spread rumors about London that suggested that the new oligarchy was medically incompetent. On May 30, 1693, for example, Robert Brady, a fellow since 1680 and Regius Professor of Physic at Cambridge, angrily reported that he was "calumniated" by four members of the College who were opposed to the new regime.[43] He had prescribed an ointment to a Mrs. Campneis for a red face, but she had died six or seven weeks afterward and on her death the four fellows "who had been concerned with the said patient after him" put it about that the ointment had caused her death.[44] Issues of proper

---

[42]Annals, 6:37, 56–59, 62–64. In the last instance, Baynard rather lamely explained that he told Mr. Swan, "You run about with a false list: tell the president you are the son of a whore." Baynard's name does not appear in the College list published in 1694, either (B.L. 777.1.2 [5,6]).

[43]The four fellows were How, Blackmore, Gibbons, and Gould.

[44]Annals, 6:66, 67–68.

medical practice were being brought into association with issues of authority; both issues divided the College.

Far more serious for the College than boycotts, slander, and rumor was the plotting of some members with illicit practitioners and the Society of Apothecaries against the "new College." Dr. Francis Bernard, who had served on the committees trying to reconcile the new and the old members and to get the new charter ratified in Parliament, apparently did not like the recent turn of events in the College. He had a Lambeth degree, which he incorporated at Cambridge in 1678 at age fifty-one; he had earlier been recommended as the apothecary to St. Bartholomew's Hospital but in 1678 gained the appointment there as assistant physician. In 1680 he became an honorary fellow, and then a fellow by virtue of the new charter in 1687. A Tory and an astrological physician, he also collected books, assembling what is said to have been the largest collection of medical books ever made in England.[45] Bernard made common cause with the Society of Apothecaries, which feared the new statutes, by employing the pen of a disgruntled practitioner, Dr. John Badger, in a public attack on the College.

Badger believed that by rights he ought to be a fellow of the College but that the new statutes had been used to deny him admission. Badger had begun as an apothecary, later taking an M.B. In July, August, and September of 1683 he had been examined in Latin and approved by the College as a licentiate. But he was told that if he held off joining the College until he had his M.D. and quit the practice of apothecary, his examination would serve to make him a candidate, "The more honorable station in their Society, and which I better deserved," he later reported.[46] His M.D. completed in July 1687, Badger went to the College several times to be admitted a candidate. Each time he was put off, however, since the College had just been reorganized under the charter of James II and new statutes were being drawn up. He finally obtained a hearing but was again refused admission, this time because the new statutes forbade entrance on a previous examination.

Badger argued that the new statutes could not apply to him, since

---

[45]See *A Catalogue of the Library of the late learned Dr. Francis Bernard* (1698); I estimate the number of medical books alone at over 4,500 titles, and he collected books in many other areas, as well. Samuel Garth refers to Bernard as "Horoscope" in *The Dispensary, A Poem* (1699); many of his medico-astrological manuscripts remain in the Sloane collection.

[46]John Badger, *The Case Between the Doctor John Badger and the Colledge of Physicians London* (1693), p. 1.

he had been admitted to the College previously. The College officers replied that he would have to abjure the Society of Apothecaries formally and bring them a notarized statement to that effect. (Badger claimed to have "quitted [his] employment in pharmacy in the year 1684.")[47] In 1693 the master, wardens, court of assistants, and other members of the Society of Apothecaries together with Bernard urged Badger to publish the College's "new illogical and unjust" statutes (supplied by Bernard) in English for all the world to see. The apothecaries also promised to support the venture by buying twenty or thirty copies apiece for distribution, which Badger later complained that they had failed to do.[48]

Along with the statutes, Badger brought out a short account of *The Case Between the Doctor John Badger and the Colledge of Physicians London* in 1693, claiming that on the basis of the College's statutes and published pamphlets "it manifestly follows that Doctor John Badger is and has been legally and duly a member of the College of Physicians London these ten years past." As the College tried to reassert its power in 1693 and to publish a list of all its members that excluded Badger, among others, he proclaimed: "The College [is] guilty of publishing to the world most notorious falsehood; and to use their own words, is very far from being any other than a perfect monopoly and confederacy."[49]

Disagreements in the College over the actions of its officers continued in 1694. There were disputes over fining William Cole for giving the anatomy lecture at Surgeons' Hall without the permission of the president, over the behavior of the censors, and over the visitations of the apothecaries' shops.[50] Suits by the officers against members and nonmembers continued.

By the end of the year, the apothecaries felt threatened enough to try to get legal protection for their practices. Rather than act directly against the College, however, the Society of Apothecaries astutely tried to raise its own prestige, indirectly asserting the professional equality of apothecaries with physicians.

The strategy of the Society of Apothecaries was to bring a bill to the House of Commons in mid-December 1694 to excuse apothecaries from serving in several parish offices. A law of that sort would

[47]Ibid., pp. 2, 3.
[48]"Letter [from Dr. Badger] to the Apothecaries Company," Sloane 4026, fol. 386. Also see John Badger, *Doctor Badger's Vindication of Himself, from the Groundless Calumnies and Malicious Slanders of some London-Apothecaries* (1701). Cf. Clark, p. 467.
[49]Badger, *Case Between the Doctor John Badger and the Colledge,* p. 4.
[50]Annals, 6:119–20, 132–33, 140.

formally elevate the apothecaries above ordinary craftsmen and artisans in London and give them a professionlike standing. The officers of the College were worried, and by the end of December they were trying to insert clauses into the bill that guaranteed what they viewed as their own rights and privileges.[51] In this instance, the College found itself allied with the leaders of the City of London, who believed some of their own authority would be questioned by such a bill. The Society of Apothecaries, the College, and the City carried their arguments to the public once again by publishing pamphlets.

The apothecaries openly admitted that they were very busy medical practitioners, being called day and night by patients, especially the "poorer sort" who could not afford to call in physicians. As such, they could not afford the time to serve on parish offices such as churchwarden, overseer of the poor, constable, scavenger, and inquestman. They usually paid a fine when called rather than serve, but these fines were being spent on the local vestrymen rather than on the public that they were serving, the apothecaries argued. The physicians had been excused many decades before on the grounds that serving on parish offices would interfere in their public business. Lawyers, attorneys, and clerks had also been exempted. They, too, then, should be exempt from such onerous offices; moreover, adding an exception for the apothecaries would not be setting a precedent for other crafts, since the apothecaries were not a trade group but a profession, serving the health of the community. A ringing declaration sealed the apothecaries' argument: since life and liberty are more valuable than property, and since those who defended property (the legal profession) were exempt from many parish duties, the apothecaries, who defended life, should be exempt as well.[52]

The City, however, argued that the fines taken from the apothecaries for not serving on parish offices, amounting to £100 per annum, went to help the poor of the parishes. If the apothecaries were exempt from office, the parishes would lose that part of their income. Should the apothecaries gain their exemption, it might well set a precedent for other companies of London and so further deplete the

[51] Annals, 6:179–80.

[52] Reasons, Humbly Offered to the Honourable House of Commons; by the . . . Society of . . . Apothecaries . . . For the Exempting them from Certain Offices and Duties (1694); Considerations Humbly Offered to the Lords Spiritual and Temporal, in Relation to the Apothecaries Bill (1694); Reasons on Behalf of the Apothecaries Bill . . . In Answer to the City of London's Petition against the said Bill (1694); The Apothecaries' Reply to the City's Printed Reasons Against their Bill (1694).

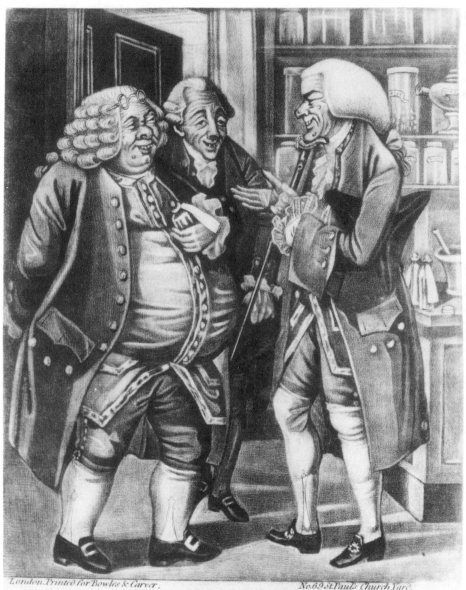

How merrily we live that Doctor's be
We humbug the Public and pocket the Fee.

Plate 10. "Scene in an apothecary's shop." Anonymous mezzotint after Robert Dighton, eighteenth century. Courtesy of the Wellcome Institute Library, London. In this satire, three obviously well-to-do apothecaries are gloating over making money by cheating the public.

parishes' treasuries. More to the point, the apothecaries had been chartered to make and compound medicines in their houses and shops, not to go about treating the ill: they were supposed to be tradesmen, not professionals. They sought higher City offices, such as alderman, deputy, common-councilman, governor of the City hospitals, commissioner of the lieutenancy and sewers, military office in the militia, and so forth. Therefore, the apothecaries did not wish to be exempted from all public offices, just from those of lower prestige—or from the fines if they refused to serve. There was a need for a law obliging citizens to serve in the parish offices, the City argued, rather than a need for a law exempting one more group from serving.[53]

The College in turn tried to rebut the notion that practicing apothecaries benefited the public. In fact, the exorbitant prices apothecaries charged for their medicines led many people to seek out cheaper "quacks," and the practicing apothecaries did not treat the poor (whom the physicians were required by statute to serve *gratis*), but instead ingratiated themselves with the wealthy. The apothecaries' argument that they knew medicine better than the physicians because they saw many prescriptions of the physicians came in for forthright counterargument, too:

> Indeed had they any true foundation in the grounds of physic, did they understand the true philosophic anatomy, the seat of diseases, with their symptoms, and the reasons of them, this might be of advantage to them, as it is to the young physicians, who improve themselves in the universities, in their travels, here in town, by visiting hospitals, consulting files, and frequenting the company of the most eminent practitioners.

But the apothecaries' claims, the physicians said, were like saying that the clerk at St. Paul's was better than the learned divines who preached there because he had heard them all. "In short, what they pretend, is charity, unwearied diligence to the sick, and public good, like generous and disinterested men; whereas pull off the mask, and you'll find a liberty to practice is all they aim at; the rest is sham and banter." For the good of the science of physic and for the future employment of the younger sons of the gentry, the College pleaded

[53]*Reasons Humbly Offered Against Passing the Bill, for Exempting Apothecaries from serving . . . Parish and Ward Offices* (1694).

with the Parliament not to give the apothecaries this right, disguised as an exemption from holding parish offices.[54]

But the opposition of the City and the College was unavailing in the House of Commons, which sent the bill to the House of Lords on January 25, 1695. During debate, the counsel for the Society of Apothecaries used words against the College such as "negligent," "careless," and "uncharitable" and declared it to be "of little use, in comparison with the apothecaries," since the apothecaries corrected physicians' prescriptions, took care of all the sick poor, and had nineteen out of twenty parts of medical practice in London. Fellows in league with the apothecaries further undermined the efforts of the College officers and the City to stop the apothecaries' bill. William Gibbons, for instance, passed along to the apothecaries all strategy being developed by the College. He even declared outright that he was promoting the apothecaries' bill.[55]

In the end, such internal divisions made it impossible for the officers either to stop the bill or to get a clause inserted in it "to secure the rights of the College." But they did halt the passage of a rider to the bill that would have given the apothecaries the clear ability to practice physic on the "poor" and in cases of "necessity." The Lords acted quickly, holding a second reading of the bill on February 4 and reporting it out of committee with minor revisions on February 9, when it passed its third reading. On February 11, the amended bill gained the assent of the Commons and the Crown.[56]

The act declared that "whereas the art of the apothecary is of great and general use and benefit, by reason of their constant and necessary assistance to His Majesty's subjects, which should oblige them solely to attend the duty of their professions," the apothecaries were exempt from parish duties.[57] For the physicians, the act contained a dangerous implication: the apothecaries were laying legal claim to medical practice and usurping the role of the College as an instrument of the public good. The House of Lords was beginning to side with the physicians' main corporate rivals. Something had to be done.

The first step taken by the officers of the College in the wake of the apothecaries' act was toward solidifying the new alliance with the

---

[54]Ibid.

[55]*House of Lords Journals*, vol. 15, pp. 471, 472; Annals, 6:185, 193–97, 186; *Manuscripts of the House of Lords, 1694–95*, p. 457.

[56]Annals, 6:193–97; *House of Lords Journals*, vol. 15, pp. 477–78, 485, 487, 488.

[57]John Raithby, ed., *The Statutes at Large, of England and Great Britain* (London, 1811), vol. 3, pp. 367–68.

City of London. The City had a constantly growing poor population that was already too large for the local parishes to support. In March of 1695, the College therefore appointed a committee to "revive" and present to the City the order of 1687 that stated that members of the College were to diagnose and prescribe to the local poor for nothing. In June a copy of the order was made and discussions were held in secret on ways to further influence the City. As discussions proceeded, a new project took shape: the College would not simply require the charity of individual members, but would act as a corporation to benefit the poor while at the same time undermining the Society of Apothecaries. The College decided to create the dispensary, first openly proposed in July.[58]

The dispensary, as originally proposed, provided for a stock of drugs to be kept on hand, paid for by a levy on members of the College, that could be either given to the poor or sold to them at cost. The physicians could then diagnose and prescribe to the poor for nothing and administer drugs out of their own repository. In the process, a list of the dispensary's drugs and their low prices would be made known to the public. This would benefit the poor and gain the applause of the City fathers and other influential men. It would also take some business from the apothecaries. Most importantly, it was believed that the dispensary would verify the physicians' charge that the apothecaries were both overprescribing and charging too much for their medicines. Consequently, the dispensary would help place the blame for the current state of medical practice squarely on the shoulders of the apothecaries, not the physicians.

The idea of something like the dispensary had been around for many decades. In the mid-1660s, a number of "scientific" fellows had argued that physicians should make their own medicines in order to improve physic and to attack the practicing apothecaries. In 1670 Jonathan Goddard had gone so far as to propose the setting up of a dispensary.[59] Others had proposed that the physicians give free advice to the poor and that the apothecaries give free medicines: "Wonderful charity at other men's cost!" Adrian Huyberts had sneered.[60] In 1675 and 1687 the College had proposed statutes making it incum-

---

[58]Annals, 6:196, 210, 217–21. For a somewhat different account of what follows, see Frank H. Ellis, "The Background of the London Dispensary," *JHM* 20 (1965): 197–212; Clark, pp. 428–47.

[59]Jonathan Goddard, *A Discourse Setting forth the Unhappy Condition of the Practice of Physic in London* (1670), p. 10.

[60]Adrian Huyberts, *A Corner-stone laid towards the Building of a New Colledge . . . in London* (1675), p. 35.

bent on all members to give free advice to the deserving poor. All of these ideas were seen as ways for the physicians to gain the public esteem while undermining the position of illicit practitioners, especially the apothecaries. As the College found itself in an increasingly untenable situation in the 1690s, it began to revive ideas of practicing charitably. But it did so with an important difference: the acts of charity would no longer be private—they would be public and they would clearly be linked to the College of Physicians as an institution. If opposition came from any quarter, blame could not be pinned on the College for obstructing the public good. The moral position of the College would be greatly strengthened by such a public stance.

But when the dispensary was first proposed to the College in July 1695, some fellows who opposed the officers' assertive policies wanted time to consider the idea. The idea was adopted at the special meeting in August, despite opposition. A list of subscribers who contributed twenty shillings each was drawn up—fifty-seven men all together. By the fourth of September, the new strategy seemed to be paying off. The City offered its thanks to the College for the dispensary and suggested that the churchwardens, overseers of the poor, rectors, vicars, and curates of the parishes certify the poor who would be allowed to receive the benefits of the dispensary. The City also suggested that the College might publish a list of its members with their addresses so that the poor and others could seek them out— excellent publicity.[61]

The formation of the dispensary set up an issue that heightened the already strong tensions within the College, however. Some fellows of the College had no wish to attack the apothecaries, being friends enough with the apothecaries and others or empirical enough in their own practices to wish to promote a free medical marketplace. They refused to subscribe to the dispensary.

The result was a further attempt on the part of the officers to discipline members and others. A document was drawn up noting that "divers good and wholesome laws and statutes of the College of Physicians have been heretofore had and made" to benefit the subjects of England as well as the College, but that some had not been acted on because the officers "were apprehensive [that] divers suits and controversies might arise and be prosecuted . . . the costs and damage as well as the trouble whereof they might in their own particular persons be subject to and yet not sufficiently indemnified by the

[61] Annals, 6:217–21, 223–27.

said College." To remedy this, the paper declared that "we the sub-scribers thereto, fellows or members of the said College, do hereby . . . each of us severally . . . oblige himself to the other of us in the penal sum of £50 . . . to assist, support, and maintain the President and Censors of the said College." Thus the members of the College pledged to support, morally and financially, the actions of their of-ficers. To this pledge, at least thirteen fellows refused to put their hands.[62]

As the College consulted with the City in late 1694 about setting up the dispensary, Francis Bernard and the Society of Apothecaries again tried to stop the officers' plans and enlisted John Badger in the fray. Bernard supplied Badger with a list of those who signed the new agreement: the "dispensary physicians." The master and wardens of the Society of Apothecaries promised that they would bear any print-ing charges and that Badger would be remunerated.[63]

Badger therefore published two broadsides in 1695. One was an "Alphabetical Catalogue of all [who] have taken the Degree of Doc-tor of Physic in our Two Universities from the year 1659, to this present year 1695. Published for the Benefit of all Englishmen, Par-ticularly to Inform the People of London; who are Honest and Reg-ular Physicians." With such a list, Badger could show that the Col-lege was not simply an association of physicians but that it excluded many physicians who were university educated while incorporating as fellows others who were not. As Badger wrote at the top of his list: "The monopoly and new association of physicians in Warwick Lane, who vulgarly call themselves the College, was the fourth of October, 1695, made up of 130 members, most of whom are no doctors; and scarce forty of them regular doctors in either of our universities, as will appear by comparing their catalogue to this."

Badger brought out another catalogue, this one indicating mem-bers of the College who had gained their degrees at a foreign univer-sity and then incorporated them at Oxford or Cambridge and mem-bers who had earned their degrees before the Restoration.[64] At the

---

[62]"Draft Agreement between Fellows and members of R.C.P. to support President and Censors of College in the Execution of the laws and statutes, 1695," R.C.P., 2012/9; Annals, 7:12–14. Those listed as refusing to sign the document were: Tyson, Pitt, Bernard, Baynard, Blackburne, How, Blackmore, Tancred Robinson, Gelsthorpe, Gibbons, Cham-berlen, Cole, and Cade. Almost all of these men had been in trouble with the officers of the College on previous occasions; some supported academic physic but not the current pol-icies or membership of the corporation.

[63]Badger, *Doctor Badger's Vindication;* "Letter [from Dr. Badger]," fol. 386.

[64]John Badger, *The Catalogue of Fellows and Other Members of the Royal College of Physi-cians, London, Dated October 4, 1695* (1695).

bottom of the list was a series of "queries." It led off with "Whether this present medley of physicians, who call themselves the College, hath not justly forfeited their charter, having notoriously violated the fundamental statutes of their own society" by admitting non-English-university physicians. The queries also labeled the College a monopoly, since it excluded some, including Badger, who had earned proper English M.D.s. The College could no longer easily retain the moral authority of being first and foremost a group of the most academically qualified physicians in London.

Hard pressed at the bar of public opinion (a force that counted for more and more) while weakened by internal disputes, the College suffered another severe blow to its authority when it lost control of the supply and inspections of medicines and the appointments of medical officers to the army and navy, which were rapidly growing in size and importance during the Nine Years War.

The lords of the admiralty had asked the College to nominate physicians to be in charge of the health of naval expeditions on several occasions (in 1692, 1693, 1694, and 1697). But differences between the two groups were already apparent in 1692, when the admiralty wanted the College to recommend three or four physicians to take care of the sick and wounded at Portsmouth, of whom they would choose one. The College decided that its recommending "so many might be a prejudice to Their Majesties' affairs, by discouraging fit and able physicians from proferring themselves for the future," and sent up only one recommendation. But the lords knew a struggle for precedence and patronage when they saw one and insisted on three names from which to choose.[65]

On the other hand, early in William's reign, the College had also inspected the drugs for the army in Flanders. John Hutton, the physician general and a fellow of the College, had written to the College's officers: "I think and am morally sure at present [that] nothing is done by the contract made twixt the public and the apothecaries for furnishing medicines to serve the army [in the] next campaign that does in any manner touch [on] or can lessen our privileges." The College demanded the right to be informed when large amounts of medicines were to be supplied by the Society of Apothecaries, so that its members could inspect them and so retain the College's supervision of the supply of medicines in England. Hutton agreed to order the apothecaries to give the College notice of requests for medical supplies.[66]

[65]Annals, 6:42–44, 45–47.
[66]Annals, 6:6–7.

But then in the autumn of 1695, during the troubles over the dispensary and the new document supporting the officers of the College, the officers and the lords of the admiralty had a falling out. The lords were interested only in running a war; the College was interested in protecting its privileges. As the case of Colbatch was also demonstrating, experimental medicine appealed to the military if it held out the promise of healthier troops; but medicine of that kind outside the control of the College undermined the College's prestige, not to mention its authority.

The lords had sent the College a letter complaining that the medicines furnished to the ships' surgeons by the apothecaries were not doing much good. They therefore wanted the College to recommend "a scheme of the several species of medicines, which in your opinion are more proper for the care of the sick and wounded men in the fleet" and to recommend how much of each medicine should be supplied in a chest for the care of 200 men. The president and the censors took the opportunity to wait on the Lords with a recommendation for reforming the abuses of which they wrote: no doubt they complained of adulterated drugs and wanted more power to supervise the apothecaries. The lords, however, replied that they only wanted an invoice of medicines for 200 men for six months. The president and the censors answered that there seemed to have been a problem with bad medicines in the chests and that they wished to prevent the problem in the future. The lords said that they could take care of that problem by themselves. The president and the censors replied yet again that

> they humbly conceived, that making a bad invoice would be of no service or use to attain the ends their Lordships aimed at, and that they, in discharge of the duty, as became them, whom the laws of the land had entirely, and more properly trusted with the care, and inspection of medicines, as well as physicians, were ready to give their Lordships the best information they could, on the ways and methods most proper in this case, which, if pursued by their Lordships, they were of opinion would prove more effectual.

The lords of the admiralty, however, refused to get involved in disputes over medical regulation. Captain Preutiman angrily told the physicians that their lordships only wanted a list of medicines and that if the College was not prepared to give them one, the physicians could all clear out. The physicians stood their ground and replied that they were there to serve His Majesty; they would also have to know where the ships were going in order to prepare a list of medicines proper for the climate. Sir Robert Rich "answered 'an invoice for 200 men was an invoice, and a fever was a fever all the world over.'" When the censors replied that there were different diseases in different places and climates, the lords told them to leave.[67] The admiralty continued to seek recommendations from the College for physicians to the fleets, but the physicians lost all de facto control over medical supplies to the military after the incident of 1695.

Trying to enforce internal discipline before turning against other rivals, the officers of the College tried yet another scheme. On the advice of counsel, they began to translate their statutes into English in the spring of 1696. In three special meetings at the end of September and the beginning of November, the statutes were read and approved. But when at the end of November the College decided to promulgate the statutes—obviously to make recalcitrant members more obedient—Josiah Clerk (an elect) and others dissented, saying that the statutes had been changed in the process of translation and had been adopted without due process, as well. The fines for disobedience had in fact been raised, among other changes. The licentiates, "in a very rude and tumultuous manner, pretend to a right in the making of the statutes," was the way the registrar put it. When the president replied that the Annals showed the statutes to have been approved at the "foundation" of the College (in 1688) and that the College's counsel thought the same, the opposing faction walked out. Those who walked out also claimed that they could not be fined for their behavior since the statutes had not yet been read in English to the whole College (meaning to them). They also refused to subscribe more money to the dispensary, which in December of 1696 was, ironically, running into financial trouble due to the costs of the drugs.[68]

For despite the objections of some members and many nonmembers, the dispensary had gone forward. By the end of June 1696, the medicines for the dispensary had been examined and approved and the workings of the dispensary had been placed under two stewards, since the committee originally appointed to oversee it spent too much time quarreling.[69] Publicity in the form of several pamphlets and

---

[67]Annals, 7:6, 7–8.

[68]Annals, 7:20–21, 35–36, 36–80, 84, 85–86, 89, 90–92. For a list of the specific complaints of these members, see the "Abridgment of the Statutes of the College of Physicians," by Thomas Gill, Sloane, 3914, fols. 61 ff.

[69]Annals, 7:29; "Report from the Committee appointed to make a Collection of Materia Medica 1696?" R.C.P., box 9, env. 191.

broadsides was put out to show how much the College had the public interest in mind and how little the apothecaries cared for anything but money, and defending the physicians from the charge that they were using the dispensary only to attack the Society of Apothecaries.[70] The College also ordered the apothecaries to start presenting their apprentices for examination and began to visit the apothecaries' shops again.[71]

But the antiauthoritarian group did not give up, either. In January 1697 these physicians sent a letter to the "visitors" of the College that had been established by the charter of Charles II: Sir John Somers (lord keeper of the Great Seal), Sir John Holt (lord chief justice of the King's Bench and former counsel to the College), Sir George Treby (lord chief justice of the Common Pleas), and Sir Edward Warden (lord chief baron of the Court of Exchequer). It declared

> That a prevailing party of the said College of Physicians have combined together, and in a fraudulent and surreptitious manner have lately passed and made as we conceive several grievous, impracticable, and illegal statutes or bylaws to which they have annexed very rigorous penalties, fines, and amercement, and that notwithstanding, your petitioners . . . have several times earnestly desired that the said statutes or bylaws should be offered to be confirmed [by a vote of a regular meeting of the whole College] according to the statute made in that behalf as it is expressly provided in the charter of King Charles the Second; your petitioners declaring at the same time their readiness to comply with the bylaws so confirmed, yet the proposal, which they conceive to be very just and reasonable, hath been still rejected.

The visitors took up their official duties and began to look into the affairs of the College but soon stopped, apparently not believing that they had the right to do so (since the charter of James II, under which the officers continued to govern, did not provide for their visitation).[72]

Despite all, the officers of the College went ahead with the dispensary and advertised its existence in several newspapers.[73] They also

---

[70]*A Briefe Account of the Dispensary* (1696); *A Further Account of the Dispensary* (1696); *A Farther Account of the Dispensaries* (1696); *The Dispensaries and Dispensary Physicians Vindicated, etc.* (1696).

[71]Annals, 7:20–21, 30–31.

[72]Annals, 7:93–96, 97; Clark, pp. 470–71. James's charter had made the king himself the "visitor" of the College. The letter was signed by J. Clerk, Stokeham, Bernard, Pitt, How, Blackmore, and Gibbons.

[73]See, for example, the *London Post-Boy,* April 14–16, 1697.

publicly attacked the Society of Apothecaries for opposing the College and for setting up a "party" within the College to frustrate their public actions.[74] The College also presented a list of the membership to the clerk of the lieutenancy and published a new catalogue of members. But on the occasion of the quarterly meeting of the full College in December 1697, only eighteen members showed up, not enough to make a quorum, and so the meeting had to be cancelled.[75]

A Partial Ending: The Groenvelt and Rose Cases

Eyes now turned to a test in the courts of the College's coercive powers. The censors had decided to act vigorously against one of the College's own: Johannes Groenvelt (otherwise known as John Greenfield), a physician with an M.D. from Utrecht (1670) who had immigrated to London about 1677 and gained licentiate status in 1681. Specializing in treating and cutting for bladder stones and the gravel, Groenvelt had also joined in the "repository" practice with John Pechey and others in 1685. He not only associated with empirics, but had good friends among the fellows in Francis Bernard, Richard Blackmore, and William Gibbons, all of whom opposed the College's current policies.[76]

In July of 1694 the censors had heard testimony against Groenvelt's practice from Susanna Withall, who brought other witnesses to corroborate her testimony.[77] Behind-the-scenes maneuvering seems likely, since her testimony was unusual: she was very exact on the therapy used by Groenvelt, while only complaining that it had "weakened" her, and Groenvelt later claimed that she did not bring

---

[74]*A Short Account of the Proceedings of the College of Physicians . . . in relation to the Sick Poor* (1697).

[75]Annals, 7:123, 124.

[76]See Groenvelt's dedication in his *De tuto cantharidum in medicina usu interno* (1698), authorized translation in 1706, as *A Treatise of the Safe, Internal Use of Cantharides in the Practice of Physick.*

[77]Groenvelt had been complained of in another case, in August 1693, by Mrs. Catherine Hawes. On August 18, the *comitia* heard her testimony with Groenvelt present: she said that he had cut her husband for the stone for £20, getting £8 in advance. He had given her a written note promising that if her husband died within the month, he would return the down payment. The husband died in five days, but Groenvelt submitted a bill for the remainder of his fee plus £3 6s. for the surgeon's fee, and he refused to consult with or allow Mrs. Hawes to consult with other physicians. The *comitia* decided to order both parties to sign releases and to get Groenvelt to pay the surgeon's bill and to return 40s. of the £8 Hawes had already paid. This satisfied both parties (Annals, 6:76–78, 78–80).

her complaint until two years after the treatment.[78] The registrar also kept unusually exact and extensive records of the testimony.

Withall claimed that she had had pains in her "lower parts" after giving birth. Groenvelt had been called, and he diagnosed an ulcer of the bladder, saying that he could cure it in three days for four pounds (of which he got half in hand) and that if he did not cure it, she could complain to the College. He then gave her eighteen pills to take. She took fifteen of them, which caused her great pain and made her evacuate bloody urine said to be in the amount of six quarts. Withall said that the pills were made of "Spanish flies" (Groenvelt used the Latin name, *cantharides*). She continued that she had grown very weak from the pills and had called Groenvelt back. He told her that if other physicians knew what was in the pills, they would esteem them very much, but he threw the remaining three pills into the fire. (One of the women present managed to save one of them.)[79]

Groenvelt testified on his own behalf in November of 1694, claiming that the internal use of cantharides was justified and had cured Withall of her ulcer. Moreover, according to his own later account, she had taken "stimulating" pills made only of cantharides rather than the pills made up by him, which contained camphor, as well, and by doing so had disobeyed his written instructions; beside which, she had kept to her bed for a long time before sending for him and was much weakened by a difficult recent childbirth. And yet she had still been cured by his treatment.

The censors, however, judged the internal use of cantharides to be bad and found him guilty of malpractice.[80] The majority of the censors voted to punish Groenvelt, but by the time they declared themselves in 1695 the College had been deeply split. One of the censors, Edward Tyson, refused to go along with the others, saying that "he questioned the power" of the College to judge Groenvelt's practice. Tyson, who had himself been harassed by the College (even though he was professor of physic at Gresham College and physician to Bridwell and Bethlehem hospitals, as well as a fellow of the Royal Society), had signed the petition to Parliament in 1689 trying to block the College from acting under James II's charter. He clearly did not believe that the College ought to be acting as a court to judge potentially therapeutic medical practices. Without Tyson's vote, Groenvelt's case could not result in a punishment. But it was heard all over

[78]Groenvelt, *De tuto,* preface.
[79]Annals, 6:153–57.
[80]Groenvelt, *De tuto,* preface; Annals, 6:175–77.

again in 1696 and 1697, when Tyson no longer sat as censor. The rehearing of his case Groenvelt attributed to "some sharp words" that he had with Richard Torlesse, a censor and an advocate of the College's new policies.[81]

In 1697 the censors once again found Groenvelt guilty of malpractice for the inward use of cantharides. A lawyer drew up a long document committing Groenvelt to Newgate prison (and fining him twenty pounds) and holding him there at the will of the president and the censors. Groenvelt blamed his imprisonment on the ill will of the censors combined with the "railings and calumnies" of the three women who testified against him. He had not been given a chance to hear their testimony or to answer their charges in 1697 but had nevertheless been sent to "the common gaol for thieves and rogues." He soon got out on habeas corpus, however, and he both sued the College in return and published a Latin tract defending his use of cantharides and accusing the censors of despotic power.[82] According to one source, the Society of Apothecaries contributed fifteen pounds to keep Groenvelt's suit going against the censors.[83] The case continued into the eighteenth century, although in the end Groenvelt lost.[84]

Again, the public was informed about Groenvelt's case. In addition to Groenvelt's own book, a pamphlet written by someone under the pseudonym of Lysiponius Celer declared that the proceedings showed that the censors were both poor physicians and not very bright, being the only members of the College who had time enough on their hands to hold office, and so they maliciously vented their sour grapes at "Greenfield." This brought all of physic into question and made all physicians judged by the "mob."[85] Charles Goodall employed Richard Boulton, an M.A. of Brascnose College, Oxford, to reply to Celer and Groenvelt (as well as Colbatch), although in the course of writing some of these pamphlets Boulton found that Good-

[81]Annals, 6:230–31; 7:3–4, 5, 9–10, 97, 100–109; Groenvelt, *De tuto,* preface.

[82]"Warrant for Commitment of J. Groenvelt to Newgate," Sloane 1786, fols. 157–58; Annals, 7:110–11, 112–13; Groenvelt, *De tuto,* preface.

[83]Badger, *Doctor Badger's Vindication.*

[84]"Groenvelt vs. Burwell et al.," 1 Ld. Raym. 454–72, *English Reports* 91; "Dr. Groenvelt versus Dr. Burnell [sic] et al.," Carthew, 421, 491–95, *English Reports* 90; "Groenvelt versus Burwell et al.," 1 Salkeld, 145, 263, 396–97, *English Reports* 91; "Groenvelt versus Burwell et al.," Holt, K.B., 184, 395, 536–37, *English Reports* 90.

[85]Lysiponius Celer, *The Late Censors Deservedly Censured; and Their Spurious Litter of Libels Against Dr. Greenfield and Others, Justly Expos'd to Contempt* (1698), p. 38. If the apothecaries were in fact supporting Groenvelt against the College, they may have commissioned this tract as they had commissioned Badger's.

all was knifing him in the back, as well, and took his case to the public in turn.[86]

Not content with stirring a hornet's nest of public ridicule against the censors, in the spring of 1698 Groenvelt brought to the Crown's attention the fact that the censors had not taken the oaths of allegiance and supremacy. Since the officers were acting as sitting judges in prosecuting others, such an omission could place them in jeopardy, especially since the end of the Nine Years War and the Whig Junto in late 1697 brought into being "one of the most confused periods in English political history."[87] The censors tried to gain more time to qualify themselves for the oaths. In May they sent a petition to the Parliament asking for the same. But a suit came against them nevertheless, and the president and censors petitioned the king for a nolle prosequi, claiming that they "find that no Censor ever did or ever thought themselves obliged to take the said oaths as not [thinking] themselves to have an office or employment within the words and meanings of the said act." The suit was dragged into the House of Lords in 1699, apparently finally dying there.[88]

The leadership of the College, then, came under increasing fire as it tried to discipline members internally, to continue prosecutions against others, and to pressure the Society of Apothecaries through the dispensary. One London wit, Ned Ward, had this to say about the College:

> They [of the College] lately committed a more able physician than themselves without bail or mainprize, for malpractice in curing a woman of a dangerous ulcer in her bladder by the use of cantharides, which they affirm not fit for internal application, though the patient's life was saved by taking it; which shows they hold it a greater crime to cure out of the common method, than it is to kill in it. And in persecuting their antagonist for the contempt of Galen and Hippocrates, they charged him for the doing that good which themselves wanted either will or knowledge to perform, and this made themselves all fools in attempt-

[86]Richard Boulton, *Letter to Dr. Charles Goodall* (1699). Also see the letters of Goodall to Hans Sloane, Oct. 26 and Dec. 11, 1698, Sloane 4037, fols. 140, 143.

[87]James R. Jones, *Country and Court: England, 1658–1714*, p. 302.

[88]Annals, 7:132, 133; "Censors Petition to the King re their omission to take the oaths of Allegiance and Supremacy . . . 1698," R.C.P., 2003/27–28; Johannes Groenvelt, *Reasons Humbly Offer'd . . . why Dr Thomas Burwell . . . [et al.] . . . should not be excused from the penalty of the Act of 25 Car. II* (1700). The College replied with *The Oath Taken by the Censors* (1700).

ing to prove the other a knave, who now sues them for false imprisonment; having also informed against them in the Crown office, as common disturbers.[89]

Moreover, the continuing controversy over the dispensary drew more public attention with the publication of Samuel Garth's *The Dispensary, A Poem* (1699). The dispensary was in turn defended by the College and by important members of the College.[90]

At the end of the decade, internal divisions and external pressures seemed about to dissolve the College as a viable institution. Two quarterly meetings in 1699 had to be cancelled due to a dearth of members in attendance, as did several meetings in the following years. A number of fellows refused to sign bonds that would oblige them to observe the statutes of the College.[91] Others being sued by the College, such as William Salmon, continued to call the College a dangerous monopoly.[92] One wit wrote about a controversy in Hell between the lawyers and the physicians over which profession was the worst—perhaps the physicians could take some cold comfort from the fact that the lawyers won their case and were declared more malicious.[93]

But the leadership would not stop prosecuting outsiders, nor would it back down on the issues that divided the College. At the end of 1702, a number of members who opposed the College's policies presented a "Petition of Grievances" in which they attempted to reach a reconciliation. "We whose names are underwritten," it began, "having a due zeal and sincere concern for the honor, and interest of our profession, cannot without being sensibly touched, reflect on the low and languishing state to which the College is at this time reduced." So a proposal was set forth:

[89]Ned Ward, *The London Spy* (1703), ed. Kenneth Fenwick, pp. 98–99.

[90]*The Necessity and Usefulness of the Dispensaries* (1702); *The Necessity of the Dispensary Asserted by the College of Physicians* (1702); Robert Pitt, *The Craft and Frauds of Physick Expos'd* (1702).

[91]*Annals*, 7:170, 172–73, 175, 180–81.

[92]William Salmon, *A Rebuke to the Authors of a Blew-Book; call'd The State of Physick in London* (1698); "College of Physicians vs Salmon," 5 Mod. 327–28, *English Reports* 87; "The President and College of Physicians, London, versus Salmon," 2 Salkeld, 451, *English Reports* 91; "The President and College of Physicians versus Salmon," 1 Ld. Raym., 680–81, *English Reports* 91. Also see James Younge, *Sidrophel Vapulans: Or, the Quack-Astrologer toss'd in a Blanket* (1699), versus Salmon; and *The State of Physick in London* (1698).

[93]*Hell in an Uproar, Occasioned by a Scuffle that Happened between the Lawyers and the Physicians* (1700).

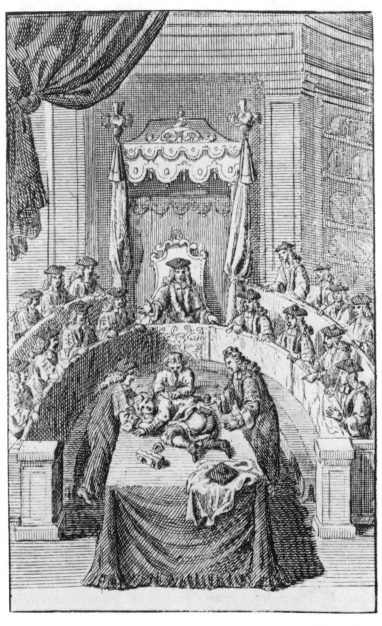

Plate 11. "A Description of the Coledge of Physicians." Engraving in Thomas Brown's "Physic Lies a-Bleeding," 1697, pp. 1419. iam; from Brown's *Works,* vol. 3, after p. 90. By permission of the British Library. In this satire, the fellows of the College of Physicians are assembled to watch an attempt to extract a knife from the bowels of a servant boy who has swallowed one, by applying a magnet to his rear end.

Upon mature and impartial consideration of the whole matter, 'tis our unanimous opinion, which we believe to be founded on just reason, that the new statutes are the principal cause of our unhappy circumstances, these having not only divided the members of our society, but by narrowing our bottom [i.e., by causing a drop in recruitment], have kept many worthy practitioners of physic in this City from entering into it, whereby our debts increase without prospect of remedy, and our body diminished without hopes of repair.

A number of statutes were then recommended for removal.[94] But after much dispute, a vote upheld the statutes. The College was split so deeply that it seemed impossible to reconcile the parties.

Moreover, the influence of the Society of Apothecaries continued to grow. In 1702 the apothecaries got the explicit right to supply medicines to the fleets without the supervision of the College. The petition of the College to the lord high admiral in February of 1703, stating that the physicians and not the apothecaries should examine the medicines, was unavailing.[95] With the growing importance of the military in English affairs, especially in affairs of state, the College found its political position greatly damaged by the loss of its rights to supervise the supply of medicines to the army and navy.

The final blow to the College's authority came with a decision in the House of Lords that gave the apothecaries the right to practice medicine. The decision was unexpected by the officers of the College, for they had carefully prepared a case against William Rose, an apothecary, and had won the case in a special verdict jury trial in the King's Bench before their former counsel, Chief Justice Holt.[96] But the House of Lords overturned the decision, apparently on grounds of anticollegiate sentiment. The implications of the House of Lords' reversal of a century of precedents on this point was truly significant for medical regulation.

William Rose, an apothecary in St. Nicholas Lane, had been complained of to the censors in 1700 by John Seale, a butcher of Hungerford Market in St. Martins in the Fields. Seale told the *comitia* that Rose had given him physic from December 5, 1699, to January 1700,

---

[94]Annals, 7:198; the document was signed by Tyson, Slare, Dawes, Welman, How, Blackmore, T. Robinson, Gibbons, Carr, Gelsthorpe, Chamberlen, Cole, and Cade.

[95]*Calendar of State Papers, Domestic,* 1702, "About 8 Dec."; Barrett, *History of the Society of Apothecaries;* Cecil Wall, "Postscript," *Chemist and Druggist* 133 (1940): 10; Annals, 7:201–2.

[96]"College of Physicians versus Rose," 3 Salkeld, 17, *English Reports* 91; "The College of Physicians against Rose," 6 Mod., 44, *English Reports* 87.

but that instead of getting better, he got much worse. This occurred despite the fact that Rose "had received of him a great deal of money, and [Seale] was to pay him yet more, as by a large bill he had brought with him it doth appear." The *comitia* ordered Mr. Swift, its attorney, to prosecute Rose "in law."[97]

Rose believed that he was being singled out for action unfairly. He sought out Seale and "railed against the College, and was very troublesome to him."[98] As Rose later explained to Hans Sloane (a fellow of the College, the physician to Christ's Hospital, and a fellow of the Royal Society), Rose had known Seale for a very long time and had done him a favor. According to Rose, Seale had been "a very loose liver, and very much addicted to women, the effects of which [in the form of syphilis, apparently] fell upon him in the last years." Seale had sought the help of a practitioner in Aldersgate Street, but the results of the treatment were a great spitting and a cough (commonly the result of mercury treatments), and Seale was wasting away. Seale therefore sought out Rose and wheedled Rose into giving him a diet drink, which made him a little better, until he relapsed. Rose stated that he had told Seale to get other advice but Seale had replied that he would have no money until the winter "when his customs came to town." Rose could not shake Seale, and anyhow, he complained, "I never yet could find that a doctor of physic cared to be burdened with such patients, especially of that distemper," so he treated Seale. But Seale had then tried to cheat him of his fee by complaining to the College: "The complaint made to the College by him and his wife, was made to defraud me of my due." Rose hoped that Sloane could help him get the College to stop the suit.[99] Sloane seems to have favored the antiauthoritarian physicians, but others controlled the College. Its officers therefore continued the prosecution on the grounds that Rose had been practicing physic, and it won the case and received a five-pound fine in King's Bench.

The verdict in King's Bench seemed to be manifestly unjust from Rose's point of view, and he petitioned the Privy Council, claiming that "he is advised there is a manifest error, and that he is properly relievable by bringing a writ of error returnable in Your Majesty's high court of Parliament." In November 1703 the new queen supplied Rose with his writ, and in February 1704, when the House of Lords next met, the writ was entered there, the final court of re-

[97]Annals, 7:171–72.
[98]Annals, 7:172.
[99]"William Rose to Hans Sloane, May 24, 1701," Sloane 4038, fol. 169.

view.[100] Early in March, having been informed of Rose's proceedings, the College formed a committee to oppose him and managed to get a petition accepted that allowed the case to be heard in a full session of the House of Lords rather than decided on in committee.[101]

The College lobbied hard for its position. It printed five hundred copies of a three-page pamphlet arguing its side of the case.[102] And printed form letters were sent to all members of the College urging them to use what influence they could: "You are desired by the President and Censors to be present at the hearing of our case against Rose the apothecary for practicing physic, before the Lords at their bar upon the [thirteenth] day of March about 10 o'clock; in the meantime, to solicit what lords you know on behalf of the College and to interest them to be there."[103]

The Lords, however, on hearing the case, "contrary to the expectation of the bystanders [deleted] as several of them since acknowledge, reversed the judgement of the Court of King's Bench."[104]

Sir Thomas Powys and Mr. Samuel Dodd represented the Society of Apothecaries in the case. Powys argued that "this is not a complaint by the people, but is a single prosecution of the physicians." He also brought out Goodall's book to quote from it statements showing that the College of Physicians had never been meant to "restrain any man in his trade." Mr. Dodd was even more direct:

"Several physicians (not so much educated in, or graduates of our own famous universities) being for the sakes of their fines, or other considerations, lately admitted into the College, are now so numerous, as to take on them the government thereof, and have fallen into divers methods for monopolizing the whole business of physic."

The physicians, he went one, "are setting up to enforce everyone to buy their advice (whether they like it or not) and this without the consent, and contrary to the will of the most eminent and best esteemed of their own profession." Additionally, he complained about the dispensary and argued that Rose had been practicing charitably. Powys also argued in reply to the College's lawyers that the case concerned one person, not the whole profession, and that the physi-

[100]S.P. 44/239/184; *House of Lords Journals,* vol. 17, p. 468.
[101]Annals, 7:213; *House of Lords Journals,* vol. 17, p. 468.
[102]*The Case of the College of Physicians London, Wherein they are Defendants* (1704).
[103]Annals, 7:213–14.
[104]*House of Lords Journals,* vol. 17, p. 482.

cians had not even found what Seale had been sick of (and so did not even know if Rose had cured him).[105]

Naturally, the College's lawyers argued that the statutes of Henry VIII gave the College the power to fine for illicit practice. "There is no pretender to physic but he will practice upon the same account" as Rose, Mr. Cooper declared; the apothecaries of London also "pretend to greater privilege than any other." The law was clear, and Their Lordships ought to affirm the judgment of the court. Mr. Browne also argued the clarity of the law and reminded the Lords that the judgment had been "only for £5," after all. After these arguments "a doctor proposed to speak" but was not allowed to do so.[106] The House of Lords, apparently disturbed by the rumors that had been reported for some years that the College officers were not the best physicians and were not enforcing a consensus of medical opinion, an idea strongly promoted by the apothecaries' attorney, reversed the law and declared for Rose.

In trying to discern the exact reasons for the Lords' decision, it may help to note that in January of 1704 the Whig-dominated House of Lords had been stage managing "populist" actions to thwart a Tory House of Commons. They tended to decide cases before them on the basis of the "rights of Englishmen" (particularly the case of *Ashby* versus *White*) and so would be tempted to decide against any "arbitrary" monopoly.[107] Moreover, in 1695 they had already granted the apothecaries an exemption from serving on parish offices, apparently because they were convinced that the apothecaries were legitimate medical practitioners who should be given the rights of other professions. The controversies of the College with the lords of the admiralty, with the Society of Apothecaries over the dispensary, and among its own members no doubt made it appear even more that the College officers were simply trying to maintain their outmoded rights and privileges in a era in which their learning and prestige were increasingly questioned. The College had largely failed to drive out of practice the dangerous quacks and instead seemed to be singling out those who most seriously competed with physicians.

Other practitioners were numerous and had found a public voice.

[105]*Manuscripts of the House of Lords*, 1703–1704, p. 54; *Observations upon the Case of William Rose an Apothecary, As represented by him To the Most Honourable House of Lords* (1704), pp. 3–6.

[106]*Manuscripts of the House of Lords*, 1703–1704, p. 54; *Observations upon the Case of William Rose*, pp. 3–6.

[107]Eveline Cruickshanks, "*Ashby* versus *White*: The Case of the Men of Aylesbury, 1701–4," in *Party and Management in Parliament, 1660–1784*, ed. Clyve Jones, pp. 87–104.

Public debates raged over systems of medical treatment. In such a milieu how could the College officers, especially when they were no longer uniformly educated in the academic traditions of physic at one of the two English universities, pretend to represent anything but an elite and narrow interest group? As the contemporary wit Ned Ward put it:

> They rail mightily in their writings against the ignorance of quacks and mountebanks, yet for the sake of lucre they license all the cozening pretenders about town, or they could not practice. This shows that it is by their toleration that the people are cheated out of their lives and money. Yet they think themselves so honest as to be in no way answerable for this public injury, as if they could not kill people fast enough themselves but must depute all the physical knaves in the town to be Death's journeymen. Thus do they license what they ought carefully to suppress, and practice themselves what they blame and condemn in others.[108]

The House of Lords decided that the law had not intended to make the College an arbitrary monopoly in its behavior, and so threw out Rose's case, despite the law.

Many people saw this victory of William Rose as the final admission that the learned traditions of physic no longer reigned supreme. Those who studied the ancient texts to understand how the human frame could best be preserved in health had come to be replaced by those both inside and outside the College who tried to invent new cures for specific illnesses and to get wealthy doing so. In Samuel Garth's *Dispensary,* Dr. John Bateman is sent down to the underworld to talk to William Harvey's shade about how to restore the prestige of the College. Harvey rebukes the contemporary physicians:

> With just Resentment and Contempt you see
> The foul Dissentions of the faculty;
> How your sad sick-ning Art now hangs her Head,
> And once a Science, become a Trade.
> Her Sons ne'er rifle her Mysterious Store,
> But study Nature less, and lucre more.[109]

---

[108]Ward, *London Spy,* p. 99.
[109]Garth, *Dispensary,* p. 69.

Robert Pitt, too, complained that "it is therefore most certain" that because of the alliances between empirical physicians and apothecaries, surgeons, and others to get money by prescribing expensive remedies, "our physicians bred up after the present mode are not deeply learn'd, but superficial pretenders to the knowledge of all diseases and their medicines."[110] On the other hand, an opponent of Pitt's, Joseph Browne, wrote that since the physicians were no longer "deeply learn'd," the officers of the College "support a private interest and arbitrary monopoly, [and] throw their scandalous and false aspersions upon the best and most eminent men of the profession, and tyrannize over the rest with the oppressive treatment of fines and imprisonment."[111]

As Browne went on to point out, the issues stood similarly to the way the issues of thirty or forty years earlier had, when Coxe, Merrett, and Goddard were writing. Like then, the physicians could not agree on what learned medicine was. Most of the old-fashioned Galenists had disappeared from the College, but the ancient texts still had their honored place in the university curricula of Oxford and Cambridge. Moreover, the "scientific" theories that were replacing the ancient traditions were many and diverse, among them, corpuscularianism, vitalism, and the "Newtonianism" of Pitcairn and others.[112]

At the root of the disputes lay a basic issue of medical practice: would the practitioner use empirically discovered remedies that had worked in previous cases, would he use a rationalist system, or would he let academic theory be his guide to the enormous individuality of different cases? The economic and social pressures to sell remedies, to develop an exclusive "method," and to play to the latest public fashions all pushed many physicians, like other practitioners, toward the first two choices. Only a vigorous defense by academically trained physicians of the juridical system that made them judges

[110]Robert Pitt, *The Frauds and Villanies of the Common Practice of Physick* (1705), preface.
[111]Joseph Browne, *The Modern Practice of Physick Vindicated* (1703), dedication.
[112] Theodore Brown believes Pitcairne obtained the "official recognition" of the College by getting its imprimatur on his books in 1694 and 1696, and he argues for the College's "reluctant but steady acceptance of 'Newtonian' medicine" after 1703 through the "striking pattern" of books "endorsed" by the Censors (Brown, *The Mechanical Philosophy and the "Animal Oeconomy": A Study in the Development of English Physiology in the Seventeenth and Early Eighteenth Centuries*, pp. 241, 267). Brown's remarks about how the censors "freely granted the *Imprimatur* to treatises maintaining a wide range of theoretical views" seems more important to me (p. 240).

of practice could allow learning to retain its preeminence. That is why Garth, in the *Dispensary*, has Harvey tell Bateman to fall at the feet of William III (the "visitor" of the College according to James II's charter):

> To him you must your sickly State refer
> Your Charter claims him as your Visitor
> Your Wounds he'll close, and sov'reignly restore
> Your science to the height it had before.[113]

Unfortunately for the College, Garth's suggestion of 1699 proved impracticable; the Parliament now counted for a great deal, and the majority of the "dispensary physicians" were no longer clearly superior in their academic training (and hence in their moral authority) to other practitioners. The House of Lords decided that despite the law, apothecaries who practiced empirical medicine were offering a service not so different from the kind being offered by the physicians, a service that should not be prohibited. The medical "profession," already moving toward cooperation among certain practitioners despite the more conservative physicians, would have to find a way to co-opt or displace empirical healers before it could emerge triumphant in the public eye two centuries later.

The medical marketplace had expanded since the early seventeenth century, and public opinion counted for more and more. Intellectual life had to an important extent grown away from the seriousness of academic, philosophical reasoning and toward wit, "science," and empiricism. The issues surrounding medical regulation by a corporate group had not changed significantly, but the political and intellectual situations had changed a great deal from James I's reign to that of Queen Anne's. No strong and independent Crown sought to control people through creating or co-opting a corporate structure in 1703, and so the College of Physicians had no important political ally. No academic elite clearly defined the framework of intellectual discussion.

The House of Lords, although it was an elite branch of government, represented public opinion more closely than the Privy Council of the early Stuarts had, a public opinion with different cultural values. Although no doubt influenced somewhat by the pleadings of the College, the Lords had no political or cultural reasons to support

---

[113]Garth, *Dispensary*, p. 69.

the College's power. In the end, then, two things undercut the regulatory authority of the College: the changed political situation, which was becoming more responsive to public opinion and to the influence of new, competitive professional and business classes with more market-oriented values; and the changed intellectual climate, which placed "common sense" and "hard-headed" empirical and "scientific" values above deeply learned academic training in the texts. The new medical order of liberty to practice, the era of the "medicine show," was publicly endorsed.

Conclusion

Many will say, a story of my own time would have pleased better:
But I say: He who in a modern story shall follow truth too near the
heels, it may chance to strike out his teeth.

Sir Walter Raleigh,
History of the World

The Rose case did not end attempts by the officers of the College of
Physicians to regulate the medical milieu in London, although it did
end their attempts to eliminate medical practice by apothecaries. Not
long after the Rose case, the officers even wrote and published a
broadside warning the fellows of the College who "countenanced
and encouraged" illicit practitioners that they, too, were subject to
penalties that would be "impartially inflicted."[1] For yet a few years,
the censors heard complaints and handed down sentences (see appendix
2, tables 1 and 2).

Yet increasingly these complaints were directed either at physicians
who were practicing without the College license or at those who
were believed to be overcharging for advice.[2] The *comitia censorum*
became more and more a body concerned with fee arbitration. An
attempt to restore to the College some real supervision of medical
practice came in 1725, when a number of physicians were told to be
examined for membership or to leave London and when a new
charter was applied for. But after failing to obtain a new charter, the
censors let lapse virtually all interest in regulation, and in the dispensary,
as well. The College of Physicians (often referred to at this time

[1] "Whereas divers Persons do illegally practice Physick . . .," B.L. 777.1.1(6).
[2] The fact that the censors heard and adjudicated cases in which apothecaries were charging
for their advice forces us to rethink the conclusion that the Rose case allowed apothecaries
to give advice but not to charge fees for it.

as the Royal College of Physicians) gradually became something rather new: a professional organization.

It is ironic that just as professional men were becoming more influential in the English state at the end of the seventeenth century, one group of professional men lost much of their former power.[3] But the influence of the liberal professionals on the state and the decline of corporate controls went hand-in-hand in the creation of the new liberal, laissez-faire system that began to take shape at the end of William III's reign and lasted well into the nineteenth century. Adam Smith had to write some tortuous passages in order to justify the influence and wealth of the professions; Adam Ferguson wrote of the professional men as being like the citizens of the Athenian state, tied to no task, left free to cultivate the mind and public pursuits.[4] Gentility became more a moral quality than a clear status based on landed wealth, a quality men of money and learning could attain even if they possessed no estates.

The physicians, in this new order far more than in the old, individually gained in social influence. They therefore had less need to protect themselves behind the barrier of corporate power. At the same time, after their coercive powers were taken from them, they could participate in public affairs without the visible marks of a monopoly. The end of the Crown's direct control of public life through chartered corporations and the rise of Parliament in its place after the Glorious Revolution remains a fact of fundamental importance to the development of England.[5]

The failure of the old medical order in London, then, was a failure of the learned physicians to maintain their place as judges of other medical practitioners. The College of Physicians had been formed by men trained in the texts, men we might today call medical philoso-

[3]See Geoffrey S. Holmes, *Augustan England: Professions, State, and Society, 1680–1730*; see pp. 163–235 for his views of the medical "profession."

[4]Adam Smith, *The Wealth of Nations* (1776; reprint ed., Chicago: University of Chicago Press, 1976), pp. 118–20; Adam Ferguson, "Of Subordination Consequent to the Separation of Arts and Professions," in *An Essay on the History of Civil Society* (1819), excerpted in *The Enlightenment: A Comprehensive Anthology*, ed. Peter Gay (New York: Simon and Schuster, 1973), pp. 567–70.

[5]For some recent defenses of the view that the Glorious Revolution did fundamentally change English political life, see: Clayton Roberts, "The Constitutional Significance of the Financial Settlement of 1690," *Historical Journal* 20 (1977): 59–76; Angus McInnes, "When Was the English Revolution?" *History* 67 (1982): 377–92; David Hayton, "The 'Country' Interest and the Party System, 1689–c.1720," in *Party and Management in Parliament, 1660–1784*, ed. Clyve Jones, pp. 37–85.

phers. Because of the broad learning these men possessed, they could give studied advice on matters of individual health and sickness, and of public policy when the "common good" touched on issues of public health. Therefore, the College had been chartered and supported by the Crown, and its members had been given juridical powers to judge other practitioners' activities by their learned standards. Their academic knowledge became the institutionalized criterion by which medical practice was gauged. The learned physicians and the Crown together established a de jure medical hierarchy in London and its environs. But by the end of the seventeenth century, that medical order was falling apart.

Part of the explanation for the fall of the College's juridical power is political. A centralizing monarchy might well support subordinate corporations like the College as a means of acting for the perceived public good as well as a means of expanding its own power and influence. The public good was not perceived in the same way by other groups in the realm, however, as two revolutions in the century proved. The revolution of 1688 cleared the way for the gradual establishment of firm parliamentary control, leading to the collapse of the juridical power of monarchically dependent corporations such as the College of Physicians. The College was not alone in this: close parallels can be drawn between the fortunes of the College and those of other corporations that depended on the Crown's support to regulate others, such as the Stationers' Company, the Distillers' Company (both guilds), and the Eastland Company (a joint-stock company).[6] The parallels further underline the importance of political institutions in shaping the frameworks that govern lives.

The Parliament had no particular stake in supporting corporations like the College, which had little voice in electing members. It did have some interest in supporting City guilds like the Society of Apothecaries. Moreover, petitioning the more public forum of Parliament for favors had publicly brought out divisions in the ranks of the fellows of the College throughout the seventeenth century. The officers of the College could govern their members less firmly when they needed public unanimity to get their will done in Parliament than when they could direct their appeals to officers of the Crown

---

[6]Cyprian Blagden, *The Stationers' Company: A History, 1403–1959* (London: George Allen and Unwin, 1960); Distillers' Company, "Court Minute Books," vols. 1–3, 1663–1683, Guildhall MS no. 6208; idem, "List of Members Admitted, 1638–1708," Guildhall MS no. 6215; and R. W. K. Hinton, *The Eastland Trade and the Common Weal in the Seventeenth Century*.

without getting assurances of support from all factions of the fellowship. Disputes within the College undermined the prestige of the body when they were aired in public. So the history of medical regulation in seventeenth-century London has a strong political component.

But in medicine, as in other fields of activity, political changes alone were not responsible for change; they occurred because people quarreled over various alternatives, alternatives involving differing notions of the public good. In terms of medical practice, the continuing debate on this topic in the seventeenth century set out a contrast: was medical practice best when governed by a group that upheld the importance of broad and ancient learning, or was it best when practitioners were allowed freedom to practice as they wished, even when their practices were based on narrower, empirical trials? The answer depended not only on the political structures of the day, but also on the intellectual, economic, and, most particularly, cultural, assumptions made by those responsible for granting authority to institutions like the College.

Intellectually, the development of the "new science" undercut the preeminence of the humanistic physic of the founders and officers of the College. The "anti-intellectualism" of the new philosophy became ever more important in setting the tone for physic and medicine—not just among the practices of empirics or licentiates such as Sydenham, but even among fellows of the College itself.

For example, John Freind's *History of Physick* (1725), often cited as a sign of the continued prestige of academic learning in physic, held views that many of his learned predecessors would have abhorred. In his first volume, he attributes the ability of the ancients in physic to their "experience and practice" rather than to their philosophy. Thus, reading the ancients gave great advantages to someone who would practice physic, but the advantages were due to the way in which the ancient testimonies could supplement one's own experiences: "Every physician will make, and ought to make observations from his own experience; but he will be able to make a better judgment and just observations, by comparing what he reads and what he sees together." Moreover, no one need worry about being misled by the ancients, since "no one is tied up from judging for himself, or obliged to give in to the notions of any author, any further than he finds them agreeable to reason, and reducible to practice." The reason Freind returns to again and again is that reading the ancient medical authors will make the reader a better practical physician: "The searcher of authors has the benefit of other men's experience together with his own, and it is from the joint-concurrence of these, that we can hope for any considerable advancement in knowledge." Concluding his argument, Freind reiterates:

> After all, I am far from thinking, that reading all the books of the Faculty, without proper observations, and good judgement, can furnish a man with such knowledge, as is required of a physician: . . . all I contend for is, that the dignity of the faculty may be maintained, which can only be done by men of suitable knowledge; which knowledge can never be obtain'd in the degree it ought to be, without reading and comparing together the ancient and modern writers, and applying each of them as they serve best for any general notion, or present exigency. And 'tis the manner of this application, which does and must make one physician excel another.[7]

A mid-seventeenth-century learned physician such as Baldwin Hamey would have been appalled at this "defense" of ancient learning. It amounted to little more than saying that reading books was good for sharpening one's empirical skills and for upholding the "dignity" of physic.

We might assume that the empirical "advancements" in medicine Freind knew about were the cause for this shift from an "ancient" to a "modern" view. But larger cultural values undoubtedly played an important part in this shift, as well. By the end of the seventeenth century, the deep learning and studied gravity of the physicians of a century before were subjects of jest. "Wit" was more highly valued than learning. Collecting antiquities, books, and objets d'art seemed a more appropriate pastime for gentlemen than the serious study of philosophical texts. "Splitting hairs" was for dusty, old scholars who would accomplish nothing necessary for life. The result was a new kind of "learned" physician, best represented by Sir Hans Sloane, president of the Royal College of Physicians and the Royal Society. Sloane was one of those who had been made a fellow of the College by the charter of James II; his collections of books, manuscripts, antiquities, and objects of natural history became the foundation for the British Museum, but his own published works were of an empirical rather than a philosophical nature.

The political changes in England therefore created a situation in

---

[7]John Freind, *The History of Physick; From the Time of Galen, to the Beginning of the Sixteenth Century* (1725), vol. I, pp. 301, 302, 303, 309–10.

which new as well as suppressed cultural and intellectual attitudes came to the surface. Without legal regulatory power over their rivals (or one another), the members of the College of Physicians found their practices subject more than ever to the demands of the public. Changed public values about what constituted proper knowledge played a very significant role in undercutting the authority of the physicians to judge medical practice. Old-fashioned learning became devalued in favor of a more utilitarian empiricism. As a result, the physicians gradually gave in to their patients' wishes and came up with their own unique theories and therapies oriented toward curing disease, not explaining it with synthetic theories.

In an important article, medical sociologist N. D. Jewson has stressed how, in the absence of a regulatory body like the College, patients came to dominate the formation of medical ideas and practices in the eighteenth century.[8] In the early twentieth century, at the end of the patient-dominated medical age, George Bernard Shaw made the same point:

> In the main, then, the doctor learns that if he gets ahead of the superstitions of his patients he is a ruined man; and the result is that he instinctively takes care not to get ahead of them. That is why all the changes [in medical practice and fashions] come from the laity.[9]

Shaw and Jewson may exaggerate the dependence of physicians on their patients' ideas when the medical marketplace loosens the bonds of medical regulation. But it is clear that when the learned physicians lost their ability to intimidate other practitioners, the doors were wide open to changing further the intellectual basis of medical practice in accord with the new values of the public.

Why did such a shift of values take place? Here one can only offer speculations. Perhaps, as Keith Thomas wrote in a similar context, the changes are ultimately "mysterious."[10] But one part of the explanation is economic.

As the money economy was more and more diffused throughout England, people increasingly began to pay money for medical services. The number of empirics as well as the number of physicians

---

[8]N. D. Jewson, "Medical Knowledge and the Patronage System in Eighteenth-Century England," *Sociology* 8 (1974): 369–85.

[9]George Bernard Shaw, "Preface on Doctors," introducing *The Doctor's Dilemma* (1911; reprint ed., London: Constable, 1930), p. lxxiv.

[10]Keith Thomas, *Religion and the Decline of Magic*, p. 663.

grew rapidly. In the process, competition for patients increased. It was no mystery that a diagnosis of a disease as an ontological entity, as a thing-in-itself rather than as the result of some defect in a person or a person's habits, could be made quickly, because it involved less knowledge of and time spent with the patient. It could also result in quickly selling a remedy said to be appropriate for the disease. A practitioner could see and treat more patients if he took an empirical rather than an academic view of medicine.

But there is a danger of circular argument here, for if the public had valued academic physic over "mere medicine," then practitioners would have supplied it. What needs to be uncovered is why the public came to value empirical medicine so much that practitioners could make good livings supplying it rather than learned physic.

Perhaps even more significant than the creation of a market for medical skills and products, then, new values may have been introduced into English society by the money economy. It is possible that as the material standards of living improved for many people, and as the threat of plague and famine became less immediate, people began to value material things more than explanations for events. A belief that a person's activities could yield benefits or ameliorate troubles might mean that people spent more thought on how to accomplish "productive" ends than on how to explain things that happened to them.[11] If so, the change would have obvious connections to the move from broadly conceived, learned explanations of health and disease to a more result-oriented, empirically derived medicine. The growing "materialism" of the society may have been reflected in increasingly "materialistic" ideas of disease and cure.

Economic changes, however, were accompanied by educational ones. In the seventeenth century, a gentry that had much experience in the universities could couch its worldly values in intellectually respectable terms. As people with utilitarian and empirical attitudes who had some appreciation for the world of learning, their views also began to be found in the mouths of intellectuals. Sir Francis Bacon, to mention the most prominent example, was trained as a jurist, not a cleric. As such, he had not much patience with what could be called the contemporary "ivory tower" intellectuals. He and others wanted useful knowledge and were willing to support endeavors that promised to produce it.

A number of significant changes in religious spirituality in Europe

---

[11]Such is the main thrust of Thomas's concluding speculations in *Religion and the Decline of Magic*.

may have helped move the public away from valuing synthetic views of the world and toward valuing more particularized and detailed understandings of events. An emphasis on God's mysterious ways and the secret "intuitions" He sometimes gives to a conscience, on His early revelations to mankind rather than on rationalistic theology derived from philosophy—these and other changes in religious thought influenced many brands of Protestantism as well as those orders of the Catholic church most touched by humanism. A radical emphasis on the human conscience alone might not result in medically or scientifically interesting ideas. But a more general scepticism about complete explanations pronounced by learned men or about the evidences on which they were based might well be tied to critical and empirical approaches to the world.

Whether these values were "caused" by Protestantism may be questioned. An argument recently made very strongly by Svetlana Alpers distinguishes between "northern" and "southern" European traditions of art and learning. To the northerners, art was a mirror of nature rather than a window to the world; it was to portray nature in all her detail rather than to portray the (literary, historical, and philosophical) meanings to be found there.[12]

This argument might suggest that deeper cultural values affected the way in which various places adapted to the new religious possibilities rather than that the cultural values were caused by any particular confession. Applied to learned physic, the argument would stress the "imported" nature of humanistic medical learning, the academic dimensions of which were rare among English practitioners before the sixteenth century. And this argument brings us again to politics: as the "renaissance" monarchy flourished in England, so too did the humanistic medicine of the learned physicians; with the end of this monarchy came the end of the preeminence of learned physic.

No single cause, then, can account for the decline of the old medical regime in seventeenth-century London, but causes enough there were. Political, social, economic, religious, and educational changes all played a part in affecting the shift of values exhibited in medical practice and regulation. Similar changes were reflected in the religious institutions of England, for as these same new values influenced the church, the significance of theology declined in favor of a more utilitarian toleration. As happened among the physicians, some ministers participated in these changes and obtained promotions for it

[12]Svetlana Alpers, *The Art of Describing: Dutch Art in the Seventeenth Century.*

while others tried to hold the gates. And as happened to the College, the established church's ability to "monopolize" religious practice was affected by the political changes of the day.

For, like their learned counterparts in the church, the fellows of the College of Physicians might have succeeded in maintaining the supremacy of medical theory for a longer time had not their regulatory power been broken because of changes in the English constitution. The College's coercive powers had been disturbed by the political transformation of England in the seventeenth century. The importance of that transformation must not be underestimated.

A brief comparison with the *Faculté de médecine de Paris* is helpful. The economy and the culture of France were subject to similar, if not identical, changes over the course of the seventeenth century, and religious movements such as Jansenism in some ways paralleled the "Puritan" theologies across the channel. Changing public values about medical practice in France caused Louis XIV to create a *Chambre royale* (1673 to 1694), a corporation composed of *médecins du roi* not of the *faculté,* at about the same time that Charles II openly supported empirics associated with the court.[13] Molière's critical treatment of physicians had its parallels on the London stage.[14] The corporations of apothecaries and surgeons in France and England both gained increasing prominence as the armies and navies attained political power and as hospital medicine grew in importance.[15]

But unlike the London College, the Paris *faculté* held on to its regulatory powers and through them continued to preserve the "dignity" of learned physic. Probably the most important reasons were that it had the support of the powerful university of Paris and that it was located in a "corporate" state with a more continuously authoritarian monarchy. Despite occasional quarrels between the university and the Crown, then, the *faculté* continued to cause other practitioners trouble in the eighteenth century as it and the London College had in the seventeenth. The *Société de correspondence royale de médecine,* created in 1776 and chartered in 1778, was perceived as a threat to the "patrimony" and "dignity" of physic.[16] But it was not

[13]L. W. B. Brockliss, "Medical Teaching at the University of Paris, 1600–1720," *Annals of Science* 35 (1978): 250.

[14]Molière, *La malade imaginaire* (1673) and *Le médecine malgré lui* (1666); Herbert Silvette, *The Doctor on Stage: Medicine and Medical Men in Seventeenth-Century England,* ed. Francelia Butler (Knoxville: University of Tennessee Press, 1967).

[15]Toby Gelfand, *Professionalizing Modern Medicine: Paris Surgeons and Medical Science and Institutions in the Eighteenth Century.*

[16]Charles Gillispie, *Science and Polity in France at the End of the Old Regime,* pp. 194–244.

until the French Revolution that the old order in French medicine was disestablished as it had been in London around the turn of the previous century.[17]

In the end, we have seen that, left to patients and healers, medical practice responds quickly to the latest public fashions. But legal institutions can change this relationship and so influence the content of medical practice. Those who were interested in medical theory—in medical learning, to use the seventeenth-century term—needed some protection from the competitive medical marketplace; they got it in the authority of the College of Physicians. The growth and decline of various institutions was crucial to the development of medical practice and medical ideas. Some shreds of the legacy of the learned physicians remain in the study of the humanities in undergraduate and graduate medical education. But perhaps our modern physicians owe a greater debt to the ordinary practitioners, who by the first years of the eighteenth century had dislodged ancient learning from its medical throne.

[17]David M. Vess, *Medical Revolution in France, 1789–1796* (Gainsville: University Presses of Florida, 1975); Michel Foucault, *The Birth of the Clinic: An Archaeology of Medical Perception,* trans. A. M. Sheridan Smith.

Appendix 1.
The College of Physicians

Unless otherwise specified, the following lists are compiled from the Annals of the College of Physicians. Munk's *Roll of the Royal College* contains errors. Elections were usually held on September 29.

Table 1: Officers, 1630–1710

	President	consiliarii		Registrar	Treasurer	Censors			
1630	Argent*	Paddy*	Atkins*	Clement*	Fox*	Clement*	Winston	Spicer	Crooke
1631		Giffard*				Fox*		Hodson	
1632								Mever.	Spicer
1633	Fox*		Paddy*		Giffard*	Fludd*	Clement*	Basker.	Ridgley
1634			Argent*			Baskerv.*	Winston	Hodson	Spicer
1635				xHodson*					
1636							*	*	
1637						Meverall			
1638				xMeverall*		*	Smith	Wright	Goddard
1639								Prujean	Clarke
1640	Meverall*		Baskerv.				Hamey	Rant	*
1641			xFox*	Prujean		Bathurst	Smith	Goddard	
1642			Clarke*		Clarke*	Prujean	Hamey	Alston	
1643								DeLau.*	Sheaf
1644								Goddard	Clarke*
1645	Clarke*		Meverall*		Meverall*		Ent	Bate	Rant
1646		Wright*							Hamey
1647				*				Mickle.	Rant
1648					Alston*	Williams		Hamey	Bate
1649			xClarke*	Hamey				Mickle.	Regimo.
1650	Prujean*					Smith*	Rant	Bathur.	Trench
1651			xAlston*				Ent	Mickle.	King
1652				*			Hamey	Emily	Coxe
1653			Harvey*			Hamey*	Ent		Stanley
1654				Ent				Wilson	Bennet
1655	Alston*				Prujean*	Williams*		Trench	Scarbu.
1656						Glisson*		Mickle.	Wilson
1657		xWill.*	xPrujean*			Paget	Trench	Whist.	
1658		Hamey*				Mickle.*		Wharton	Merrett

Year								
1659	Collins	King	Paget	Ent*				
1660	Baber	Merrett	Goddard					Glisson*
1661	Wharton							
1662	Whistl.							
1663								xGlisson*
1664	Croydon	Scarbur.	Mickle*		Hamey*			Ent*
1665							xGlisson*	Gliss.*
1666	Wharton	Staines*	Goddard	Staines*	Mickleth.*			Mickle.*
1667	Croydon	Whistler	Coxe	Coxe			Alston*	xStaines*
1668	Collins	Merrett	Goddard	Goddard				xCoxe*
1669	Croydon	Stanley	Paget*	Wharton				Whistler*
1670	Collins	Merrett	Goddard	Coxe		Staines*	xStaines*	Coxe*
1671	Dacres	Betts	Whistl.	*				xScarburgh
1672	Needham	Croydon						
1673	Allen	Betts				Whistler		
1674	Frankl.	Barwick						
1675	Coysh	Brookes						
1676	Clerk	Lawson	Charle.	Rogers	Coxe*		Ent*	Charl.*
1677	Brown	Needham	Col., Jr	Staines*				Scarb.*
1678	Croone	Milling.	Col., Sr	Paget*				
1679	Brooke	Allen	Col., Jr	Whistler*	Whistler*			
1680	?	Milling.						
1681		?	?	?		Collins, Sr		xEnt*
1682	Hulse	Hodges	Allen	Charleton	Rogers*	Whistler*		Coxe*
1683	Alvey	Brown	Atfield	Witherly*		Coxe*		Whist.*
1684	Brooke	Milling.	Barwick	Burwell*		xScarburgh		Witherly*
1685	Briggs	Dawkins	Browne	Betts*	Millington	xBurwell*	[Knight]	
1686								
1687	Bateman	Pitt	Elliott	Barwick*			Rogers*	Charl.*
1688	Blackb.	Harris	Griffi.	Johnson			Witherley*	Scarb.*
1689	Gill	Davis	Gordon	Burwell*			Burwell*	
1690	Bateman	Morton	Griffi.	Collins*	Burwell*	Griffith		Charleton

Table 1 —continued

Year	President	consiliarii		Registrar	Treasurer	Censors			
1691		Mill.*	Betts*	Bateman			Hulse		
1692	Burwell*	Collins*	Witherly*	Gill	Lawson*	Brook*	Clerk	Briggs	Slare
1693			xBrooke*			Collins*	Slare	Dawes	
1694	Lawson*	Browne*	Burwell*		Browne*	Burwell*	Torles.	Tyson	Lister
1695	Collins*	Millington*						Dawes	Gill
1696	Milling.*	Collins*					*		
1697		Browne*				Collins*	Hulse*	Morton	Goodall
1698		Burwell*					Browne*	Charlet.	Harris
1699									Hulse
1700		Collins*							Harris
1701		Lawson*				Browne*	Torlesse*	*	Torle.*
1702	x/Browne.*	Charleton*		Bateman		Pitt			Brooke
1703					/Hulse	Goodall*	Garth		Woodwa.
1704						Harris*	Bateman		Hawys
1705		Collins*				Goodall*	Vaughan		Braith.
1706							Sloane	xColl.*	Gill
1707	x/Clerk*	Goodall*	Clerk/			How	Bateman		Chambe.
1708	C/Good.*	G./Clerk*			/Clerk	Slare*		Gould	Colebr.
1709		/Harris*				Gill	*	Sloane	Darnel.
1710		Dawes*						Dawes*	Colebr.

x = predecessor deceased.
/ = elected mid-year.
* = elect.
? = unknown.

Table 2: Elects, 1630–1710

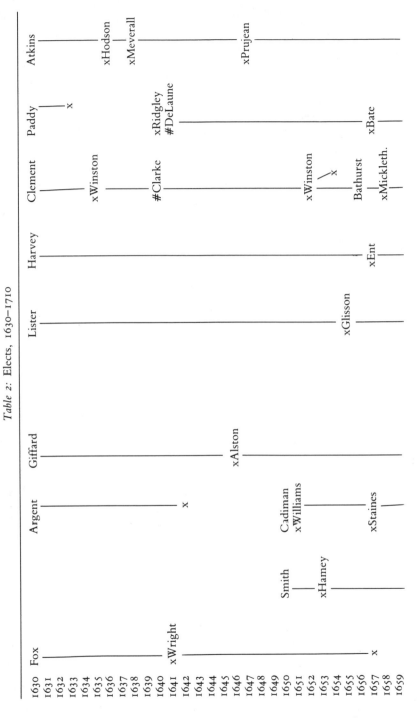

Table 2—*continued*

xFrazier   x   Charleton

xPaget   xWitherly

xRogers   #Lawson

xCollins

xScarburgh   #

Brooke

xClarke
xGoddard
xCoxe
xBetts

xKing   xBarwick   #Milling.

xWhistler
xBurwell

1660
1661
1662
1663
1664
1665
1666
1667
1668
1669
1670
1671
1672
1673
1674
1675
1676
1677
1678
1679
1680
1681
1682
1683
1684
1685
1686
1687
1688
1689
1690
1691

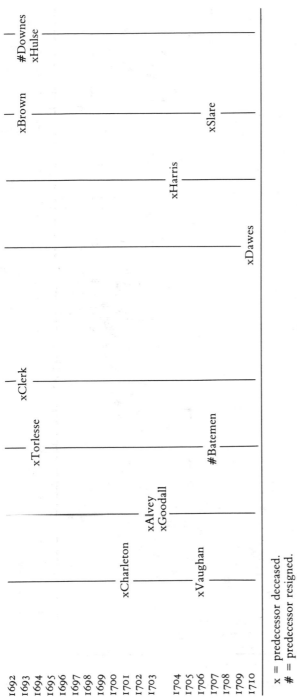

1692
1693
1694
1695
1696
1697
1698
1699
1700
1701
1702
1703
1704
1705
1706
1707
1708
1709
1710

xCharleton

xTorlesse

xClerk

xBrown

#Downes
xHulse

xAlvey
xGoodall

#Batemen

xDawes

xHarris

xSlare

xVaughan

x = predecessor deceased.
# = predecessor resigned.

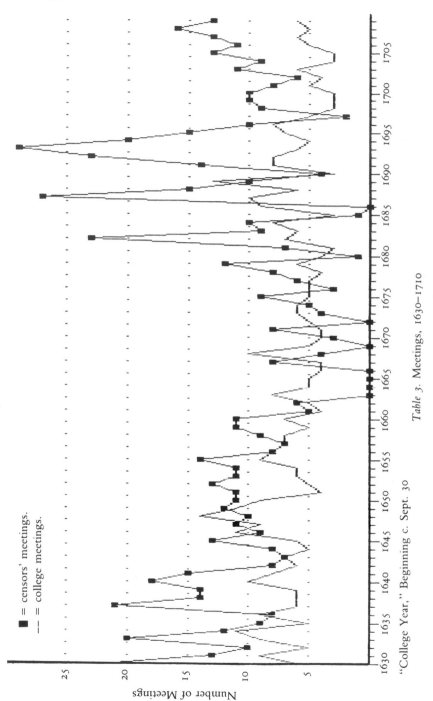

= censors' meetings.
-- = college meetings.

Number of Meetings

25

20

15

10

5

"College Year," Beginning c. Sept. 30

1630   1635   1640   1645   1650   1655   1660   1665   1670   1675   1680   1685   1690   1695   1700   1705

Table 3. Meetings, 1630–1710

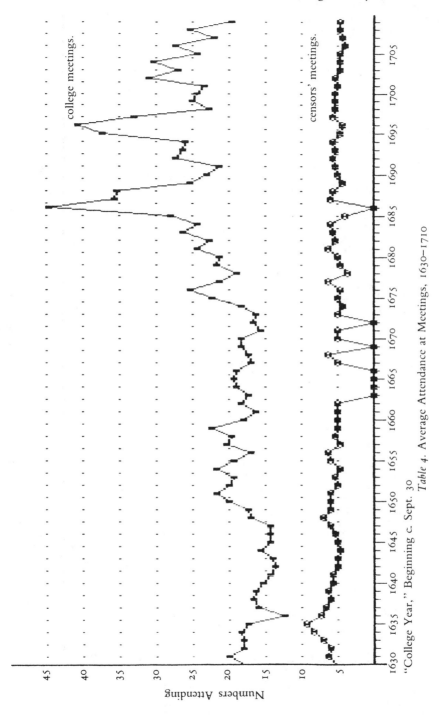

college meetings.

censors' meetings.

Table 4. Average Attendance at Meetings, 1630–1710

"College Year," Beginning c. Sept. 30

Numbers Attending

45
40
35
30
25
20
15
10
5

1630 1635 1640 1645 1650 1655 1660 1665 1670 1675 1680 1685 1690 1695 1700 1705

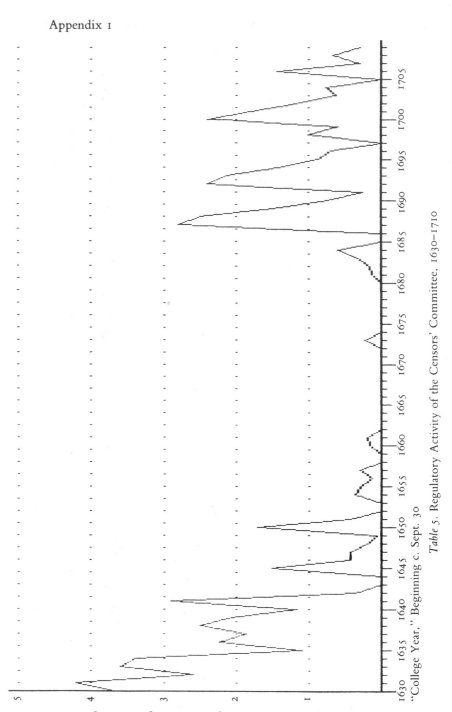

Table 5. Regulatory Activity of the Censors' Committee, 1630–1710

Table 6: Number of Members, 1628–1705

	Fellows	Candidates	Licentiates	Honorary Fellows	Total
1628*	37	6	7		50
1630*	36	8	10		54
1635*	38	1	7		46
1636*	37	1	7		45
1647*	34	13	5		52
1650*	37	10	7		54
1654(c.)*	36	12	10		58
1669^	43	23	8	69	143
1676#	53	17	6	46	122
1683#	45	8	15	29	97
1688#	79	2	28	17	126
1693#	74	5	37	13	129
1694#	73	5	40	11	129
1695#	70	5	41	11	127
1704#	65	5	37	4	111
1705#	63	8	36	3	110

* = From Annals.
^ = From list on flyleaf, *Anglia Notitiae* (1669), B.L. P.P.3360.
# = From printed lists of members, B.L. 777.1.2.

Appendix 2.
College Regulatory Activity

The following tables are compiled from the Annals of the College of Physicians. All cases recorded in the Annals are given in these tables, but not every action is recorded in the Annals. The tables are therefore intended to give a full account of the College's *recorded* actions, which may be taken to be indications of the variations in regulatory activity from year to year, presuming that the number of unrecorded actions (which seems to have been slight) did not vary significantly over time. The variations in activity recorded cannot be correlated with changes in holders of the office of registrar. Information on activity before 1640 is in the possession of the Oxford Wellcome Unit for the History of Medicine.

276

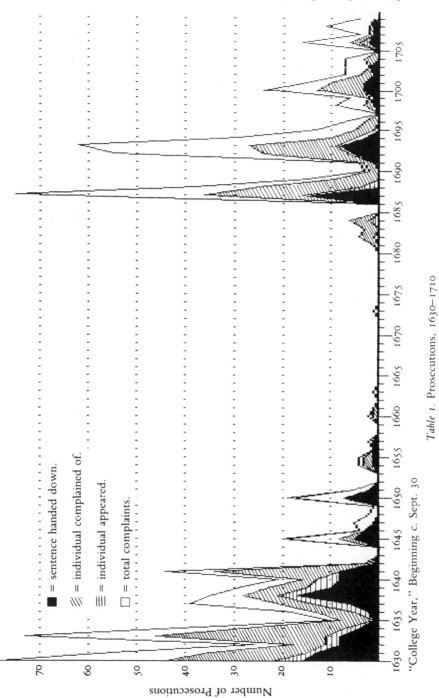

■ = sentence handed down.

\\\\ = individual complained of.

≣ = individual appeared.

☐ = total complaints.

Number of Prosecutions

"College Year," Beginning c. Sept. 30

Table 1. Prosecutions, 1630–1710

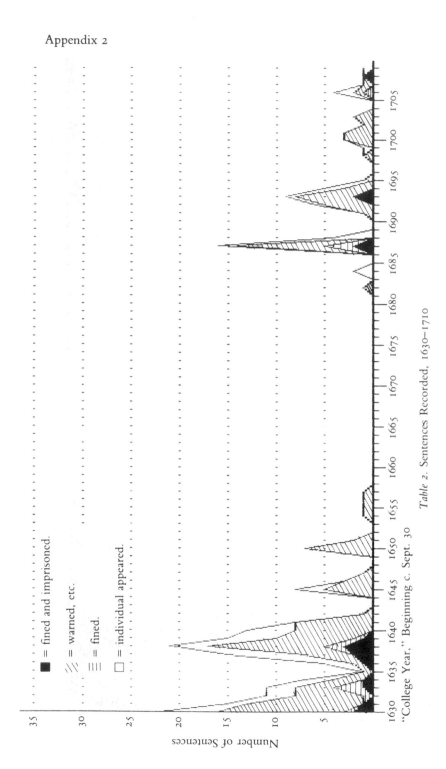

Table 2. Sentences Recorded, 1630–1710

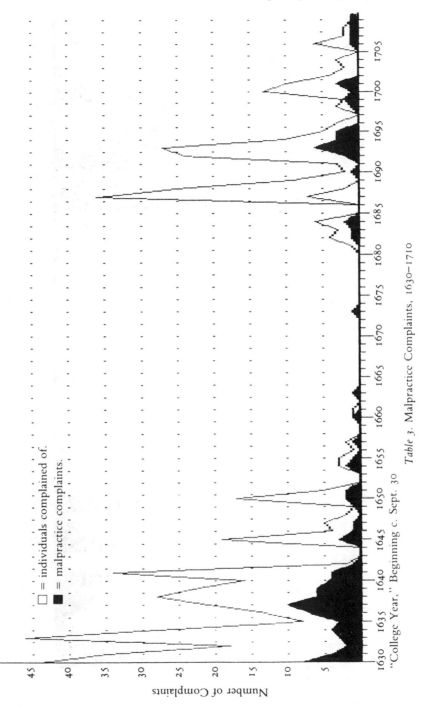

Table 3. Malpractice Complaints, 1630–1710

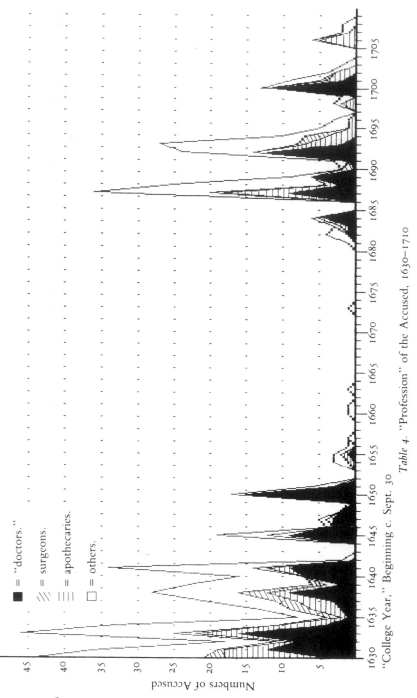

Appendix 3.
English Royal Physicians

No attempt has ever been made to list precisely the holders of the office of English royal physician in the seventeenth century (although the Scottish royal physicians—not the same persons—have been listed by the Scottish Record Office). There were two kinds of royal physician—first physician and physician-in-ordinary—and one of the former and several of the latter (normally three or four) served at any one time. They held salaried positions under appointment by the Privy Seal (although the extant records of payment indicate that they often drew little of their salary, and that almost always in arrears).

Other physicians or ordinary practitioners might be consulted in particular cases by the king and members of his family but did not have standing appointments: these men were sometimes called royal physicians extraordinary (that is, without regular salary). Many of the royal physicians extraordinary called themselves royal physicians, so there is confusion about who held the official posts. The following list includes only those who can with certainty be known to have held a position as royal physician under the Privy Seal. It is undoubtedly therefore incomplete at some points, but caution is imperative in beginning to sort out the real from the pretended "royal" physicians.

James I:
    First Physician:
        J. Craige, Jr.
        T. de Mayerne
    Physicians-in-Ordinary:
        Sir S. Baskerville
        J. Hammond
        J. Maccolo

H. Atkins
Wm. Harvey

Charles I:

First Physician:
Sir T. de Mayerne
Physicians-in-Ordinary:
M. Lister
Sir S. Baskerville
J. Craige, Jr.
A. Ramsey
D. Beton
Wm. Denton
H. Atkins
Wm. Harvey

During the war, 1642–49:
First Physician:
Wm. Harvey
Physicians-in-Ordinary:
Edm. Smith
S. Turner
Wm. Denton
E. Greaves

(Cromwell):

"State's Chief Physician":
G. Bate
Physicians-in-Ordinary:
J. Bathurst
J. Goddard
L. Wright

Charles II:

First Physician:
Sir A. Fraizer
G. Bate
C. Scarburgh
Physicians-in-Ordinary:
T. Witherley
T. Clarke
T. Whitaker
J. Micklethwaite
J. Baber
E. Greaves
Wm. Quartermaine
J. Colladon

J. Hinton
T. Waldron
E. Dickinson
James II:
First Physician:
C. Scarburgh
Physicians-in-Ordinary:
E. Dickinson
R. Brady
F. Bernard
C. Fraiser
Sir T. Witherley
William III:
First Physician:
C. Scarburgh
T. Millington
J. Hutton
Physicians-in-Ordinary:
W. Harris
R. Blackmore
C. Fraiser
T. Goodman
C. Harrell
Lawrence
Stockolm

Appendix 4. Statutes and Court Cases re the College of Physicians

Statutes:

"An Act concerning Phesicions and Surgeons," 3 Hen. VIII, c. 11.

"An Acte Concerning Phisicions," 14 and 15 Hen. VIII, c. 5.

"Concerning Phisicians," 32 Hen. VIII, c. 40.

"Concerning Barbers and Chirurgians," 32 Hen. VIII, c. 42.

"An Acte that persons being no commen surgeons maie mynistre medicines owtwarde," 34 and 35 Hen. VIII, c. 8.

"An Acte touching thincorporation of the Phisitions in London," 1 Mariae, St. 2, c. 9.

Court Cases:

"Dr. Laughton against Gardiner," Trinity Term, 4 Jac. 1; Cro. Jac. 121.

"Dr. Atkins against Gardiner," Easter Term, 5 Jac. 1; Cro. Jac. 159.

"Dr. Bonham's Case," Mich. 6 Jacobi 1; 8 Co. Rep. 107a.

"College of Physician's Case," Trinty 7 Jacobi; 2 Brownl. and Golds., 255.

"The corporation of Physitians Plaintiff, against Doctor Tenant for practising of Physick," Hillar., 11 Jac.; 2 Bulstrode, 185.

"Doctor Alphonso, and the Colledge of Physitians in London," Mich. 12 Jac.; 2 Bulstrode, 259.

"Butler against The President of the College of Physicians," Easter Term, 7 Car. I; Cro. Car. 256.

"Colledge de Physicians versus Butler," Trin. An. VIII Caroli Regis; Jones, W. 261.

"Doctor Goddard's Case," 12 Car. II; 1 Sid. 29.

"Dr. Goddard's Case," Hill. 12 & 13 Car. II; 1 Lev. 19.

"Dr. Goddard's Case in Assize Br. 76," Trin. 13 Car. II; 1 Keble, 75, 84.

"Roy versus Pordich," 21 Car. II; 1 Sid., 431.

"Doctor Poordage," 21 Car. 2; 1 Mod. 22.

"Dr. Pordage," 21 Car. II; 2 Keble, 578.

"Colledge of Physitians and Cooper or Hubert," 27 Car. II; 3 Keble 587.

"The Colledge of Physitians and Needham," 28 Car. II; 3 Keble, 672.

"The College of Physicians against Bush," 3 William and Mary; 4 Mod. 47.

"The College of Physicians against Basset," 3 Will. and Mary; 12 Mod. 10.

"The College of Physicians against Salmon," 8 Will. 3; 5 Mod. 327.

"The President and College of Physicians vers. Talbois," 8 & 9 Will. 3; 1 Ld. Raym., 153.

"Groenvelt versus Burnell [sic] & al'," Pasch. vel Mich. 9 W. 3.; Holt, K.B., 536.

"Groenvelt versus Dr. Burnell [sic] & al'," S. Mich. 9 Will. 3; Carthew, 421.

"Groenvelt versus Burwell," Trin. 10 Will. 3; 1 Salkeld, 263.

"Dr. Groenvelt versus Dr. Burnell [sic] & al'," Pasch. 11 Wm. 3; Carthew, 491.

"College of Physicians vers. Levett," Easter Term, 11 Will. 3; 1 Ld. Raym., 472.

"Dr. Groenvelt v. Dr. Burwell et al', Censors of the College of Physicians," Easter Term, 11 Will. 3; 1 Ld. Raym., 454.

"Groenvelt versus Burwell & al," Trin. 12 Will. 3; 1 Salkeld, 144, 396.

"Groenvelt versus Burwell & al'," Trin. 12 W. 3; Holt, K.B. 395.

"Groenwelt versus Burwell," Trin. 12 W. 3; Holt, K.B. 184.

"The President and College of Physicians vers. Salmon," Trin. 13 Will. 3; 1 Ld. Raym. 680.

"The President and College of Physicians, London, versus Salmon," Trin. 13 Will. 3; 2 Salkeld, 451.

"College of Physicians versus Rose," Hill. 1703; 3 Salkeld 17.

"The College of Physicians against Rose," Michaelmas term, 2 Queen Anne; 6 Mod. 44.

Selected Bibliography

Manuscripts Cited

Royal College of Physicians, London

For a brief description of the holdings of the Royal College of Physicians, see *Historical Manuscripts Commission, 8th Report*. London, 1882. App. 1, pp. 225b–234b.

Annals: *Annales Collegii Medicorum*. English as well as Latin typescripts exist for the first five volumes. Vol. 1: 1518–1572; Vol. 2: 1581–1608; Vol. 3: 1608–1647; Vol. 4: 1647–1682; Vol. 5: 1682–1690; Vol. 6: 1691–1695 (beginning with this volume, all entries are in English); Vol. 7: 1695–1710.

"An Answer to the Exceptions of the Surgeons, 1641." Box 4, env. 40.

"A Briefe of the Apothecaries Cause against the Colledge of Physitians and new Patent of Distillers and the College Answer, 1640." Box 4, env. 33.

"Censors Petition to the King re their omission to take the oaths of Allegiance and Supremacy . . ., 1698." 2003/27–28.

"A Deduction of the Apothecaries Behaviour Toward the College, 1640." Box 4, env. 31.

"Draft Agreement between Fellows and members of R.C.P. to support President and Censors of College in the Execution of the laws and statutes, 1695." 2012/9.

"Exceptions by the Chirurgeons to the Bill preferred by the College, 1641." Box 4, env. 40.

"Legal Opinion on several cases relating to the College of Physicians . . ., 1682." 2012/54–55.

"Legal Opinions [of Serj. Creswell Levinz] re confirmation of College statutes, etc., 1688." 2012/6–8.

"Legal Opinion re Power of College over Extra-Licentiates, 1683." 2014/2.

Bibliography

"Legal Opinion re propriety of College of Physicians issuing licenses to practice outside of London, 1682." 2014/1.

"Opinion of Counsel on the power of the College to constitute different orders of men. . . , 1680." Box 9, env. 172.

"Opinions on Legal Powers of the Censors, 1688." 2003/22–26.

Palmer, Ralph. "The Life of the Most Eminent Dr. Baldwin Hamey," 1733. 337.

"Petition of the Apothecaries [with] the Answere of the Doctors thereunto, 1640." 340/25.

"Petition of the College to Parliament for Suppression of Ignorant Practitioners, 1689[?]." Box 4, env. 48.

"Rationes Accepti et Expensi in Collegio Medico. Londonensium." 2073.

"Report from the Committee appointed to make a Collection of Materia Medica, 1696[?]." Box 9, env. 191.

Whistler, Daniel. "Inventory of his goods, chattles, and debts, 1684." Box 9, env. 109.

British Library, Sloane Collection

"A. N. to T. O." Sloane 631, fols. 168–77.

"Abridgment of the Statutes of the College of Physicians." By Thomas Gill. Sloane 3914, fols. 61 ff.

"Advyse to a young physitian. to one who intends to studie medicine and live thereby." Sloane 163, fols. 1–5.

"At the Committee of the College November 12 1689." Sloane 1789, fol. 160.

[Goodall, Charles]. "Information on the College of Physicians." Sloane 3914.

"A Just and Necessarie Complaint concerning Physicke." Sloane 2563, fols. 1–19.

"Letter from C. Bernard to Colbatch." Sloane 1783, fols. 80–81.

"Letter [from Dr. Badger] to the Apothecaries Company." Sloane 4026, fols. 386–87.

"Letters and Papers of Glisson." Sloane 2251.

"Qualifications of a Physician." Sloane 3216, fols. 42–91.

Untitled notes [of H. Stubbe?]. Sloane 1786, fols. 116–28.

"Warrant for Commitment of J. Groenvelt to Newgate." Sloane 1786, fols. 157–58.

"William Rose to Hans Sloane, May 24, 1701." Sloane 4038, fol. 169.

Wittie, R. "Letter to 'brother' [physician], March 21, 1671/2." Sloane 1393, fol. 12.

————. "Letter to Yarborough." Sloane 1393, fols. 15–16.

Guildhall Library

"Collection of Copy Acts and Ordinances, together with other papers relating to the regulation of the Apothecary Society, 1618–1743." Guildhall MS no. 8293.

Diocese of London. "Certificates and Testimonials." Guildhall MS no. 10,116 (boxes 1–4), no. 10,116A.
Distillers' Company. "Charter and Statutes, 15 Charles I, 1639." Guildhall MS no. 6228.
———. "Court Minute Books." Vols. 1–3, 1663–1683. Guildhall MS no. 6208.
———. "List of Members Admitted, 1638–1708." Guildhall MS no. 6215.
"Draft Bill of Proceedings in Court of Star Chamber by the Society of Apothecaries against several persons carrying on apothecaries trade for making and selling defective and inferior medicine, 1621–2." Guildhall MS no. 8285.
"Mayoral Precepts and Orders to the Apothecaries Company, 1661–1747." Guildhall MS no. 8296.
"Miscelleaneous Papers of the Barber-Surgeons' Company, 1612–1763." Guildhall MS no. 9833.
"Papers Relating to Disputes and Suits Between the Society of Apothecaries and the Barber-Surgeons' Company, 1640–1708." Guildhall MS no. 8290.
"Sundry Account and Memoranda Book, Apothecaries Company." Guildhall MS no. 8204.

Primary Sources Cited, Printed Before 1740

Occasionally, I have dated a source or made an attribution that differs from the entry in the catalogue of the British Library. All sources were published in London unless otherwise indicated.

Answers to the Objections Against the College Bill. 1689.
The Apothecaries' Reply to the City's Printed Reasons Against their Bill. 1694.
Badger, John. *The Case Between Doctor John Badger and the Colledge of Physicians London.* 1693.
———. *The Catalogue of the Fellows and Other Members of the Royal College of Physicians, London, Dated October 4, 1695.*
———. *Doctor Badger's Vindication of Himself, from the Groundless Calumnies and Malicious Slanders of some London-Apothecaries.* 1701.
Biggs, Noah. *'Mataeotechnia medicinae praxeos.' The Vanity of the Craft of Physick.* 1651.
Bolnest, Edward. *Medicina Instaurata: or, A Brief Account of the True Grounds and Principles of the Art of Physick.* 1665.
Boulton, Richard. *An Answer to Dr. Leigh's Remarks.* 1698.
———. *An Examination of Mr. John Colbatch his Treatise of the Gout.* 1699. [fragment]
———. *A Letter to Dr. Charles Goodall.* 1699.
Boyle, Robert. *Some Considerations Touching the Usefulnesse of Experimental Naturall Philosophy.* Oxford, 1663.
Brian, Thomas. *The Pisse-Prophet or, Certaine pisse-pot Lectures.* 1637.
A Brief Account of the Dispensary. 1696.
Brown, Thomas. *Physick Lies a Bleeding, or the Apothecary turned Doctor.* 1697.
Browne, Joseph. *The Modern Practice of Physick Vindicated.* 1703.

Bibliography

Buckworth, Theophilus. "Gentlemen, Take Notice. . . ." B.L. L.R. 404.a. 4(42). 1680(?).

The Case of the College of Physicians, London. 1689.

The Case of the College of Physicians London, Wherein they are Defendants. 1704.

Castle, George. *The Chymical Galenist: A Treatise Wherein the Practise of the Ancients is reconcil'd to the new Discoveries in the Theory of Physick.* 1667.

"A Catalogue of Chymical Medicines sold by R. Rotteram at the Golden Bull. . . ." S.P. 29/408/126.

A Catalogue of the Library of the late learned Dr. Francis Bernard. 1698.

Celer, Lysiponius. *The Late Censors Deservedly Censured; and Their Spurious Litter of Libels Against Dr. Greenfield and Others, Justly Expos'd to Contempt.* 1698.

Certain Necessary Directions as well for the Cure of the Plague, as for preventing the Infection. 1636; another ed., 1665.

Chamberlayne, Edward. *Angliae Notitia, Or the Present State of England.* 14th ed., 1682.

Chamberlen, Hugh. *A Proposal for the Better Securing of Health. Humbly Offered to the Consideration of the Honourable Houses of Parliament.* 1689.

Chamberlen, Peter. *To the Honourable House of Commons Assembled in Parliament, the Humble Petition of Peter Chamberlen, Doctor in Physick.* 1648.

––––––. *A Voice in Rhama: or, The Crie of Women and Children.* 1647.

Coke, Edward. *The Fourth Part of the Institutes of the Laws of England: Concerning the Jurisdictions of Courts.* (1st ed., 1644.) 1648.

Colbatch, John. *The Doctrine of Acids in the Cure of Diseases Farther Asserted.* 1698.

––––––. *Novum Lumen Chirurgicum: Or, A New Light of Chirurgery.* 1695.

––––––. *A Physico Medical Essay, Concerning Alkaly and Acid.* 1696.

––––––. *A Relation of a very Sudden and Extraordinary Cure.* 1698.

––––––. *Some Farther Considerations Concerning Alkaly and Acid.* 1696.

––––––. *A Treatise of the Gout.* 1697.

Collegii Medicorum Londinensium Fundatores et Benefactores. 1662.

Considerations Humbly Offered to the Lords Spiritual and Temporal, in Relation to the Apothecaries Bill. 1694.

Cook[e], John. *Unum Necessarium: Or, the Poore Mans Case: Being an Expedient to Make Provision for all poore People in the Kingdome.* 1648.

Cotta, John. *A Short Discoverie of the Unobserved dangers of severall sorts of ignorant and unconsiderate Practisers of Physicke in England.* 1612.

Coward, William. *Alcali Vindicatum: Or, The Acid Opiniator not guilty of Truth.* 1698.

[Coxe, Daniel]. *A Discourse, wherein The Interest of the Patient in Reference to Physick and Physicians is Soberly Debated.* 1669.

D., C. *Some Reasons, of the Present Decay of the Practise of Physick in Learned and Approved Doctors, in an Answer to a letter lately Received from A. B. Doctor of Physick . . . with some Remedies Proposed to Amend it.* 1675.

DeLaune, Thomas. *Angliae Metropolis: or, The Present State of London.* 1690.

"Directions for the Sugar Plums. . . ." S.P. 31/1/245.

The Dispensaries and Dispensary Physicians Vindicated, etc. 1696.

Emes, Thomas. *A Dialogue Between Alkali and Acid.* 1698.

An Essay for the Regulation of the Practice of Physick, Upon which Regulation Are grounded the Composure of all Differences Between Physicians and Apothecaries. 1673.

Fage, John. *Speculum Aegrotorum: the sicke mens glasse.* 1606.

A Farther Account of the Dispensaries. 1696.

Freind, John. *The History of Physick; From the Time of Galen, to the Beginning of the Sixteenth Century.* 1725.

A Further Account of the Dispensary. 1696.

Gadbury, John. *London's Deliverance Predicted.* 1665.

Garencières, Theophilus de. *A Mite Cast into the Treasury of the Famous City of London.* 1665.

Garth, Samuel. *The Dispensary, A Poem.* 1699.

Glanvill, Joseph. *Plus Ultra; Or the Progress and Advancement of Knowledge Since the Days of Aristotle.* 1668.

———. *A praefatory answer to Mr. Henry Stubbe.* 1671.

Goddard, Jonathan. *A Discourse Setting forth the Unhappy Condition of the Practice of Physick in London.* 1670.

Goodall, Charles. *The Royal College of Physicians of London Founded and Established by Law.* 2 vols. 1684.

[Goodall, Charles]. *A Short Account of the Institution and Nature of the College of Physicians, London. Publish'd by Themselves.* 1686.

Groenvelt, Johannes. *De tuto cantharidum in medicina usu interno.* 1698.

———. *Reasons Humbly Offer'd . . . why Dr. Thomas Burwell . . . [et al.] . . . should not be excused from the penalty of the Act of 25 Car. II.* 1700.

———. *A Treatise of the Safe, Internal Use of Cantharides, in the Practice of Physick.* 1706.

Groenvelt, Johannes, Richard Browne, Christopher Crelle, John Pechey, and Philip Guide. *The Oracle for the Sick.* 1685.

H., J. "A Most excellent and rare Drink. . . ." 1650(?).

Hart, James. *'Klinike', Or, the Diet of the Diseased.* 1633.

Harvey, Gideon. *The Accomplisht Physician.* 1670.

———. *A Discourse of the Plague.* 1665.

Hell in an Uproar, Occasioned by a Scuffle that Happened between the Lawyers and the Physicians. 1700.

Heydon, John. *A New Method of Rosie Crucian Physick.* 1658.

———. *A Quintuple Rosie-Crucian Scourge for the due Correction of . . . Geo. Thomson.* 1605.

Hodges, Nathaniel. *Vindiciae Medicinae et Medicorum: Or, An Apology for the Profession and Professors of Physick.* 1666.

Huyberts, Adrian. *A Corner-stone laid towards the Building of a New Colledge . . . in London.* 1675.

The Intelligencer. 1665.

Johnson, William. *'Agurto-Mastix,' or, Some Brief Animadversions Upon two late Treatises; . . . Galeno-Pale; . . . the Poor Man's Physitian.* 1665.

———. *Short Amimadversions [sic] upon the Book lately published by one who stiles himself Noah Biggs, Helmonti Psittacum.* Prefix to L. Fioravanti, *There Exact Pieces.* 1652.

Kephale, Richard. *Medela Pestilentiae.* 1665.

Leigh, Charles. *A Reply to John Colbatch, Upon his late Piece, Concerning the curing the Biting of a Viper by Acids.* 1698.

Lex Talionis; Sive Vindiciae Pharmacoporum: Or a Short Reply to Dr. Merrett's Book; And Others written against the Apothecaries. 1670.

Lockier, Lionel. *An Advertisement, Concerning those most Excellent Pills Called Pillulae Radiis Solis Extractae.* 1665.

M., T. *A Letter Concerning the Present State of Physick, and the Regulation of the Practice of it in this Kingdom. Written to a Doctor here in London.* 1665.

Medice Cura Teipsum! or the Apothecaries Plea . . . from a Real Well-wisher to both Societies. 1671.

Mercurius Politicus. 1650–59.

Merrett, Christopher. *Catalogus librorum, instrumentorum chirurgicorum, rerum curiosarum, exoticarumque Coll. Med. Lond. quae habentur in Musaeo Harveano.* 1660.

[———]. *The character of a compleat physician, or naturalist.* 1680(?).

———. *A Collection of Acts of Parliament, Charters, Trials at Law, and Judges Opinions Concerning Those Grants to the Colledge of Physicians London.* 1660.

———. *Self-Conviction; or an Enumeration of the Absurdities, Railings against the College, and Physicians in general . . . and also an Answer to the Rest of Lex Talionis.* 1670.

———. *A Short Reply to the Postscript, etc., of H[enry] S[tubbe].* 1670.

———. *A Short View of the Frauds, and Abuses Committed by Apothecaries.* 1669.

[Merry, Nathaniel.] *A Plea of the Chymists or Non-Colegiats: Or, Considerations Natural, Rational, and Legal, in Relation to Medicine.* 1683.

The Necessity and Usefulness of the Dispensaries. 1702.

The Necessity of the Dispensary Asserted by the College of Physicians. 1702.

Nedham, Marchamont. "Epistolary Discourse." Prefix to Edward Bolnest, *Medicina Instaurata.* 1665.

———. *Medela Medicinae. A Plea for the free Profession, and a Renovation of the Art of Physick.* 1665.

News from the Coffee-House . . . Poem. 1667.

The Oath Taken by the Censors. 1700.

Observations upon the Case of William Rose an Apothecary, As represented by him To the Most Honourable House of Lords. 1704.

O'Dowde, Thomas. *The Poor Man's Physician.* 3d ed. 1665.

A Paper Delivered in by Dr. Alston, Dr. Bates, Dr. Hamens, Dr. Micklethwait . . . to the Honourable Committee for Bathes and Bath-Stoves . . . together with an Answer thereunto by Peter Chamberlen. 1648.

Pechey, John. *The Store house of Physical Practice.* 1695.

Petty, William. *The Advice of W. P. to Mr. Samuel Hartlib for the Advancement of Some Particular Parts of Learning.* 1648.

Philosophical Transactions. 1665– .

The Physicians Reply to the Surgeons Answer. 1689.

Pitt, Robert. *The Craft and Frauds of Physick Expos'd.* 1702.

———. *The Frauds and Villanies of the Common Practice of Physick.* 1705.

Primrose, J[ames]. *Popular Errours, or the Errours of the People in Physick.* Trans. Robert Wittie. 1651.

Reasons for Passing the Physicians Bill. 1689.

Reasons Humbly Offered Against Passing the Bill, for Exempting Apothecaries from serving . . . Parish and Ward Offices. 1694.

Reasons, Humbly Offered to the Honourable House of Commons; by the . . . Society of . . . Apothecaries . . . For the Exempting them from Certain Offices and Duties. 1694.

Reasons on Behalf of the Apothecaries Bill . . . In Answer to the City of London's Petition against the said Bill. 1694.

Rogers, George. *Oratio anniversaria . . . in commemorationem beneficiorum a Doctore Harveio.* 1682.

Salmon, William. *A Rebuke to the Authors of a Blew-Book; call'd The State of Physick in London.* 1698.

Sermon, William. *An Advertisement Concerning those most Famous and Safe Cathartique and Diuretique Pills.* 1672.

Shepheard, William. *Of Corporations, Fraternities, and Guilds.* 1659.

A Short Account of the Proceedings of the College of Physicians . . . in relation to the Sick Poor. 1697.

A Short State of the Case Between the Physicians and Surgeons. 1690.

"Smart's Aurum Purgans." B.L. 546.d.44(2). 1664(?).

Sprackling, Robert. *Medela Ignorantiae: Or a Just and Plain Vindication of Hippocrates and Galen from the Groundless Imputations of M. N.* 1665.

Sprat, Thomas. *The History of the Royal Society of London.* 1667.

Starkey, George. *Nature's Explication and Helmont's Vindication.* 1657.

————. *A Smart Scourge for a Silly, Sawcy Fool.* 1665.

The State of Physick in London. 1698.

Stubbe, Henry. *Campanella Revived.* 1670.

————. *A Censure upon certain passages contained in the History of the Royal Society.* Oxford, 1671.

————. *An Epistolary Discourse Concerning Phlebotomy.* 1671.

————. *Legends no Histories: or, A Specimen of Some Animadversions Upon the History of the Royal Society.* 1670.

————. *The Lord Bacons relation of the sweating-sickness examined.* 1671.

————. *The Plus Ultra Reduced to a Non Plus.* 1670.

T., C., Dr. [Timothy Clarke?]. *Some Papers Writ in the Year 1664. In Answer to a Letter, Concerning the Practice of Physick in England.* 1670.

Thomson, George. *'Aimatiasis', or, The True Way of Preserving the Bloud.* 1670.

————. *Galeno-Pale: Or, A Chymical Trial of the Galenists.* 1665.

————. *A Letter Sent to Mr. Henry Stubbe.* 1672.

————. *'Loimotomia'; Or, The Pest Anatomized.* 1666.

————. *'Misokumias Helegkos'; or, A Check Given to the insolent Garrulity of Henry Stubbe.* 1671.

————. *'Plano-Pnigmos', or, A Gag for Johnson, That Published Animadversions upon Galeno-Pale. And a Scourge for that Pitiful Fellow Mr. Galen.* 1665.

Trye, Mary. *Medicatrix, or the Woman-Physician: Vindicating Thomas O'Dowde . . . against . . . Henry Stubbe.* 1675.

Tuthill, Francis. *A Vindication of some Objections Lately Raised against Dr. John Colbatch his Hipothesis.* 1698.

Twysden, John. *Medicina Veterum Vindicata: Or An Answer To a Book, entituled Medela Medicinae.* 1666.

Bibliography

V., J. *Golgotha; or, A Looking-Glass for London.* 1665.
W., C. *Reflections on a Libel, Intituled, A Plea for the Apothecaries.* 1671.
W., S. *An Examination of the Late Treatise of the Gout.* 1698.
Webster, John. *Academiarum Examen.* 1654.
Wood, Owen. *An alphabetical book of physicall secrets.* 1639.
Younge, James. *Sidrophel Vapulans: Or, the Quack-Astrologer toss'd in a Blanket.* 1699.

PRIMARY SOURCES CITED PRINTED SINCE 1740.

Acts of the Privy Council. HMSO.
Calendar of State Papers, Domestic. HMSO.
Commons Journals. HMSO.
Cromwell, Oliver. *Original Letters and Papers of State Addressed to Oliver Cromwell.* Ed. John Nickolls. London, 1743.
Evelyn, John. *The Diary of John Evelyn.* Ed. E. S. DeBeer. 6 vols. Oxford: Clarendon Press, 1955.
Glanvill, Joseph. *The Vanity of Dogmatizing: The Three Versions.* With critical introduction by Stephen Medcalf. Hove, Sussex: Harvester Press, 1970.
House of Lords Journals. HMSO.
Josselin, Ralph. *The Diary of Ralph Josselin: 1616–1683.* Ed. Alan MacFarlane. London: Published for the British Academy by Oxford University Press, 1976.
Manuscripts of the House of Lords. HMSO.
Moryson, Fynes. *An Itinerary.* 1617. Reprint. New York: MacMillan, 1908.
Oldenburg, Henry. *The Correspondence of Henry Oldenburg.* Ed. A. Rupert and Marie Boas Hall. Madison: University of Wisconsin Press, 1966–73; London: Mansell, 1975–.
Paracelsus: Selected Writings. Ed. Jolande Jacobi. Princeton: Princeton University Press, 1951.
Petty, William. *The Petty Papers.* Ed. Marquis of Lansdowne. 2 vols. London: Constable, 1927.
"Proposed Act of 1689." In *Historical Manuscripts Commission, 12th Report.* London, 1890. App. 6, pp. 121–29.
Raithby, John, ed. *The Statutes at Large, of England and Great Britain.* London, 1811.
Royal Commission on Historical Manuscripts, 6th Report. London: HMSO, 1877.
Shadwell, Thomas. "The Virtuoso." In *The Complete Works,* ed. Montague Summers. London: Fortune Press, 1927. Vol. 3, pp. 95–182.
Stuart Royal Proclamations. Vol. I. Ed. James Larkin and Paul Hughes. Oxford: Clarendon Press, 1973.
Ward, Ned. *The London Spy.* First printed in serial form, London, 1698–1700; printed as a book in 1703. Ed. Kenneth Fenwick. London: Folio Society, 1955.
Willughby, Percival. *Observations in Midwifery (1640–70).* Ed. Henry Blenkinsop in 1863, with a new introduction by John L. Thornton. East Ardsley, Wakefield, Yorkshire: S. R. Publishers, 1972.

SELECTED SECONDARY SOURCES

The Medical Community

Allen, Phyllis. "Medical Education in Seventeenth Century England." *JHM* 1 (1946): 115–43.

Aveling, J. H. *English Midwives: Their History and Prospects*. London: Churchill, 1872.

Axtell, James L. "Education and Status in Stuart England: The London Physician." *History of Education Quarterly* 10 (1970): 141–59.

Birken, William J. "The Fellows of the Royal College of Physicians of London, 1603–1643: A Social Study." Ph.D. diss. University North Carolina, Chapel Hill, 1977.

––––––. "The Puritan Connexions of Sir Edward Alston, President of the Royal College of Physicians, 1655–1666." *MH* 18 (1974): 370–74.

––––––. "The Royal College of Physicians of London and Its Support of the Parliamentary Cause in the English Civil War." *Journal of British Studies* 23 (1983): 47–62.

Black, William G. *Folk–Medicine: A Chapter in the History of Culture*. London: Published for the Folk-Lore Society by E. Stock, 1883.

Bloom, J. Harvey, and R. Rutson James. *Medical Practitioners in the Diocese of London, Licensed under the Act of 3 Henry VIII, c. 11: An Annotated List, 1529–1725*. Cambridge: Cambridge University Press, 1935.

Brockliss, L. W. B. "Medical Teaching at the University of Paris, 1600–1720." *Annals of Science* 35 (1978): 221–51.

Bylebyl, Jerome J., ed. *William Harvey and His Age*. Baltimore: Johns Hopkins University Press, 1979.

Cipolla, Carlo M. *Public Health and the Medical Profession in the Renaissance*. Cambridge: Cambridge University Press, 1976.

Clark, George N. *A History of the Royal College of Physicians of London*. 2 vols. Oxford: Clarendon Press, 1964–66.

Debus, Allen G., ed. *Medicine in Seventeenth-Century England: A Symposium Held at UCLA in Honor of C. D. O'Malley*. Berkeley and Los Angeles: University of California Press, 1974.

Dittrick, Howard. "Fees in Medical History." *Annals of Medical History* 10 (1928): 90–101.

Donnison, Jean. *Midwives and Medical Men: A History of Inter-Professional Rivalries and Women's Rights*. New York: Schocken Books, 1977.

Forbes, Thomas R. *Chronicle from Aldgate: Life and Death in Shakespeare's London*. New Haven: Yale University Press, 1971.

Foster, Joseph. *Alumni Oxonienses, 1500–1714*. 4 vols. Oxford: Parker, 1891–92.

Foucault, Michel. *The Birth of the Clinic: An Archaeology of Medical Perception*. Trans. A. M. Sheridan Smith. New York: Vintage Books, 1973.

Frank, Robert G., Jr. "The John Ward Diaries: Mirror of Seventeenth Century Science and Medicine." *JHM* 29 (1974): 147–79.

––––––. "Science, Medicine and the Universities of Early Modern England: Background and Sources." *History of Science* 11 (1973): 194–216, 239–69.

Bibliography

Freidson, Eliot. "Client Control and Medical Practice." *American Journal of Sociology* 65 (1959–60): 374–82.

Gelfand, Toby. *Professionalizing Modern Medicine: Paris Surgeons and Medical Science and Institutions in the Eighteenth Century.* Westport, Conn.: Greenwood Press, 1980.

Hamilton, Bernice. "The Medical Professions in the Eighteenth Century." *Economic History Review* 4 (1951): 141–69.

Hand, Wayland D. *Magical Medicine: The Folkloric Component of Medicine in the Folk Belief, Custom, and Ritual of the Peoples of Europe and America.* Berkeley and Los Angeles: University of California Press, 1980.

Hill, Christopher. "The Medical Profession and Its Radical Critics." In *Change and Continuity in Seventeenth-Century England,* pp. 157–78. Cambridge: Harvard University Press, 1975.

Innes Smith, R. W. *English-Speaking Students of Medicine at the University of Leyden.* Edinburgh: Iver and Boyd, 1932.

Jewson, N. D. "Medical Knowledge and the Patronage System in Eighteenth Century England." *Sociology* 8 (1974): 369–85.

Keevil, John J. "The Seventeenth Century English Medical Background." *BHM* 31 (1957): 408–24.

—————. *The Stranger's Son.* London: G. Bles, 1953.

Keynes, Geoffrey. *The Life of William Harvey.* Oxford: Clarendon Press, 1966.

Kocher, Paul H. "Paracelsian Medicine in England: The First Thirty Years." *JHM* 2 (1947): 451–80.

Kudlien, Fridolf. "Medicine as a 'Liberal Art' and the Question of the Physician's Income." *JHM* 31 (1976): 448–59.

Levine, Joseph M. *Doctor Woodward's Shield: History, Science and Satire in Augustan England.* Berkeley and Los Angeles: University of California Press, 1977.

MacDonald, Michael. *Mystical Bedlam: Madness, Anxiety, and Healing in Seventeenth-Century England.* Cambridge: Cambridge University Press, 1981.

Mathias, Peter. "Swords and Ploughshares: The Armed Forces, Medicine and Public Health in the Late Eighteenth Century." In *War and Economic Development: Essays in Memory of David Joslin,* ed. J. M. Winter, pp. 73–90. Cambridge: Cambridge University Press, 1975.

Mullett, Charles F. "Physician vs. Apothecary, 1669–1671: An Episode in an Age-Long Controversy." *Scientific Monthly* 49 (1939): 558–65.

Munk, W. R. *The Roll of the Royal College of Physicians,* vol. 1, 1518–1700. London: Longman, 1861.

O'Hara-May, Jane. *Elizabethan Dyetary of Health.* Lawrence, Kans.: Coronado Press, 1977.

O'Malley, Charles D., ed. *The History of Medical Education.* Berkeley and Los Angeles: University of California Press, 1970.

Porter, Roy. "Was There a Medical Enlightenment in Eighteenth-Century England?" *British Journal of Eighteenth-Century Studies* 5 (1982): 49–63.

Poynter, F. N. L., ed. *The Evolution of Medical Education in Britain.* London: Pitman, 1966.

—————. *The Evolution of Medical Practice in Britain.* London: Pitman, 1961.

—————. *The Evolution of Pharmacy in Britain.* London: Pitman, 1965.

Rattansi, P. M. "The Helmontian-Galenist Controversy in Restoration England." *Ambix* 12 (1964): 1–23.

———. "Paracelsus and the Puritan Revolution." *Ambix* 11 (1963): 24–32.

Roberts, Robert S. "The London Apothecaries and Medical Practice in Tudor and Stuart London." Ph.D. diss., University of London, 1964.

———. "The Personnel and Practice of Medicine in Tudor and Stuart England." *MH* 6 (1962): 363–82; 8 (1964): 217–34.

Rousseau, G. S. "'Sowing the Wind, and Reaping the Whirlwind': Aspects of Change in Eighteenth-Century Medicine." In *Studies in Change and Revolution: Aspects of English Intellectual History, 1640–1800*, ed. Paul J. Korshin, pp. 129–59. Menston, Yorkshire: Scolar Press, 1972.

Russell, Andrew W., ed. *The Town and State Physician in Europe from the Middle Ages to the Enlightenment*. Wolfenbüttel: Herzog August Bibliothek, 1981.

Sharp, Lindsay. "The Royal College of Physicians and Interregnum Politics." *MH* 19 (1975): 107–28.

Stevenson, Lloyd G. "The Siege of Warwick Lane: Together with a Brief History of the Society of Collegiate Physicians (1767–1798)." *JHM* 7 (1952): 105–21.

Thomas, Henry. "The Society of Chymical Physitians: An Echo of the Great Plague of London, 1665." In *Science, Medicine, and History*, ed. E. Ashworth Underwood, vol. 2, pp. 55–71. New York: Oxford University Press, 1953.

Thompson, Charles J. S. *The Quacks of Old London*. London: Brentano's, 1928.

Underwood, E. A., ed. C. Wall, H. C. Cameron. *A History of the Worshipful Society of Apothecaries of London: vol. 1: 1617–1815*. London: Oxford University Press, 1963.

Venn, John, and J. A. Venn. *Alumni Cantabrigienses*. 2 vols. Cambridge: Cambridge University Press, 1924–27.

Waddington, Ivan. "The Role of the Hospital in the Development of Modern Medicine: A Sociological Analysis." *Sociology* 7 (1983): 211–24.

———. "The Struggle to Reform the Royal College of Physicians, 1767–1771: A Sociological Analysis." *MH* 17 (1973): 107–26.

Wake, C. H. H. "The Changing Pattern of Europe's Pepper and Spice Imports, ca. 1400–1700." *Journal of European Economic History* 8 (1979): 361–403.

Webster, Charles. "The College of Physicians: 'Solomon's House' in Commonwealth England." *BHM* 41 (1967): 393–412.

———. "English Medical Reformers of the Puritan Revolution: A Background to the 'Society of Chymical Physitians.'" *Ambix* 14 (1967): 16–41.

———. *Health, Medicine and Mortality in the Sixteenth Century*. Cambridge: Cambridge University Press, 1979.

Willcock, John W. *The Laws Relating to the Medical Profession*. London: J. and W. T. Clarke, 1830.

Medical and Scientific Ideas

Alpers, Svetlana. *The Art of Describing: Dutch Art in the Seventeenth Century*. Chicago: University of Chicago Press, 1983.

Bibliography

Arber, Agnes. *Herbals, Their Origins and Evolution; A Chapter in the History of Botany, 1470–1670.* Cambridge: Cambridge University Press, 1912.

Brown, Harcourt. *Scientific Organizations in Seventeenth Century France (1620–1680).* 1934. Reprint. New York: Russell and Russell, 1967.

Brown, Theodore M. "The College of Physicians and the Acceptance of Iatromechanism in England, 1665–1695." *BHM* 44 (1970): 12–30.

———. *The Mechanical Philosophy and the 'Animal Oeconomy': A Study in the Development of English Physiology in the Seventeenth and Early Eighteenth Centuries.* New York: Arno Press, 1981.

———. "Physiology and the Mechanical Philosophy in Mid-Seventeenth Century England." *BHM* 51 (1977): 25–54.

Bylebyl, Jerome J. "The Medical Side of Harvey's Discovery: The Normal and the Abnormal." In *William Harvey and His Age,* ed. Bylebyl, pp. 28–102. Baltimore: Johns Hopkins University Press, 1979.

Davis, Audrey B. *Circulation Physiology and Medical Chemistry in England, 1650–1680.* Lawrence, Kans.: Coronado Press, 1973.

Dear, Peter. "*Totius in verba*: Rhetoric and Authority in the Early Royal Society," *Isis* 76 (1985): 145–61.

Debus, Allen G. *The Chemical Philosophy: Paracelsian Science and Medicine in the Sixteenth and Seventeenth Centuries.* 2 vols. New York: Science History Publications, 1977.

Frank, Robert G., Jr. *Harvey and the Oxford Physiologists: Scientific Ideas and Social Interaction.* Berkeley and Los Angeles: University of California Press, 1980.

———. "Institutional Structure and Scientific Activity in the Early Royal Society." *Proceedings of the XIVth International Congress of the History of Science,* vol. 4, pp. 82–101. Tokyo, 1975.

———. "The Physician as Virtuoso in Seventeenth–Century England." In *English Virtuosi in the Sixteenth and Seventeenth Centuries,* pp. 59–114. Los Angeles: William Andrews Clark Memorial Library, 1979.

Gillispie, Charles. *Science and Polity in France at the End of the Old Regime.* Princeton: Princeton University Press, 1980.

Hannaway, Owen. *The Chemists and the Word: The Didactic Origins of Chemistry.* Baltimore: Johns Hopkins University Press, 1975.

Hill, Christopher. *Intellectual Origins of the English Revolution.* Oxford: Clarendon Press, 1965.

Hunter, Michael. *John Aubrey and the Realm of Learning.* London: Duckworth, 1975.

———. "Reconstructing Restoration Science: Problems and Pitfalls in Institutional History." *Social Studies of Science* 12 (1982): 451–66.

———. *The Royal Society and Its Fellows, 1660–1700.* Chalfont St. Giles, Bucks.: British Society for the History of Science, 1982.

———. *Science and Society in Restoration England.* Cambridge: Cambridge University Press, 1981.

Jacob, James R. *Henry Stubbe, Radical Protestantism, and the Early Enlightenment.* Cambridge: Cambridge University Press, 1983.

———. *Robert Boyle and the English Revolution: A Study in Social and Intellectual Change.* New York: Burt Franklin, 1977.

Jacob, J. R. and Margaret C. Jacob. "The Anglican Origins of Modern Science: The Metaphysical Foundations of the Whig Constitution." *Isis* 71 (1980): 251–67.

Jones, Richard F. *Ancients and Moderns: A Study of the Rise of the Scientific Movement in Seventeenth-Century England*. 1936. 2d ed. St. Louis: Washington University Press, 1961.

Kargon, Robert H. *Atomism in England from Hariot to Newton*. Oxford: Clarendon Press, 1966.

King, Lester S. *The Road to Medical Enlightenment, 1650–1695*. New York: American Elsevier, 1970.

Levine, Joseph M. "Ancients and Moderns Reconsidered." *Eighteenth-Century Studies* 15 (1981): 72–89.

Mulligan, Lotte and Glenn. "Reconstructing Restoration Science: Styles of Leadership and Social Composition of the Early Royal Society." *Social Studies of Science* 11 (1981): 327–64.

Niebyl, Peter H. "Science and Metaphor in the Medicine of Restoration England." *BHM* 47 (1973): 356–74.

Pagel, Walter. *Jean Baptista Van Helmont: Reformer of Science and Medicine*. Cambridge: Cambridge University Press, 1982.

––––––. *Paracelsus: An Introduction to Philosophical Medicine in the End of the Renaissance*. New York: S. Karger, 1958.

––––––. "Religious Motives in the Medical Biology of the Seventeenth Century." *BHM* 3 (1935): 97–128, 213–31, 265–312.

––––––. *William Harvey's Biological Ideas: Selected Aspects and Historical Background*. New York: Hafner, 1967.

Purver, Margery. *The Royal Society: Concept and Creation*. London: Routledge and Kegan Paul, 1967.

Stearns, R. P. "The Relations between Science and Society in the Later Seventeenth Century." In *The Restoration of the Stuarts: Blessing or Disaster?* pp. 67–75. Washington, D.C.: Folger Shakespeare Library, 1960.

Steneck, Nicholas H. " 'The Ballad of Robert Crosse and Joseph Glanvill' and the Background to *Plus Ultra*." *British Journal for the History of Science* 14 (1981): 59–74.

Stevenson, Lloyd G. " 'New Diseases' in the Seventeenth Century." *BHM* 39 (1965): 1–21.

Syfret, R. H. "Some Early Critics of the Royal Society." *Notes and Records of the Royal Society* 8 (1950): 20–64.

––––––. "Some Early Reactions to the Royal Society." *Notes and Records of the Royal Society* 8 (1950): 207–58.

Thomas, Keith. *Religion and the Decline of Magic*. New York: Charles Scribner's Sons, 1971.

Wear, Andrew. "William Harvey and the 'Way of the Anatomists.' " *History of Science* 21 (1983): 223–49.

Webster, Charles. *From Paracelsus to Newton: Magic and the Making of Modern Science*. Cambridge: Cambridge University Press, 1982.

––––––. *The Great Instauration: Science, Medicine and Reform, 1626–1660*. New York: Holmes and Meier, 1975.

Bibliography

Stuart England

Ashton, Robert. *The City and the Court, 1603–1643*. Cambridge: Cambridge University Press, 1979.

———. *The English Civil War: Conservatism and Revolution, 1603–1649*. London: Weidenfeld and Nicolson, 1978.

Clark, Alice. *The Working Life of Women in the Seventeenth Century*. New York: Harcourt, Brace and Howe, 1920.

Curtis, Mark H. "The Alienated Intellectuals of Early Stuart England." *Past and Present*, no. 23 (1962): 25–63.

Dawson, J. P. "The Privy Council and Private Law in the Tudor and Stuart Periods." *Michigan Law Review* 48 (1950): 393–428, 627–56.

Fisher, F. J. "The Development of London as a Centre of Conspicuous Consumption in the Sixteenth and Seventeenth Centuries." *Transactions of the Royal Historical Society*, 4th series, 30 (1948): 37–50.

———, ed. *Essays in the Economic and Social History of Tudor and Stuart England: In Honour of R. H. Tawney*. Cambridge: Cambridge University Press, 1961.

Grassby, Richard. "Social Mobility and Business Enterprise in Seventeenth-Century England." In *Puritans and Revolutionaries: Essays in Seventeenth-Century History Presented to Christopher Hill*, ed. Donald Pennington and Keith Thomas, pp. 355–81. Oxford: Clarendon Press, 1978.

Herrup, Cynthia. "Law and Morality in Seventeenth-Century England." *Past and Present*, no. 106 (1985): 102–23.

Hexter, J. H. "The Education of the Aristocracy in the Renaissance." *Journal of Modern History* 22 (1950): 1–20.

Hibbard, Caroline M. *Charles I and the Popish Plot*. Chapel Hill: University of North Carolina Press, 1983.

Hinton, R. W. K. *The Eastland Trade and the Common Weal in the Seventeenth Century*. Cambridge: Cambridge University Press, 1959.

Hirst, Derek. "The Privy Council and Problems of Enforcement in the 1620s." *Journal of British Studies* 18 (1978): 46–66.

Holmes, Geoffrey S. *Augustan England: Professions, State and Society, 1680–1730*. London: George Allen and Unwin, 1982.

Hunt, William. *The Puritan Moment: The Coming of Revolution to an English County*. Cambridge: Harvard University Press, 1983.

Jones, Clyve, ed. *Party and Management in Parliament, 1660–1784*. New York: St. Martin's, 1984.

Jones, James R. *Country and Court: England, 1658–1714*. Cambridge: Harvard University Press, 1978.

———. *The Revolution of 1688 in England*. London: Weidenfeld and Nicholson, 1972.

Jordan, W. K. *The Charities of London, 1480–1660: The Aspirations and Achievements of the Urban Society*. London: Allen and Unwin, 1960.

Laslett, Peter. *The World We Have Lost: England before the Industrial Age*. New York: Charles Scribners' Sons, 1965.

Levin, Jennifer. *The Charter Controversy in the City of London, 1660–1688, and Its Consequences*. London: Athlone Press, 1969.

McInnes, Angus. "When Was the English Revolution?" *History* 67 (1982): 377–92.

McKendrick, Neil, John Brewer, and J. H. Plumb. *The Birth of a Consumer Society: The Commercialization of Eighteenth-Century England.* London: Europa Publications, 1982.

Miller, John Leslie. "The Crown and the Borough Charters in the Reign of Charles II." *English Historical Review* 100 (1985): 53–84.

————. *James II: A Study in Kingship.* Hove, East Sussex: Wayland Publishers, 1978.

————. "The Potential for 'Absolutism' in Later Stuart England." *History* 69 (1984): 187–207.

Patten, John. *English Towns, 1500–1700.* Hamden, Conn.: Archon Books, 1978.

Roberts, Clayton. "The Constitutional Significance of the Financial Settlement of 1690." *Historical Journal* 20 (1977): 59–76.

Russell, Conrad. "Why Did Charles I Call the Long Parliament?" *History* 69 (1984): 375–83.

Sharpe, J. A. "The History of Crime in Late Medieval and Early Modern England: A Review of the Field." *Social History* 7 (1982): 187–203.

Slack, Paul. "Books of Orders: The Making of English Social Policy, 1577–1631." *Transactions of the Royal Historical Society,* 5th series, 30 (1980): 1–22.

Spufford, Margaret. *Contrasting Communities: English Villagers in the Sixteenth and Seventeenth Centuries.* Cambridge: Cambridge University Press, 1974.

————. *The Great Reclothing of Rural England: Petty Chapmen and Their Wares in the Seventeenth Century.* London: Hambleton Press, 1984.

————. *Small Books and Pleasant Histories: Popular Fiction and Its Readership in Seventeenth-Century England.* London: Methuen, 1981.

Stone, Lawrence. "The Educational Revolution in England, 1560–1640." *Past and Present,* no. 28 (1964): 41–80.

————. "Social Mobility in England, 1500–1700." *Past and Present,* no. 33 (1966): 16–55.

Tawney, R. H. *The Agrarian Problem in the Sixteenth Century.* 1912. Reprint. New York: Harper Torchbooks, 1967.

Thirsk, Joan. *Economic Policy and Projects: The Development of a Consumer Society in Early Modern England.* Oxford: Clarendon Press, 1978.

————. "Younger Sons in the Seventeenth Century." *History* 54 (1969): 358–77.

Worden, Blair. "Classical Republicanism and the Puritan Revolution." In *History and Imagination,* ed. H. Lloyd-Jones, V. Pearl, and B. Worden, pp. 182–200. London: Duckworth, 1981.

Wrightson, Keith, and David Levine. *Poverty and Piety in an English Village: Terling, 1525–1700.* New York: Academic Press, 1979.

Wrigley, E. A., and Roger Schofield. *The Population History of England, 1541–1871: A Reconstruction.* Cambridge: Harvard University Press, 1981.

Index

Albemarle: George Monck, Duke of, 47–48, 53, 149, 153
Allen, Thomas, 186, 194, 267
Alston, Edward, 104, 127, 134, 140, 162–163, 266, 267, 269
Alvey, Thomas, 219, 267, 271
anatomy, 33, 61, 120, 123, 142, 145, 151, 186, 189, 228, 231
Anglesey, Earl of, 149
Argent, John, 266, 269
Arlington, Earl of, 149, 191, 196
Atfield, John, 219, 267
Atkins, Henry, 97, 266, 269, 282
Atwell, Hugh, 32
Aubrey, John, 48, 166

Baber, John, 136, 137, 144, 267, 282
Bacon, Francis, 97, 119, 150, 181, 185, 189, 260
Badger, John, 210, 227–228, 235–236
Badiley, Richard, 122
Baines, Thomas, 144
Barber-Surgeons' Company, 33, 46, 70, 105, 184, 208, 222, 228; and Bill of 1663, 140; Petition of 1641, 101
Barker, Richard, 129, 131
Barnaby, Henry, 86
Barrett, William, 83
Bartlot, Richard, 201
Barton, Giles, 82, 84, 136
Barwick, Peter, 202, 223, 267, 270
Baskerville, Simon, 103, 266, 281, 282
Bastwick, John, 100
Bate, George, 104, 108, 112, 127, 136, 163, 266, 269, 282
Bateman, John, 206, 212, 220, 221, 250, 252, 267, 268, 270
Bathurst, John, 266, 269, 282

Baynard, Edward, 226, 235
Beale, John, 172
Bennet, Christopher, 266
Bentley, Jane, 82
Bernard, Francis, 195, 220, 221, 227, 228, 235, 239, 240, 283
Beton, David, 282
Betts, Edward (Jr), 217
Betts, John (Sr), 192, 202, 206, 217, 267, 268, 270
Bigges, Henry, 122
Bigges, Noah, 122–124, 125, 154, 186
Bigges, Thomas, 122
Bird, John, 83
Birdwell, Mary, 82
Bishop, Ralph, 105
Blackburne, Richard, 220, 221, 222, 235, 267
Blackmore, Richard, 54, 215, 220, 221, 226, 235, 239, 240, 246, 283
Blagrave, Charles, 196
Blank, William, 129, 131
board of health, 98
Bolnest, Edward, 152, 153, 159
Bonham, Thomas, 20, 79, 131, 136, 201
Books of Orders, 98
Borelli, Gian Alfonso, 195
Boulton, Richard, 242
Bourne, John, 187, 188
Boyle, Robert, 60, 110, 129, 166, 175, 190, 214
Brady, Robert, 226, 283
Brian, Thomas, 66
Briggs, William, 267, 268
Brooke, Humphrey, 219, 220, 267, 268, 270
Brouncker, Viscount William, 152
Brown, Thomas, 42, 210

Index

Browne, Edward, 219, 267, 268, 271
Browne, Joseph, 251
Browne, Thomas, 63
Brushye, John, 35
Buckingham: George Villiers, First Duke
    of, 98
Buckingham: George Villiers, Second
    Duke of, 149, 152, 162, 170, 179
Buggs, John, 87–90, 136, 201
Burnett, William, 195
Burwell, Thomas, 222, 267, 268, 270
Butler, George, 84, 201
Butler, Mary, 86
Buttler, Mary, 45

Cade, Salisbury, 235, 246
Cadyman, Thomas, 116, 269
Caius, John, 50, 201
Cambridge, 50, 51, 89, 118, 127, 147,
    219, 251; Caius College, 81; Christ's
    Church, 81, 103; Trinity, 84
Campanella, T., 179
Carlysle, Earl of, 153
Carr, Richard, 246
Casaubon, Meric, 178
Castle, George, 164
Catcher, Richard, 104, 112
Celer, Lysiponius, 242
Chamberlayne, Edward, 197
Chamberlen, Hugh, Jr., 235, 246, 268
Chamberlen, Peter, 114–115, 116
Chambre royale, 262
Chapell, Bartholomew, 58
Charles I, 95, 114, 115
Charles II, 54, 95, 120, 136, 137, 145,
    153, 190, 262
Charleton, Walter, 107, 115, 119, 127,
    190, 195, 201, 220, 222, 267, 268, 270,
    271
chemistry, 42, 109, 112, 120, 121–124,
    142, 143, 147, 148, 149, 150–154, 156–
    157, 184, 190
circulation of blood, 107, 109–110
Clarendon: Edward Hyde, Earl of, 134,
    136, 149, 160, 162
Clarke, Anne, 85
Clarke, John, 81, 85, 101, 103, 104, 105–
    106, 112, 116, 266, 269
Clarke, Timothy, 66, 140, 143, 144, 156,
    180, 282
Clarke, William, 84–85
Clayton, Thomas, 108
Clement, William, 266, 269
Clench, Andrew, 194, 207–208
Clerk, Josiah, 219, 238, 239, 267, 268, 271
Clowes, William, Jr., 87
Clowes, William, Sr., 46
Coatesworth, Caleb, 74

Coke, Edward, 104, 131, 189
Colbatch, John, 74, 214, 237, 242
Cole, William, 228, 235, 246
Colebrooke, George, 268
Colladon, John, 156, 282
College of Graduate Physicians, 128–129,
    149
College of Physicians: and attorneys, 84,
    115, 195–196, 198, 206, 212, 218, 242,
    247, 249; and Bill of 1661, 138–141; of
    1689, 217–219; of 1690, 221–222; and
    case of 1656, 129–130, 136–137, 187,
    190, 201; of 1692, 225; censoring of
    books, 206; censors' committee, 77–80,
    81–90, 90–92; and Charles I, 98–99;
    and Charles II, 191, 192, 198, 202;
    charter of 1518, 211, 218; of 1618, 199;
    of 1656, 128, 131, 137, 199; of 1663,
    137–138, 199, 211, 212, 239; of 1687,
    204–205, 211, 212, 213, 215, 217, 218,
    220, 223, 239, 241, 252; and City of
    London, 105, 233, 234; and civil war,
    103–106; and Court, 88, 135–136, 140,
    160–162; as court of record, 77; and
    critics, 113–115, 121–127, 141–143,
    152–155, 158–160, 198; and Crown, 80,
    87, 92, 97–99, 132, 160, 191–192, 196–
    197, 198, 202–205, 208–209, 256;
    decline of in 1640s, 106–107; elections,
    76; election of 1641, 102–103; of 1645,
    105; of 1650, 116; of 1655, 127; of 1667,
    162; of 1668, 162–163; of 1682, 196; of
    1684, 202; of 1692, 222; elects, 103;
    fees, 76–77, 205, 224, 254; fellowship,
    72–73, 105, 220; finances, 106, 117,
    145, 160, 184, 199, 205, 220; fines, 208,
    224, 242; and fire of London, 160;
    founding, 71–72; and Glorious
    Revolution, 211–213; Gulstonian
    lectureship, 75; Harveian Museum and
    Library, 117–118, 119, 136, 160, 163;
    Harveian oration, 75, 119, 199;
    honorary fellows, 119, 140, 143–145,
    160, 191, 195; internal discipline, 223–
    225, 234–235, 240–243; internal
    divisions, 162–165, 171, 193–195, 208,
    213, 215–220, 225–227, 228, 234–235,
    238, 239, 244–246, 250, 256–257; and
    James I, 95–97; juridical strength, 19–
    21, 78–80, 90–92, 131; and laboratory,
    112–113, 207; as learned society, 107–
    109, 135, 162; licenciates, 73–74;
    licensing of books, 204; lists of
    members, 196; and London physicians,
    78; and lords of admiralty, 236–238;
    Lumleian lectureship, 74–75; meetings,
    74; as monopoly, 46, 74, 80, 92, 113,
    114, 122, 128–129, 130, 131, 135, 189,

203, 228, 235, 248, 249, 250, 251, 255, 262; as "new college," 208, 211–213, 217, 221, 225–226, 227; numbers of members, 75–76, 205, 217, 220; officers, 76; original purposes, 72; and Parliament, 99–105; petition of 1640, 99–100; of 1641, 101–102; of 1689, 218–219; of 1702, 244; physic garden, 46; and poor, 187–188, 207, 231, 233–234; privileges of members, 75; and professional etiquette, 55; as professional organization, 255; and public, 85–86, 90; rebuilding, 162–163, 183–184; reforms of 1647, 113; regulation, 104–106, 113, 127–131, 134, 136–137, 186–191, 205–207, 223, 254, 255–256; and Restoration, 134–138; in sixteenth century, 20; statutes of 1647, 73, 107; of 1688, 205–207, 212, 218, 219, 220, 223–224, 225, 227–228; of 1693, 225; of 1696, 238, 239; of 1697, 246; and universities, 105

Collins, John, 89
Collins, Samuel, (Jr.), 163, 186, 222, 267
Collins, Samuel, (Sr.), 196, 267, 268, 270
Combes, Robert, 131
Conquest, Charles, 217
Cooke, John, 114, 115, 116, 130
courts: Chancery, 196; Common Pleas, 88, 129; Exchequer, 78, 89, 128; High Commission, 39, 100, King's Bench, 35, 46, 78, 130, 135, 188, 190, 198, 246, 247, 248; Marshalsea, 188; Star Chamber, 78, 87, 93, 98
Coxe, Daniel (the elder), 167, 169, 176, 177, 195, 251
Coxe, Thomas, 128, 138, 163, 196, 266, 267, 270
Coysh, Elisha, 267
Craige, John, Jr., 72, 281, 282
Cromwell, Oliver, 103, 120, 122, 132, 143, 158, 178
Crooke, Helkiah, 266
Croune, William, 201, 267
Crown: and corporations, 26, 93, 197, 202, 252, 255, 256; Privy Council, 36, 82, 93, 98, 146, 156, 247, 252. See also College of Physicians, and Crown
Croyden, Thomas, 138, 163, 186, 267
Culpeper, Nicholas, 121, 125–126, 154
Cutler, John, 199

Dacres, Arthur, 267
Danby: Thomas Osborne, Earl of, 187, 192
Darnelley, Richard, 268
Davis, Nicholas, 156, 157, 158, 267

Dawes, William, 246, 268, 271
Dawkins, William, 267
Dawson, Hannibal, 33
Dawson, William, 33
Deantry, Edward, 156, 157, 158
DeLaune, Gideon, 49, 97, 266, 269
DeLaune, Paul, 103, 104
Denton, William, 107, 282
Descartes, René, 110, 142, 179
Dey, Joseph, 148, 158
Dickinson, Edmund, 283
Digby, Kenelm, 89, 110
disease, 29–30, 61, 231; as acids and alkalies, 214; ague, 83, 147; bloody urine, 241; chilblains, 38; chops, 38; consumption, 41, 147; cough, 38, 247; dead palsy, 86; dropsy, 33, 41; ferments, 184; fevers, 147, 223, 238; fits, 48; gonorrhoea, 83; gout, 38, 41, 83; gravel, 38; headache, 83; heat, 38; hypochondriac winds, 41; itch, 38; jaundice, 85; king's evil, 41, 87; malignant fever, 47; measles, 147; morphew, 38; new, 108, 146; noise in the head or ears, 38; as ontological entities, 68, 186, 260; pains of teeth, 38; pestilential venom, 158; plague, 47; plague of 1518, 71; of 1625, 98; of 1630, 87, 98, 130; of 1636, 130; of 1665, 155–158; pox, 83, 147; renes, 82; rickets, 38, 108, 120, 147, 165; scabbedness, 38; scurvy, 38, 41, 147, 214; smallpox, 147, 223; sores, 38; sores or swellings in the throat, 38; stone, 38, 58, 240; surfeit, 85; syphilis, 46, 247; torment in the guts, 38; tympany, 84; ulcer of bladder, 241, 243; venereous and scorbific ferments, 146; vermination, 146; whooping cough, 31; wind, 38; of women, 147; worms, 38, 147
dispensary, 25, 233–234, 235, 237, 238–239, 244, 248, 254
Dodd, Samuel, 248
Dorchester: Henry Pierrepoint, Marquis of, 119, 144, 146, 154, 184
Downes, John, 219, 271
Drake, Roger, 110
drugs, 139, 167, 196, 231, 233; abortifacients, 145; acidic and alkaline, 214; antidote, 158; antimonial cups, 39; balsam, 38, 43; beautifying waters, 41; camphor, 241; cantharides, 241, 242, 243; cathartique and diuretique pills, 44, 48; coffee, 41; compound, 65; conserve, 142, 158; cordial, 85, 139, 158; cordial-drink, 38; cordial-pill, 43; dentifrices, 41, diet drink, 247; Dr. Gifford's water, 54; drops, 41; elaterium, 85; Goddard's

drugs (*cont.*)
drops, 54; golden elixirs, 41; imported, 34; isingeglasse, 82; lac sulphuris, 42; liquid snuff, 41; lozenges, 41; may dew, 41; mercury pills, 84, 247; milk, 82; nectar and ambrosia, 41; ointment, 226; pills, 241; plaster, 43; poisons, 145; price, 38, 231, 233; ramatroe, 105; secrets, 54, 58, 66, 83, 145, 176; simples, 65, 83, 142; Spanish wine, 88; spirit, 158; unicorn's horn, 134; water, 43. See also therapy; physic

economy, market, 33–35, 47, 259–260
Eland, Francis, 82
Elliott, John, 206, 212, 217, 267
Emily, Thomas, 119, 266
empiricism, 121–124, 252, 259, 260
Ent, George, 104, 108, 112, 118, 127, 137, 138, 145, 162, 163, 164, 201, 266, 267, 269
Evans, John, 39
Evelyn, John, 48

Faculté de Médecine, 95, 262
Finch, John, 144
fines, 85, 88–89, 130, 137, 190, 247, 251
Fioravanti, Leonard, 125
Firmin, John, 80
Fletcher, of Gutter Lane, 188
Fludd, Robert, 266
Fox, Simeon, 81, 103, 266, 269
Fraiser, Charles, 283
Fraizer, Alexander, 136, 137, 138, 156, 160, 173–174, 270, 282
Francis, Peter, 83
Frankland, Thomas, 267
Freeman, William, 201
Freind, John, 215, 257–258
Fryer, John, 83, 148

Gadbury, John, 158
Gale, Thomas, 46
Galen, 73, 154, 185, 243
Galenism. See physic
"Gallypot, Tom," 210
Gardener, 136, 201
Garencières, Theophilus, 157–158
Garrett, John, 195
Garth, Samuel, 215, 244, 250, 252, 268
Gassendi, Pierre, 110, 179
Gelsthorpe, Edward, 235, 246
Gerrard, John, 46
Gibbons, William, 226, 232, 235, 239, 240, 246
Gibson, Thomas, 195
Giffard, John, 266, 269

Gilbert, Richard, 84
Gill, Thomas, 212, 238, 267, 268
Glanvill, Joseph, 171–172
Glisson, Francis, 104, 107, 108, 127, 147, 162, 163, 164, 201, 266, 267, 269
Goddard, Jonathan, 54, 104, 107, 127, 137, 156, 163, 167, 168, 169–170, 171, 175, 176, 177, 233, 251, 266, 267, 270, 282
Goddard, William, 116, 135, 148, 220
Goodall, Charles, 80, 173, 199–201, 203, 212, 242, 248, 268, 271
Goodman, Thomas, 283
Gordon, John, 212, 267
Gould, William, 226, 268
Goulston, Theodore, 201
Gray, the Quacker, 188
Gray, Robert, 217
Greaves, Edward, 136, 138, 156, 282
Grent, Thomas, 59, 87, 104
Grent, William, 106
Gresham College, 107, 241
Grew, Nehemiah, 193, 195
Griffith, Richard, 221, 267
Groenvelt, Johannes, 240–243
Grove, John, 84
Guildford, Lord Francis, 199
Gurden, Aaron, 84

Haak, Theodore, 107, 110
Hadworth, Samuel, 208
Hale, John, 59
Hamey, Baldwin, Jr., 53, 104, 112, 117, 137, 162, 163, 173, 258, 266, 267, 269
Harder, Frederick, 196
Harrell, Christian, 283
Harris, Walter, 267, 268, 271, 283
Hartlib, Samuel, 111, 112, 120, 124, 128
Harvey, Eliab, 144
Harvey, Gideon, 158, 176, 177
Harvey, William, 51, 58, 75, 103, 108, 109, 116, 117–119, 120, 137, 143, 144, 176, 184, 201, 250, 252, 266, 269, 282
Hawes, Catherine, 240
Hawys, John, 268
Heath, Lord, 88
Helmontianism. See chemistry, Van Helmont
Henry VIII, 71, 137
Herbert, George, 32
herbs: deadly nightshade, 30; henbane, 30; pilewort, 30; sneeze wort, 30; squirting cucumber, 85; wound wort, 30
Hermeticism, 121, 149
Herring, Samuel, 130
Hester, John, 124
Heydon, John, 124, 158

Hinton, John, 283
Hippocrates, 73, 185, 243
Hobbes, Thomas, 110
Hodges, Nathaniel, 59, 150, 151–152, 156, 159, 173, 178, 186, 267
Hodson, Eleazar, 266, 269
Holland, Lord, 84
Holt, John, 195–196, 198, 212, 239, 246
hospitals, 111–112, 231; Bethlehem, 241; Bridwell, 241; Christ's, 89, 247; at Leiden, 111; military, 111; St. Bartholomew's, 227
How, George, 226, 235, 239, 246, 268
Hulse, Edward, 221, 267, 268, 271
humanism, medical, 48, 50–51, 71, 107, 109–110
Hunt, John, 83
Hutchinson, John, 136
Hutton, John, 236, 283
Huyberts, Adrian, 80, 188–190, 196, 201, 233

iatromechanism, 195
imprisonment, 85, 88, 242, 251

Jackson, Mr., 82, 86
James I, 72, 95, 252
James II, 48, 153, 183, 202, 204, 205, 207, 209
James, William, 186
Johnson, William, 113, 117, 125–126, 154, 155, 158, 173, 184
Johnstone, William, 267
Jones, of Hatton-Garden, 43
Jones, of Moor-fields, 188
Josselyn, Ralph, 29
Joubert, Laurent, 67

Kempson, William, 82
Kephale, Richard, 158
King, Edmund, 191, 266, 267, 270
Knight, John, 198, 267

Lane case, 87
Larimore, Isabella, 104
Lawson, John, 219, 223, 267, 268, 270
Le Febvre, Nicaise, 120, 148, 184
Leiden, 52, 89, 108, 109–110, 111, 128, 194, 219
Le-Neve, Robert, 42
Leverett, James, 87, 92
Levinz, Creswell, 212, 224
licensing, medical, 28, 45, 72, 79–80; by archbishop, 45; by bishops, 45, 187, 196; by university, 45, 196
Lidsam, Thomas, 58
Lilly, William, 39

Linacre, Thomas, 50, 71, 201
Lister, Martin, 98, 194, 195, 268
Lister, Matthew, 269, 282
Locke, John, 53, 185
Lockier, Lionel, 42
London: Aldersgate Street, 247; Billingsgate, 90; Canon Street, 162; Charing Cross, 124; City, 35, 47, 97, 197, 229, 231, 232, 233, 234, 235; Court of Aldermen, 105; Distillers' Company, 98, 116, 256; Eastland Company, 256; Fetter Lane, 87; Fleet Prison, 88, 129; Foster Lane, 87; Grocers' Company, 95–97, 99; Guildhall, 129, 130; guilds, medical, 45–47; Hungerford Market, 246; King's Street, 82; Knightrider Street, 131; Lord Mayor, 156; Merchant Taylor's School, 81; Newgate prison, 130, 242; Oldstreet, 83; Robin-Hood Court, 82; St. Alphage's, 83; St. Andrews Holborn, 90; St. Botolph's, 84; St. Botolph-without-Aldgate, 98; St. Lawrence Jewry, 81; St. Martin's Ludgate, 81; St. Martin-within-Ludgate, 81; St. Nicholas Lane, 246; St. Saviour's, 83; Stationers' Company, 256; Warwick Lane, 87; West Harding Street, 47; White Chapel, 84. See also Barber-Surgeons' Company; Society of Apothecaries
London Gazette, 47, 223
Lorayne, Peter, 82
Lower, Richard, 193, 201, 208, 212
Lucatello, Matthew, 84

M., T., 141–143, 150, 154, 167, 169, 170
Maddocks, Jane, 35
Malpighi, Marcello, 195
malpractice, 20, 85–86, 89, 90, 104, 106, 113, 117, 130, 131, 241, 242, 243
Manchester, Earl of, 153
Marrin, Nicholas, 87–88
Master, John, 79, 195
Mayerne, Louis Turquet de, 98
Mayerne, Theodore Turquet de, 95–97, 98–99, 116, 281, 282
Maynwaring, Everard, 167, 175
Mead, Richard, 53–54, 215
médecins du roi, 262
medical books, 43–45, 53–54, 215, 227
medical practice: advertising, 36–41, 43–45, 47, 83, 124–125, 128, 156–158, 175, 188, 224–225, 226, 239–240; astrological, 39, 121, 158, 227; and common law, 28, 85–86, 117, 187, 190; competition, 22, 28, 56, 60, 67–68; consultations, 55–56, 240; curing, 66;

medical practice (*cont.*)
  degrees, 50–52; illicit, 91, 104;
  incorporated, 51; mandated, 51; and
  patronage, 47–48
medical practitioners 91; apothecaries, 46–
  47, 84, 91, 157, 177, 187, 198, 199, 204,
  208, 224, 227, 228, 233, 234, 236, 249,
  251; attacks on, 167–170; chemists, 124,
  198; chemists, royal, 120; clergy, 32,
  91; drug pedlars, 35–41; empirics, 25,
  28, 84, 88, 122, 124, 128, 143, 145, 151,
  159, 160, 177, 196, 198, 213, 223, 240,
  262; fees, 45, 58, 83, 84–85, 86, 88, 92,
  114, 130, 188, 196, 240, 247, 248;
  income, 33, 49, 53, 59, 104; midwives,
  31, 33; mountebank, 35, 36, 39, 41,
  198, 250; nurses, 111; ordinary, 41–49,
  91, 105, 122, 198; and patrons, 89, 236;
  quack, 35; surgeons, 46, 177, 198, 204,
  240, 251; traditional, 30–33, 124; and
  war, 47, 103, 116, 122, 214, 222, 236–
  238, 246; women, 33, 198
medical research, 108–110, 117, 118–120,
  126–127, 132, 142–143, 164, 165
Mendez, Fernando, 217
Merrett, Christopher, 108, 119, 128, 131,
  136, 137, 138, 160, 162, 163, 165, 169,
  171, 175, 176, 177–178, 180, 186, 196,
  220, 251, 266, 267
Merry, Nathaniel, 198, 203
Mersenne, Marin, 107, 110, 179
Meverall, Othowell, 81, 101, 103, 104,
  105–106, 112, 266, 269
Micklethwaite, John, 104, 112, 137, 138,
  162, 163, 164, 195, 201, 266, 267, 269,
  282
Millington, Thomas, 164, 203, 212, 218,
  220, 221, 223, 267, 268, 270, 283
Mills, Walter, 194
Moore, John, 83
Moray, Robert, 152–153
More, Henry, 178
Morley, Christopher Love, 195
Morton, Richard, 80, 267, 268
Morton, Richard, Jr., 219, 220
Moryson, Fynes, 61
Murrey, Thomas, 119

Napier, Richard, 62
Napier, Sir Richard, 118
Nedham, Marchamont, 145–147, 153,
  159, 164, 176, 189, 191
Needham, ?Marchamont, 190, 201
Needham, Walter, 201, 207, 220, 221, 267
Newcastle: William Cavendish, Duke of,
  110

new philosophy, 23–24, 25, 107–110, 120,
  126–127, 141–143, 152–153, 163–167,
  170–172, 178, 213–214, 251, 252, 257–
  258; corpuscularianism, 110, 111, 119,
  251; microscope, 142; Newcastle circle,
  110–111, 120; Newtonianism, 215, 251;
  Oxford Philosophical Club, 108; 1645
  group, 107–108
Novell, Thomas, 194

Oath: of the National Covenant, 105; of
  Obedience, 192; of Supremacy, 192; of
  Supremacy and Allegiance, 217, 243
O'Dowde, Thomas, 42, 148–149, 152,
  154, 155, 156, 158, 175
Oldenburg, Henry, 172
Ormonde, Duke of, 149
Owen, George, 201
Oxford, 50, 51, 89, 194, 219, 251; All
  Souls, 146, 164; Brasenose, 242; Exeter,
  105; Magdalen Hall, 107; Merton, 83

Paddy, William, 266, 269
Padua, 50, 81, 83, 109, 110, 144, 219
Paget, Nathan, 127, 266, 267, 270
Paman, Henry, 207
Paracelsianism, 46, 109, 121–122, 124,
  150, 154, 185
Parliament, 192, 213, 252, 255; of 1610,
  97; of 1614, 97; of 1621, 47, 72, 98; of
  1624, 47, 72, 98, 100; of 1640, 99; of
  1640–, 99–103; Act of 1523, 72, 131,
  187, 188, 190, 249; Act of 1543, 85–86;
  Act of 1553, 78, 97; Act of 1661, 137;
  Act of 1695, 232; and corporations, 256;
  House of Commons, 141, 217, 219,
  222, 232, 249; House of Lords, 130,
  190, 192, 217, 219, 232, 243, 246, 247,
  249, 250, 252
patients, 66–67, 259, 263; and
  practitioners, 60–61
Pechey, John, 224–225, 240
Pell, John, 111
Pelling, Margaret, 30
Pemberton, Francis, 195, 212
Pembroke and Montgomery, Earl of, 88
Petty, William, 110–112, 127, 166
Peyton, Mary, 53
Pharmacopoeia, 47; of 1588, 97; of 1618,
  97, 121; of 1650, 112, 121
physic, 54, 61, 62, 65, 123, 124–125, 146,
  150, 151, 152, 164–165, 172, 213, 224,
  231, 242, 250, 251, 255–256, 257, 260;
  non-naturals, 61; nosology, 186;
  pathology, 61; physiology, 61, 119,
  185; prognostication, 65; uroscopy, 53,
  66, 67, 196

physicians, 122; and competition, 68; and curing, 52–54, 63–67; education of, 50–52; learned, 20; and learning, 49, 62–65, 93; and reputation, 53–56; royal, 95, 97–98, 115, 135–136, 144, 160, 195, 202, 223; status of, 56–61, 70–71, 93, 226
Pigott, William, 82
Pitcairn, William, 251
Pitt, Robert, 206, 207, 235, 239, 251, 267, 268
Plattes, Gabriel, 32
Popham, John, 46
Power, Henry, 63
Powys, Thomas, 248
prescriptions, 87, 139, 224
Preutiman, Captain, 237
Primrose, James, 125
professions, 25, 35, 58, 204, 229–232, 248, 249, 255; reform of, 104, 113, 121, 122
Prujean, Francis, 81, 104, 106, 112, 116, 127, 137, 138, 140, 160, 266, 269, 270
public good, 71, 204, 207, 256, 257
public opinion, 125, 132, 195, 215, 229, 236, 239, 242–244, 248, 250, 252, 259, 263

Quartermaine, William, 138, 140, 144, 282

Radcliffe, John, 49, 53, 193, 215
Raleigh, Walter, 254
Ramsey, Alexander, 282
Rand, William, 128–129, 149
Randal, Edward, 131
Rant, William, 104, 112, 266
Read, Alexander, 83–84
Regimorter, Assuerus, 104, 108, 266
Rich, Robert, 238
Ridgley, Thomas, 103, 266, 269
Riverius, Lazare, 154
Robinson, Richard, 207
Robinson, Tancred, 207, 235, 246
Rogers, George, 213, 215, 217, 218, 219, 223, 267, 270
Rose, William, 25, 246–249, 250, 254
Rowe, Francis (alias Vintner), 84–85
Royal Society, 24, 142, 143, 144, 151, 152–153, 163, 164, 165, 170–172, 173, 175, 176, 177, 178, 179, 180, 193–194, 207, 215, 241, 247, 258; Philosophical Transactions, 168
Russell, John, 36, 191

Saffold, Thomas, 41
Salmon, Peter, 104

Salmon, William, 244
Sampson, Henry, 195
Savory, Robert, 33
Scarburgh, Charles, 108, 118, 128, 201, 202, 208–209, 223, 266, 267, 270, 282, 283
science. See new philosophy
Seale, John, 246–247, 249
Selden, John, 137
Sennert, Daniel, 65, 154
Sermon, William, 43, 47–48, 51
Shaftesbury, Earl of, 53
Shaw, George Bernard, 259
Shaw, Hester, 33
Sheaf, Thomas, 104, 266
Sheldon, Gilbert, 149, 159, 178
Sheppard, Samuel, 39
Short, Thomas, 193
Slack, Paul, 44
Slare, Frederick, 194, 246, 268, 271
Sloane, Hans, 207, 215, 247, 258, 268
Smith, Edmund, 81, 101, 116, 266, 269, 282
Smith, Robert, 82
Smith, William, 58
social status, 255, 258; gentry, 26, 56, 58, 59–60; middling, 22. See also physicians, status
Société de correspondence royale de médecine, 262
Society of Apothecaries, 46–47, 70, 82, 88, 98, 99, 100, 129, 159, 184, 187, 190, 208, 213, 220, 227, 228, 232, 235, 242, 246, 248, 249, 256; and Bill of 1663, 138–140; of 1694, 228–232, 236, 239; and critics, 176–177; founding, 95–97
Society of Chemical Physicians, 24, 145, 147–151, 153, 154, 155, 159, 164, 169, 175, 188; and plague, 156–157
Somers, John, 239
South, Robert, 178
Southwell, John, 42
Spicer, Richard, 266
Sprackling, Robert, 147, 173
Sprat, Thomas, 170–171, 172
Sprigg, William, 120
St. John, Chief Justice, 131, 137
Stafford, Viscount, 153
Staines, William, 84, 104, 127, 162, 163, 267, 269
Stanley, Henry, 128, 138, 266, 267
Starkey, George, 42, 124, 148, 155, 158
Starlinge, Roger, 83
Steno, Nils, 195
Stokeham, William, 195, 221, 239
Story, Elizabeth, 82
Strafford, Thomas, 116

Streater, Aron, 82
Stubbe, Henry, 172–178, 180, 186
Sudell, Nicholas, 43
Sunderland: Robert Spencer, Earl of, 203
Sydenham, Thomas, 74, 185–186, 201, 224, 257
Sylvius, Franciscus de la Böe, 109

therapy, 61, 184, 189–190, 215; clister, 139; diet, 65; flux, 82, 84; ointment, 82; plaster, 83; purging, 65, 82; regimen, 60–65; royal touch, 87; touch, 87; venesection, 65, 150, 185; vomit, 83, 88
Thomas, Keith, 259
Thomson, George, 42, 150–151, 152, 155, 156, 158, 159–60, 180, 186
Tomson, Ellen, 85
Torlesse, Richard, 219, 220, 242, 268, 271
Trench, Edmund, 127, 266
Trevy, George, 239
Trigge, Thomas, 39
Trigge, William, 114, 129–131, 189, 190
Trikley, James, 82
Trye, Mary, 42, 149
Turner, Benjamin, 82
Turner, Robert, 158
Turner, Samuel, 282
Twige, Robert, 83
Twysden, John, 158–159
Tyson, Edward, 194, 195, 218, 219, 235, 241, 242, 246, 268

Usher, John, 83
Utrecht, 111, 194, 240

Van Helmont, Jean Baptista, 122, 124, 126, 150, 154, 179, 184, 185
Van Mullen, Gerard, 196
Vaughan, William, 268, 271
Vicary, Thomas, 46
virtuosi, 24, 151, 166, 170–172, 177
vitalism, 195, 251

Waldgrave, William, 217
Waldron, Thomas, 163, 283
Wale, Jan de, 110
Wall, Anna, 84
Wallis, John, 107
Ward, John, 32
Ward, Ned, 36, 41, 243, 250
Warden, Edward, 239
Warner, Edward, 148
Weale, Job, 42
Webster, Charles, 30, 90, 120
Webster, John, 124
Welman, Simon, 246
Wersley, Isabella, 88
Wharton, Thomas, 138, 156, 163, 180, 201, 266, 267
Whigs, 197, 208, 222, 243, 249
Whistler, Daniel, 108, 138, 156, 162, 196, 201, 202, 266, 267, 270
Whitaker, Tobias, 282
Whitehall Palace, 136, 153
Wilkins, John, 107, 179
William III, 53, 54, 202, 209, 252
Williams, Maurice, 116, 266, 269
Willis, Thomas, 176, 184–185, 193, 201
Wilson, Edmund, Jr., 128
Windebank, John, 195
Winston, Thomas, 103, 116, 143, 266, 269
Withall, Susanna, 240–241
Witherly, Thomas, 156, 202, 203, 206, 218, 222, 267, 268, 270, 282, 283
Wittie, Robert, 32, 42, 180, 195
Woodward, John, 215, 268
Woolwich, 122
Wotton, Josiah, 83
Wright, Laurence, Sr., 103, 104, 143, 266, 269, 282
Wright, Robert, Jr., 104
writs: habeas corpus, 88, 188, 242; nolle prosequi, 187, 243; quo warranto, 82, 197, 202; writ of error, 130, 190, 247

Yardley, John, 83
Yelverton, Henry, 97

Library of Congress Cataloging-in-Publication Data

Cook, Harold John.
 The decline of the old medical regime in Stuart London.

 Bibliography: p.
 Includes index.
   1. Medicine—England—London—History—17th century. 2. Royal College
of Physicians of London—History. 3. London (England)—History. 4. Great
Britain—History—Stuarts, 1603–1714. I. Title. [DNLM: 1. History of Medi-
cine, 17th Cent.—London. WZ 70 FE5 C7d
R488.L8C66 1986   610'.9421   85-26932
ISBN 0-8014-1850-X (alk. paper)